Depression: A Multidisciplinary Approach

Editorial Advisor

JOEL J. HEIDELBAUGH

ELSEVIER

1600 John F. Kennedy Boulevard • Suite 1800 • Philadelphia, Pennsylvania, 19103-2899

http://www.theclinics.com

CLINICS COLLECTIONS
ISSN 2352-7986, ISBN-13: 978-0-323-84862-6

Editor: John Vassallo (j.vassallo@elsevier.com)

Clinics Collections (ISSN 2352-7986) is published by Elsevier Inc., 360 Park Avenue South, New York, NY 10010-1710. Business and editorial offices: 1600 John F. Kennedy Boulevard, Suite 1800, Philadelphia, PA 19103-2899. **POSTMASTER:** Send address changes to *Clinics Collections*, Elsevier Health Sciences Division, Subscription Customer Service, 3251 Riverport Lane, Maryland Heights, MO 63043. **Customer Service: Telephone: 1-800-654-2452** (U.S. and Canada); **1-314-447-8871** (outside U.S. and Canada). **Fax: 314-447-8029. E-mail: journalscustomerserviceusa@elsevier.com** (for print support); **journalsonlinesupport-usa@elsevier.com** (for online support).

Reprints. For copies of 100 or more of articles in this publication, please contact the Commercial Reprints Department, Elsevier Inc., 360 Park Avenue South, New York, NY 10010-1710. Tel.: 212-633-3874; Fax: 212-633-3820; E-mail: reprints@elsevier.com.

Contributors

EDITOR

JOEL J. HEIDELBAUGH, MD, FAAFP, FACG
Departments of Family Medicine and Urology, University of Michigan Medical School, Ann Arbor, Michigan, USA; Ypsilanti Health Center, Ypsilanti, Michigan, USA

AUTHORS

ALKA ANEJA, MD
Medical Director, Department of Psychiatry, Fremont Hospital, Fremont, California, USA

GLORIA ANGELETTI, MD
Centro Lucio Bini, Azienda Ospedaliera Sant'Andrea, UOC di Psichiatria, NESMOS Department, Sapienza School of Medicine and Psychology, Sant'Andrea University Hospital, Rome, Italy

GERARD ANMELLA, MD
Barcelona Bipolar and Depressive Disorders Program, Hospital Clinic, University of Barcelona, Institute of Neuroscience, IDIBAPS, CIBERSAM, Barcelona, Catalonia, Spain

ARGELINDA BARONI, MD
Clinical Assistant Professor, Department of Child and Adolescent Psychiatry, Hassenfeld Children's Hospital at NYU Langone, NYU Grossman School of Medicine, NYC H 1 H/ Bellevue, Child Study Center, New York, New York, USA

REGINA BARONIA, MD
Research Associate, Department of Psychiatry, Texas Tech University Health Sciences Center, Lubbock, Texas, USA

STEPHANIE BRENNAN, MD
Senior Resident, Department of Pediatrics, Texas Tech University Health Sciences Center, Lubbock, Texas, USA

ALEXIS CHAVEZ, MD
Child and Adolescent Psychiatry Fellow, Department of Psychiatry, University of Colorado, Anschutz, Aurora, Colorado, USA

JUDITH A. COHEN, MD
Professor of Psychiatry, Drexel University College of Medicine, Allegheny Health Network, Pittsburgh, Pennsylvania, USA

MILANGEL T. CONCEPCION ZAYAS, MD, MPH
Clinical Assistant Professor of Psychiatry, Dartmouth Geisel School of Medicine, Dartmouth-Hitchcock Medical Center, Staff Psychiatrist, West Central Behavioral Health

CHRISTINE B. COSTA, DNP, PMHNP-BC
California State University Long Beach, Assistant Professor, School of Nursing, Long Beach, California, USA

LISA M. CULLINS, MD
Child and Adolescent Psychiatrist, Adjunct Assistant Professor of Behavioral Sciences and Pediatrics, George Washington University School of Medicine, Washington, DC, USA

MICHAEL D. DE BELLIS, MD, MPH
Director, Healthy Childhood Brain Development and Developmental Traumatology Research Program, Professor, Department of Psychiatry and Behavioral Sciences, Duke University Medical Center, Durham, North Carolina, USA

LAVINIA DE CHIARA, MD
NESMOS Department, Sant'Andrea Hospital, Sapienza University, School of Medicine and Psychology, Centro Lucio Bini, Rome, Italy

VALERIA DEL VECCHIO, MD, PhD
Department of Psychiatry, University of Campania "Luigi Vanvitelli," Naples, Italy

KATARINA FRIBERG FELSTED, PhD
Associate Professor, Gerontology Interdisciplinary Program, College of Nursing, University of Utah, Salt Lake City, Utah, USA

SARA N. FERNANDES, MA
Clinical Research Assistant, New York State Psychiatric Institute, Columbia University Irving Medical Center, New York, New York, USA

ANDREA FIORILLO, MD, PhD
Department of Psychiatry, University of Campania "Luigi Vanvitelli," Naples, Italy

LISA R. FORTUNA, MD, MPH
Director, Child and Adolescent Psychiatry, Boston Medical Center, Assistant Professor of Psychiatry, Boston University School of Medicine, Boston, Massachusetts, USA

VINCENZO GIALLONARDO, MD
Department of Psychiatry, University of Campania "Luigi Vanvitelli," Naples, Italy

ANNA GIMENEZ, MD
Barcelona Bipolar and Depressive Disorders Program, Hospital Clinic, University of Barcelona, Institute of Neuroscience, IDIBAPS, CIBERSAM, Barcelona, Catalonia, Spain

SUSANA GOMES-DA-COSTA, MD
Barcelona Bipolar and Depressive Disorders Program, Hospital Clinic, University of Barcelona, Institute of Neuroscience, IDIBAPS, CIBERSAM, Barcelona, Catalonia, Spain

KATHERINE GOTHAM, PhD
Assistant Professor, Department of Psychiatry and Behavioral Sciences, Vanderbilt University Medical Center, Nashville, Tennessee, USA

LINDA SUE HAMMONDS, DNP, PMHNP-BC, FNP-BC
Department of Community Mental Health, University of South Alabama, Assistant Professor, College of Nursing, Mobile, Alabama, USA

GLORIA T. HAN, MA
Doctoral Candidate, Department of Psychology, Vanderbilt University, Nashville, Tennessee, USA

SARAH E. HERBERT, MD, MSW
Clinical Associate Professor, Department of Psychiatry and Behavioral Sciences, Morehouse School of Medicine, Atlanta, Georgia, USA

DELFINA JANIRI, MD
NESMOS Department (Neuroscience, Mental Health, and Sensory Organs), School of Medicine and Psychology, Sant'Andrea Hospital, Sapienza University, UOC Psichiatria, Centro Lucio Bini, Rome, Italy; Icahn School of Medicine and Mount Sinai, New York, New York, USA

NADIA JASSIM, BS, MFA
School Mental Health Team, Division of Child and Adolescent Psychiatry, Lucile Packard Children's Hospital at Stanford, Stanford University School of Medicine, Stanford, California, USA

WEI JIANG, MD
Professor, Departments of Psychiatry and Behavioral Sciences and Medicine, Duke University Health System, Durham, North Carolina, USA

BRANDON JOHNSON, MD
Attending Psychiatrist, CARES, Director of Faculty Practice in Psychiatry, Mount Sinai St. Luke's Hospital, Assistant Professor of Psychiatry, Icahn School of Medicine at Mount Sinai, New York, New York, USA

SHASHANK V. JOSHI, MD
School Mental Health Team, Associate Professor and Director of Training, Division of Child and Adolescent Psychiatry, Lucile Packard Children's Hospital at Stanford, Stanford University School of Medicine, Stanford, California, USA

ANNE KELLY, LCSW
San Francisco VA Health Care System, San Francisco, California, USA

GIORGIO D. KOTZALIDIS, MD, PhD
Neurosciences, Mental Health, and Sensory Organs (NESMOS) Department, Faculty of Medicine and Psychology, Sapienza University, Sant'Andrea University Hospital, UOC Psichiatria, Rome, Italy

GEORGIOS D. KOTZALIDIS, MD, PhD
Centro Lucio Bini, Azienda Ospedaliera Sant'Andrea, UOC di Psichiatria, NESMOS Department, Sapienza School of Medicine and Psychology, Sant'Andrea University Hospital, Rome, Italy

ALEXIA EMILIA KOUKOPOULOS, MD, PhD
Azienda Ospedaliera Universitaria Policlinico Umberto I, Sapienza School of Medicine and Dentistry, Centro Lucio Bini, Rome, Italy

EMILY B. KROSKA, PhD
Clinical Assistant Professor, Department of Psychological and Brain Sciences, University of Iowa, Iowa City, Iowa, USA

DELPHINE LEE, LCSW
Menninger Department of Psychiatry and Behavioral Sciences, Baylor College of Medicine, Houston, Texas, USA

SCOTT LEIBOWITZ, MD
Medical Director of Behavioral Health, THRIVE Gender Development Program, Nationwide Children's Hospital, Clinical Associate Professor, The Ohio State University College of Medicine, Columbus, Ohio, USA

MARIJN LIJFFIJT, PhD
Assistant Professor, Menninger Department of Psychiatry and Behavioral Sciences,
Baylor College of Medicine, and the Research Care Line, Michael E. DeBakey VA Medical
Center, Houston, Texas, USA

CRISTIAN LLACH, MD
Barcelona Bipolar and Depressive Disorders Program, Hospital Clinic, University of
Barcelona, Institute of Neuroscience, IDIBAPS, CIBERSAM, Barcelona, Catalonia, Spain

MARIO LUCIANO, MD, PhD
Department of Psychiatry, University of Campania "Luigi Vanvitelli," Naples, Italy

JULIE LUTZ, PhD
Postdoctoral Fellow, Department of Psychiatry, University of Rochester Medical
Center, Center for the Study and Prevention of Suicide, Rochester, New York,
USA

GIOVANNI MANFREDI, MD, PhD
Centro Lucio Bini, Azienda Ospedaliera Sant'Andrea, UOC di Psichiatria, NESMOS
Department, Sapienza School of Medicine and Psychology, Sant'Andrea University
Hospital, Rome, Italy

NITHYA MANI, MD
Fellow in Child and Adolescent Psychiatry, Lucile Packard Children's Hospital at
Stanford, Stanford University School of Medicine, Stanford, California, USA

NASUH MALAS, MD, MPH
Director of Pediatric Consultation-Liaison Psychiatry, Assistant Professor, Departments
of Psychiatry, and Pediatrics and Communicable Diseases, University of Michigan
Medical School, Ann Arbor, Michigan, USA

SANJAY J. MATHEW, MD
Michael E. DeBakey VA Medical Center, Menninger Department of Psychiatry and
Behavioral Sciences, Baylor College of Medicine, Houston, Texas, USA

LORENZO MAZZARINI, MD, PhD
Neurosciences, Mental Health, and Sensory Organs (NESMOS) Department, Faculty of
Medicine and Psychology, Sapienza University, Sant'Andrea University Hospital, UOC
Psichiatria, Rome, Italy

KATHLEEN T. McCOY, DNSc, APRN, PMHNP-BC, PMHCNS-BC, FNP-BC, FAANP
Associate Professor, Department of Community Mental Health, University of South
Alabama, College of Nursing, Mobile, Alabama, USA

KANAKO Y. McKEE, MD
Associate Clinical Professor, Division of Geriatrics, Department of Medicine, University of
California, San Francisco, San Francisco VA Health Care System, San Francisco,
California, USA

SHALICE McKNIGHT, DO
Child and Adolescent Psychiatrist, Fort Belvoir Community Hospital, Fort Belvoir, Virginia,
USA

REGINA MIRANDA, PhD
Professor, Department of Psychology, Hunter College and The Graduate Center, City
University of New York, New York, New York, USA

WYNNE MORGAN, MD
Assistant Professor, Department of Psychiatry, Division of Child and Adolescent Psychiatry, University of Massachusetts Medical School, Worcester, Massachusetts, USA

ANDREA MURRU, MD, PhD
Barcelona Bipolar and Depressive Disorders Program, Hospital Clinic, University of Barcelona, Institute of Neuroscience, IDIBAPS, CIBERSAM, Barcelona, Catalonia, Spain

KEISUKE NAKAGAWA, MD
Postdoctoral Scholar, Department of Psychiatry and Behavioral Sciences, UC Davis Health, Sacramento, California, USA

MICHAEL W. NAYLOR, MD
Professor of Clinical Psychiatry, Department of Psychiatry, The University of Illinois at Chicago, Institute for Juvenile Research, Chicago, Illinois, USA

KATE B. NOONER, PhD
Director of the Trauma and Resilience Laboratory, Associate Professor, Department of Psychology, University of North Carolina Wilmington, Wilmington, North Carolina, USA

BRITTANY O'BRIEN, PhD
Michael E. DeBakey VA Medical Center, Menninger Department of Psychiatry and Behavioral Sciences, Baylor College of Medicine, Houston, Texas, USA

ISABELLA PACCHIAROTTI, MD, PhD
Barcelona Bipolar and Depressive Disorders Program, Hospital Clinic, University of Barcelona, Institute of Neuroscience, IDIBAPS, CIBERSAM, Barcelona, Catalonia, Spain

KIRSTEN PANCIONE, DNP, PMHNP-BC, FNP-BC
Department of Community Mental Health, University of South Alabama, Assistant Professor, College of Nursing, Mobile, Alabama, USA

MARYLAND PAO, MD
Chief of Psychiatry Consultation-Liaison Service, Clinical Director of the National Institute of Mental Health (NIMH), Intramural Research Program, National Institutes of Health, National Institute of Mental Health, Clinical Research Center, Bethesda, Maryland, USA

GIULIO PERUGI, MD
Associate Professor, Department of Clinical and Experimental Medicine, University of Pisa, Psychiatry Unit 2, Azienda Ospedaliero-Universitaria Pisana, Pisa, Italy

FLORENCIA PEZZIMENTI, MEd
Research Assistant, Department of Psychiatry and Behavioral Sciences, Vanderbilt University Medical Center, Nashville, Tennessee, USA

SIGITA PLIOPLYS, MD
Head of Pediatric Neuropsychiatry Program, Professor, Department of Child and Adolescent Psychiatry, Ann and Robert H. Lurie Children's Hospital of Chicago, Northwestern University Feinberg School of Medicine, Chicago, Illinois, USA

UJJWAL RAMTEKKAR, MD, MPE, MBA
Associate Medical Director, Partners for Kids, Nationwide Children's Hospital, Columbus, Ohio, USA

CHIARA RAPINESI, MD
Neurosciences, Mental Health, and Sensory Organs (NESMOS) Department, Faculty of Medicine and Psychology, Sapienza University, Sant'Andrea University Hospital, UOC Psichiatria, Rome, Italy

DAVID E. ROTH, MD, FAAP, FAPA
Medical Director, Mind & Body Works, Inc., Honolulu, Hawaii, USA

GAIA SAMPOGNA, MD
Department of Psychiatry, University of Campania "Luigi Vanvitelli," Naples, Italy

GABRIELE SANI, MD
Institute of Psychiatry, Universita' Cattolica del Sacro Cuore, Department of Psychiatry, Fondazione Policlinico Universitario "Agostino Gemelli" IRCCS, Rome, Italy

JEANETTE M. SCHEID, MD, PhD
Associate Professor, Department of Psychiatry, Michigan State University, East Lansing, Michigan, USA

CLAUDIO N. SOARES, MD, PhD, FRCPC, MBA
Professor, Department of Psychiatry, Queen's University School of Medicine, Executive Lead, Research and Innovation, Providence Care Hospital, Kingston, Ontario, Canada

MARTINE M. SOLAGES, MD
Child and Adolescent Psychiatrist, Pediatrician, Silver Spring, Maryland, USA

ZACHARY N. STOWE, MD
Professor, De, USA partment of Psychiatry, University of Wisconsin-Madison, Madison, Wisconsin, USA

ALAN C. SWANN, MD
Professor, Menninger Department of Psychiatry and Behavioral Sciences, Baylor College of Medicine, Staff Psychiatrist, Mental Health Care Line, Michael E. DeBakey VA Medical Center, Houston, Texas, USA

MARC VALENTÍ, MD, PhD
Barcelona Bipolar and Depressive Disorders Program, Hospital Clinic, University of Barcelona, Institute of Neuroscience, IDIBAPS, CIBERSAM, Barcelona, Catalonia, Spain

KIMBERLY A. VAN ORDEN, PhD
Associate Professor, Department of Psychiatry, University of Rochester Medical Center, Center for the Study and Prevention of Suicide, Rochester, New York, USA

ROMA A. VASA, MD
Associate Professor, Department of Psychiatry and Behavioral Sciences, Johns Hopkins University School of Medicine, Kennedy Krieger Institute, Baltimore, Maryland, USA

NORMA VERDOLINI, MD, PhD
Barcelona Bipolar and Depressive Disorders Program, Hospital Clinic, University of Barcelona, Institute of Neuroscience, IDIBAPS, CIBERSAM, Barcelona, Catalonia, Spain

EDUARD VIETA, MD, PhD
Barcelona Bipolar and Depressive Disorders Program, Hospital Clinic, University of Barcelona, Institute of Neuroscience, IDIBAPS, CIBERSAM, Barcelona, Catalonia, Spain

SARAH MALLARD WAKEFIELD, MD
Assistant Professor, Department of Psychiatry, School of Medicine, Texas Tech
University Health Sciences Center, Texas Tech University, Lubbock, Texas, USA

PETER M. YELLOWLEES, MBBS, MD
Professor of Psychiatry, Department of Psychiatry and Behavioral Sciences, Chief
Wellness Officer, UC Davis Health, Sacramento, California, USA

SOFIJA ZEKOVIĆ-ROTH, LAc, DOM
Clinical Director, Mind & Body Works, Inc., Honolulu, Hawaii, USA

EMILY ZUCKERMAN, BA
Research Associate, Department of Child and Adolescent Psychiatry, NYU Langone
Health, New York, New York, USA

SARAH MACLEAD WAKEFIELD, MD
Assistant Professor, Department of Psychiatry, School of Medicine, Texas Tech University Health Sciences Center, Texas Tech University, Lubbock, Texas, USA

PETER M. YELLOWLEES, MBBS, MD
Professor of Psychiatry, Department of Psychiatry and Behavioral Sciences, Chief Wellness Officer, UC Davis Health, Sacramento, California, USA

SOFIJA ZEKOVIC-ROTH, LAc DOM
Clinical Director, Mind & Body Works, Inc., Honolulu, Hawaii, USA

EMILY ZUCKERMAN, BA
Research Associate, Department of Child and Adolescent Psychiatry, NYU Langone Health, New York, New York, USA

Contents

> Depression management in primary care settings is the norm, in the United
> States and globally. As incidence and prevalence of depression continue
> to mount, there are innovative models of treatment, newer understandings,
> more open philosophies, and evidence-informed treatments that may
> address this troubling public health issue. This article attempts to succinc-
> tly examine the evidence in identifying and treating this in the United States
> in an expedient, evidence-Informed manner to assist those in need of have
> care that is patient centered, of high quality, affordable, and readily acces-
> sible across the lifespan.

> Psychiatrists have valuable training, knowledge, and experience to serve
> as champions for physician health. The prevalence of physician burnout,
> suicide, and depression negatively affects the health care system at a crit-
> ical time when the country faces a physician shortage, increasing costs,
> and a push toward higher quality of care. Psychiatrists are in prime posi-
> tion to serve as the "Physician's Physician" and lead their organizations
> to increase awareness, build capacity, and drive cultural change. New
> leadership opportunities exist for psychiatrists, including the role of chief
> wellness officer, serving on physician well-being committees, and learning
> skills required to treat other physicians as patients.

> The Diagnostic and Statistical Manual of Mental Disorders Fifth Edition
> introduced the specifier "with mixed features" including 3 or more nonover-
> lapping typical manic symptoms during a major depressive episode in bipo-
> lar disorder type I or II or unipolar major depressive disorder. Excluding
> overlapping excitatory symptoms, which are frequently observed in mixed
> depression, leaves many patients with mixed depression undiagnosed. As
> a consequence, alternative diagnostic criteria have been proposed, claim-
> ing for the inclusion in the rubric of mixed features the following symptoms:
> psychomotor agitation, mood lability, and aggressiveness. A deeper

health concern within the autism community. This article is intended to provide a brief overview of the prevalence, impact, presentation, and risk factors associated with cooccurring depression in children and adolescents with ASD. Clinical guidelines for the assessment and treatment of depression in the ASD population are offered in line with the small existing evidence base.

Sleep disturbances have been linked to suicidal ideation and behaviors in adolescents. Specifically, insomnia and nightmares are associated with current suicide risk and predict future ideation. Associations between hypersomnia, sleep apnea, and suicide remain inconclusive. Potential biological mechanisms underlying these relationships include executive functioning deficits and hyperarousal. Related psychological factors may include thwarted belongingness, perceived burdensomeness, and negative appraisals. Assessing suicide risk in patients with sleep disturbances, and vice versa, is needed. Therapeutic interventions such as cognitive behavior therapy for insomnia and imagery rehearsal treatment, as well as pharmacologic treatments, show promise in treating sleep disorders and suicidal behavior.

In this article, the authors make a compelling case that all clinicians who treat youth with depressive disorders should embrace strategies to engage with school staff to best serve their patients in the classroom. Because these disorders have a high incidence in the school population (13% of US teens experienced at least 1 major depressive episode in 2016), this can affect learning, social interactions, and classroom engagement. Several approaches are highlighted for assessment of depressive symptoms, intervention and treatment in school settings, and prevention strategies, including depression education curricula and programs promoting subjective well-being, such as positive psychology and mindfulness.

Justice-involved youth are at exceedingly high risk of trauma exposure, multisystem involvement, and mental health distress, including depression. Justice-involved youth carry with them both a high symptom burden and a high cost to society. Both could be reduced through evidence-based prevention and treatment strategies. Effective treatment of mental disorders may reduce future justice involvement, whereas lack of treatment increases likelihood of justice involvement into adulthood. Multiple effective programs exist to improve the lives of justice-involved youth and subsequently decrease the cost to society of detaining and adjudicating these youth within the juvenile justice system.

of Mental Disorders, 5th edition, mixed features specifier to these episodes risks misdiagnosis.

Perinatal care, including the management of mental health issues, often falls under the auspices of primary care providers. Postpartum depression (PPD) is a common problem that affects up to 15% of women. Most women at risk can be identified before delivery based on psychiatric history, symptoms during pregnancy, and recent psychosocial stressors. Fortunately, there have been a variety of treatment studies using antidepressants, nonpharmacologic interactions, and most recently, allopregnanolone (Brexanolone) infusion that have shown benefits. The most commonly used screening scale, Edinburgh Postnatal Depression Scale, a 10-item self-rated scale, has been translated into a variety of languages.

Windows of vulnerability for depression have been associated with increased sensitivity to hormonal changes experienced by some women during the luteal phase, postpartum, and/or menopause. Increased awareness has resulted in greater adoption of screening tools for mood and behavioral changes and tailored therapies. This article discusses study results and controversies surrounding therapies uniquely designed for menopause-related depression.

The varied physical, social, and psychological stressors that accompany advanced disease can be burdensome and cause intense emotional suffering, hindering the ability of patients and families to cope in day-today life and negatively affecting quality of life. This article addresses key concepts for the assessment and management of commonly encountered types of psychological distress in serious illness including grief, prolonged grief, major depressive disorder, death contemplation, and suicidal ideation.

Lesbian, gay, bisexual, and transgender (LGBT) youth have unique risk factors that predispose them to depression at higher rates than their non-LGBT peers. Family rejection, bullying, and lack of societal acceptance can contribute to negative health outcomes. Additionally, youth with gender dysphoria may need or benefit from medical interventions. LGBT youth also have the same risk factors as non-LGBT youth, requiring clinicians to decipher risk factors associated with sexual and gender

Katarina Friberg Felsted

Mindfulness has been applied in several adaptations, including Mindfulness-Based Stress Reduction and Mindfulness-Based Cognitive Therapy, to treat chronic conditions in older adults. Older adults may be particularly well suited for mindfulness interventions, because they bring decades of life experience to this contemplative therapy. Mindfulness is also an appealing intervention for older adults as it is inexpensive, effective over time, and easy to access. This article examines mental and physical chronic conditions proven responsive to mindfulness, including cognitive function, anxiety, depression, sleep quality, loneliness, posttraumatic stress disorder, cardiovascular conditions, diabetes, rheumatoid arthritis, Parkinson's disease, urge urinary incontinence, and chronic pain.

Preface

Clinics Review Articles have been a part of the physicians', nurses', and residents' library for nearly 100 years. This trusted resource covers more than 50 medical disciplines every year, producing thousands of articles focused on the most current concepts and techniques in medicine. This collection of articles, devoted to Depression, draws from this *Clinics* database to provide multidisciplinary teams with practical, clinical advice on diagnosis and management of many important areas in this mental health field.

A multidisciplinary perspective is key to effective team-based management. Featured articles from the *Psychiatric Clinics of North America, Child and Adolescent Psychiatric Clinics of North America, Nursing Clinics of North America, Medical Clinics of North America, Clinics in Geriatric Medicine*, and *Obstetrics and Gynecology Clinics of North America* reflect the wide range of clinicians who manage patients with depression.

I encourage you to share this issue with your colleagues in hopes that it may promote more collaboration, new perspectives, and informed, effective care for your patients.

Joel J. Heidelbaugh, MD, FAAFP, FACG
Departments of Family Medicine
and Urology
University of Michigan Medical School
Ann Arbor, MI 48103, USA

Ypsilanti Health Center
200 Arnet, Suite 200
Ypsilanti, MI 48198, USA

E-mail address:
jheidel@umich.edu

https://doi.org/10.1016/j.ccol.2020.12.049
2352-7986/21/© 2020 Published by Elsevier Inc.

Anticipating Changes for Depression Management in Primary Care

Kathleen T. McCoy, DNSc, APRN, PMHNP-BC, PMHCNS-BC, FNP-BC, FAANP[a,*],
Christine B. Costa, DNP, PMHNP-BC[b],
Kirsten Pancione, DNP, PMHNP-BC, FNP-BC[a,1],
Linda Sue Hammonds, DNP, PMHNP-BC, FNP[a,2]

KEYWORDS

- Depression • Telehealth • Wellness-based reimbursement initiative
- Measurement based care • Pharmacogenetics • Integrative care model

KEY POINTS

- Depressive clinical presentations are diverse, including lack of sad affect for various reasons, and normative for culture presentation(s).
- Measurement-based care as standard for usual practice is an emerging practice.
- There is increased drive for wellness care versus encounter-based care.
- Telehealth offers the unique ability to increase access to care.
- The integrative care model shows promising potential to avoid treatment disruption and ensure continuity of care.

INTRODUCTION

Depression is a global issue, according to the World Health Organization (WHO), exceeding 300 million people affected, an increase of 18% between 2005 and 2015.[1] As reported by Pratt and Brody in 2014,[2] US households have some 7.6% depressed persons aged 12 years and over, with moderate or severe depressive symptoms, with women more often affected than men. In that report, those living below the poverty line have increased occurrence of depression. With only 35% of those seeking treatment with mental health professionals within the last year, leaving

This article originally appeared in *Nursing Clinics*, Volume 54, Issue 4, December 2019.

Disclosure: The authors have nothing to disclose.

[a] Department of Community Mental Health, University of South Alabama, HAHN 3044, 5721 USA Drive North, Mobile, AL 36688-0002, USA; [b] College of Nursing, California State University, Long Beach, 1250 Bellflower Boulevard MS 0301, Long Beach, CA 90804, USA

[1] Present address: 13707 Ishnala Circle, Wellington, FL 33414.

[2] Present address: 287 Sunny Valley Lane, Poplar Bluff, MO 63901.

* Corresponding author. 534 Ridgecrest Drive, McMinnville, TN 37110.

E-mail address: mccoy@southalabama.edu

the remainder as untreated, or treated in primary care. Because depression has affective, cognitive, and somatic effects, it is important for providers to be able to diagnose, treat and/or refer in a timely manner for good clinical outcomes.[2] Halverson and colleagues[3] reported that most patients with depression present initially in primary care settings. Common clinical presentations, appropriate treatment, and the changing dynamics for the care of patients with depression in primary care settings are reviewed in this article.

CAUSES OF DEPRESSION

There are different biological and psychosocial theories related to the causes of depression. The course of the illness varies significantly with age of onset, biological factors, environmental and personal vulnerabilities, such as poverty, loss, or series of losses (spousal, death of loved one/significant other), or sudden physiologic/psychological insult, such as motor vehicle accident(s) and financial issues.[4] Comorbid mental and medical disorders, including those of idiopathic origin, exacerbate the clinical course of illness.

INCIDENCE

The incidence of depression in the global population, as reported by WHO in 2015, was estimated to be 4.4%.[1] Depression is more often found in women (5.1%) than in men (3.6%). Its prevalence varies from a low 2.6% among men in the Western Pacific Region to 5.9% among women in the African Region. Prevalence rates vary by age, peaking in older adulthood (above 7.5% among women, and above 5.5% among men, aged 55–74 years). Childhood depression in those under the age of 15 years is more common than in those over the age of 15 years. Globally, 322 million people suffer with depression, with almost half of these individuals residing in the South-East Asia Region and the Western Pacific Region, including India and China. This increase of 18.4% from 2005 to 2015, reflects the overall global population increase. Globally, depressive disorders are ranked as the single largest contributor to non-fatal health loss, and contribute to 7.5% of all *Years Lost to Disability* reports. Suicide is more prevalent in lower-income nations than in middle- to high-income nations, is seen in men more than in women, and peaks between the ages of 17 and 20 years, and gradually levels off across the lifespan.

Brody and Pratt[2] reported that, between 2013 and 2016, of 8.1% of adults with depression in the US, in a given 2-week period, the incidence of women with depression was twice that in men. Age did not change prevalence, but culture had a bearing: non-Hispanic Asian adults had the lowest prevalence of depression, and this prevalence did not vary significantly among other races and Hispanic-origin groups studied. The low-income variable increases the occurrence of depression in proportion to the extent of experiences of poverty at the family income level. Approximately 80% of depressed adults report functional impairments (work, home, and social activities) because of symptoms. Depression rates by sex in the US, from 2007–2008 to 2015–2016, show no significant changes. Mojtabai and colleagues[5] investigated the prevalence of major depressive disorder among school-age children aged 12 to 17 years, noting a significant increase in the previous decade: 8.7% in 2005 to 11.5% in 2014, and a 37% surge in major depressive disorder among school-age children. In 2018, WHO reported, globally, an estimated 53,000 deaths by suicide in school-age children in 2016, making suicide the third leading cause of death in 15- to 19-year-olds; second leading cause of death in women in this age group.[6]

PATHOPHYSIOLOGY

Science has moved from the pure monoamine theory of depression, as per Goldberg and colleagues[7] and McEwen's[8] publications in the Annals of the New York Academy of Science, to the theory of linked connections between elevated hypothalamic-pituitary-adrenal axis activity and protracted stress consideration. The complexity and heterogeneity of depression, as described by Duman,[9] defies a simple understanding of the pathophysiology of depression, and through new and fast-acting novel treatments, some pathways are more easily seen. Among the stress/depression associations with neuronal atrophy, with its characteristic loss of limbic and cortical synaptic connections, it is thought that concomitant decreased expression of hippocampal and prefrontal cortex brain-derived neurotrophic factor (BDNF) occurs. More recent studies have elucidated the role of glutamate and its transmission, followed by changes in BDNF, causing downstream signaling and reducing stimulation of synapses and concomitant reduction of brain functioning.

THEORY

Alterations in synaptogenesis and neural plasticity cause functional disconnections, which underly the pathophysiology (and treatment) of depression.[9] The results are neuronal atrophy, resulting in problems in the signaling pathways caused by stress and depression. Neurotrophic factors, proinflammatory cytokines, sex steroids, metabolic/feeding factors (ie, insulin/diabetes, leptin, and ghrelin), among other factors, play a role in depression and its alleviation. With several causes merging, including the stress diathesis of McEwen,[8] it is clear that there is no one straight path to depression, and depression may result from cumulative responses to multiple influences.

SOCIAL DETERMINANTS OF MENTAL HEALTH

Social context influences the development and course of mental illness. According to WHO, social determinants of health, or conditions in which individuals "are born, grow, live, work and age," are influenced by economic status, social power, and access to resources such as education, health, and safe environments.[10] Determinants for mental health include discrimination, adverse early life experiences, lack of and/or poor education, unemployment, poverty, food insecurity, housing instability, adverse housing, and poor access to health care, and these cause cumulative physical and psychological stress over time, resulting in systematic differences in mental health development and prognosis. Such factors are part and parcel of case formulations for depressed patients to reduce impacts by acting on social determinants in care planning.

Awareness of intersecting effects of race, gender, and socioeconomic status on depression is important.[11] For example, whether income operates as a risk or protective factor for patients with depression depends on these and other socioeconomic characteristics. Because higher rates of depression are seen in lower-socioeconomic populations, predictions of higher risk for these populations, as well as adverse consequences and poor treatment outcomes, are outlined below. Frameworks created to incorporate social determinants of health provide a more complete picture of why people become ill initially, and what it takes to readily access quality health care, targeted to individual health outcomes.[12]

INTERPLAY OF SOCIAL DETERMINANTS OF HEALTH ON DEPRESSION OUTCOMES

- White women benefit from higher income and the residual effect of high income (above and beyond education, employment, and marital status).

- Race (African American) and high household income has been found to be protective against risk of 12-month major depressive episode.
- Larger mental health gain from household income for women than men.
- High household income was protective for Caucasian women, and high education was protective for African American women.
- High income is a risk factor for depression in African American men after controlling for effects of other socioeconomic indicators.[12]

PRIMARY CARE SCREENING FOR SOCIAL DETERMINANTS

Screening for social determinants of health helps identify patients who may benefit from greater support in one or more areas, thus promoting a holistic, public health approach, especially for those individuals who come from marginalized and underserved backgrounds. These factors are closely linked to health outcomes. The growing body of evidence supports social screening and intervention in primary care, while recognizing the need to continue developing and refining available screening tools and interventions. It is important to take more complete health histories, screening for social and environmental determinants of mental health in primary care, including identifying factors such as: family history of depression, adverse early life experiences, maternal stress during pregnancy, unemployment, food insecurity, poor education, and homelessness/housing instability, discrimination, and domestic/intimate partner violence. Screening for social determinants of health in clinical care includes health-related behaviors such as poor nutrition, excessive drinking, substance use, and physical inactivity.[12]

POLICY CHANGE

Policy changes to alleviate social determinants of health, such as poverty, racism, violence, and lack of access to resources, can have far-reaching impacts in improving the health of a community, state, or nation. Although there are no universal screening requirements for social determinants, addressing only the symptoms of illness and ignoring root causation will not improve population health. Screening benefits include providing whole-person care and more accurate diagnosis. Understanding important information in terms of living conditions and social context, reduces recurrent emergency room visits by addressing the underlying causes of illness and decreases costs through early intervention, increasing adherence to treatment regimens, and providing more trauma-informed care. In operationalizing effective screening for social determinants of health in clinical care, good clinical outcomes move from the "margins to the mainstream."[13]

GENERAL POPULATION PRESENTATION OF MAJOR DEPRESSIVE DISORDER

There are many variations and levels of depression (**Table 1**). Major depressive disorder is the generic depression discussed. Patients presenting with less than full criteria should still be considered for appropriate therapeutic management. Symptom presentation in children/adolescents varies slightly with increased irritability being a typical presentation seen by family, friends, and providers.[28] Other high-risk populations vulnerable to depression include those with substance abuse, the elderly, and postpartum women. Postpartum depression and/or psychosis are high risk for those with a previous history of depression, as are bipolar states because of disturbances in sleep cycle, changing family dynamics, and high biological flux.[10] Depression in the elderly can often be overlooked due to somatic presentations, the ageing process,

Table 1
Across the lifespan clinical presentation/evidence for depression with developmentally appropriate evidence informed screening instrument

Lifespan Population-Based Symptoms of Depression	Screening Instruments
General population Symptoms must be present during the same 2-week period, representing a change in functioning to include either depressed mood and/or loss of interest or pleasure that are clearly not attributable to another disorder and 5 or more of the following per the American Psychological Association[14] • Depressed mood most of the day, most days, either by subjective report (sad, empty, hopeless) or observable by others • Marked diminished interest, pleasure, in all or almost all, activities most of the day, every day either by report of self/others • Significant weight loss not related to dieting (5% change in body weight/month) or appetite decrease nearly daily or weight gain • Insomnia or hypersomnia nearly daily • Psychomotor agitation or retardation nearly every day • Fatigue or loss of energy nearly every day • Feelings of worthlessness or excessive guilt nearly daily • Lowered ability to think, concentrate or indecisiveness, nearly daily • Recurrent thoughts of death, recurrent suicidal ideation without a specific plan, or attempt or a specific plan for committing suicide	Mood Disorder Questionnaire (MDQ) for adults https://www.integration.samhsa.gov/clinical-practice/screening-tools[15] PHQ-9 https://www.uspreventiveservicestaskforce.org/Home/GetFileByID/218[16] PRIME-MD Patient Health Questionnaire (PHQ) http://www.oacbdd.org/clientuploads/Docs/2010/Spring%20Handouts/Session%20220j.pdf[17]
Hallmark school-age presentation of depression[15] • Irritability • Fatigue (somatic complaints) • Insomnia or sleeping more • Decline in academic functioning	Pediatric Symptom Checklist (PSC-17) https://www.brightfutures.org/mentalhealth/pdf/professionals/ped_sympton_chklst.pdf[18] Columbia Suicide Severity Rating Scale (CSSRS) https://cssrs.columbia.edu/wp-content/uploads/C-SSRS_Pediatric-SLC_11.14.16.pdf[19]
Hallmark presentation of depression with substance use • Symptoms of depression are not due to direct physiologic effects of substance • Symptoms and history should be weighed carefully together in the diagnostic assessment	CAGE-AID http://www.integration.samhsa.gov/images/res/CAGEAID.pdf[20] Beck Depression Inventory (BDI) https://www.apa.org/pi/about/publications/caregivers/pra ctice-settings/assessment/tools/beck-depression.aspx[21]

(continued on next page)

Table 1 (continued)	
Lifespan Population-Based Symptoms of Depression	**Screening Instruments**
• Referral for treatment of substance use • 2-wk duration depressed mood/loss of interest before use of substance or abstinence free of substance[16,17]	
Hallmark presentation of depression for women of childbearing age • Non-gravid: see DSM-5 description (see **Box 1**) (excepting those with premenstrual-related disorders and other differential diagnosis) • Gravid: ○ More emotional lability per Fischer (2018) than non-gravid counterparts ○ 50% of pregnancies in the United States are unplanned as per Bonham, The Shriver Report (2018) ○ 60% of pregnancies in the bipolar population are unplanned per Rusner et al • Postpartum: ○ Spousal/family upheaval ○ Financial upheaval ○ General biological flux, hormonal, sleep, lactation, pain, weight issues • Menopausal: ○ Mood changes common ○ If more than normal, seek solutions through the North American Menopause Society ○ Screen for depression ○ Antidepressants and psychotherapy/counseling combinations recommended (NAMS)	For women of childbearing age: Massachusetts General Hospital https://womensmentalhealth.org/[22] For all pregnant women wk 26 through 6 wk postpartum: Edinburgh Postpartum Depression Scale (EPDS) https://www.knowppd.com/epds-ppd-screening/[23] For peri-menopausal women: https://www.menopause.org/for-women/menopauseflashes/mental-health-at-menopause/depression-menopause[24,25]
Hallmark elderly presentation of depression • Depressive mood • Loss of interest/desire ○ Anhedonia • Excessive feelings of guilt • Psychomotor ○ Agitation, retardation	Geriatric Depression Scale (GDS) https://consultgeri.org/try-this/general-assessment/issue-4.pdf[26]
• Vegetative symptoms Sleepiness, loss of appetite, insomnia • Somatic symptoms Headaches, backaches, gastrointestinal, pain • Cognitive symptoms Dullness, indecision	Geriatric Depression Scale-15 http://geriatrictoolkit.missouri.edu/cog/GDS_SHORT_FORM.PDF[27]

Data from Refs.[14–24,26]

Box 1	
Medication treatment implications/strategies	
Lifespan Presentations	**Psychopharmacologic**
Adult (general population)	Selective serotonin reuptake inhibitor (SSRIs), serotonin-norepinephrine reuptake inhibitor (SNRIs), buspirone, lithium, and thyroid as augmentation strategies, newer atypical antipsychotic formulations
School age	• Start low, go slow
	• First line: fluoxetine plus therapy
	• Second line: sertraline or lexapro
	• Third line: venlafaxine
	• May consider bupropion or duloxetine after venlafaxine
	• Close monitoring essential secondary to risk of bipolar exacerbation vs suicide
	Pharmacologic considerations are important in school age youth despite negative media coverage 2004–2006 and US Food and Drug Administration (FDA) initiation of black box warnings of all SSRIs of potential increased risk of suicide in youths, SSRI youth prescription rates dropped 20%, culminating in the largest increase in the Centers for Disease Control and Prevention (CDC) report on school-age suicides (2011), stressing the importance that evidence shows SSRIs are safe and effective if closely monitored. All adolescent post mortem toxicology reports are absent of antidepressants despite being prescribed.[29–31]
Substance use	• Certain SSRIs, SNRIs, buspirone, most likely patient has had previous trials, rule out bipolar mood disorder
	• Considerations of comorbid attention-deficit/ hyperactivity disorder and/or acute/chronic pain syndromes and pregnancy
	• Awareness of prescription medication abuse: gabapentin, diphenhydramine, quetiapine, carisoprodol, clonidine, and ibuprofen[32]
Women of childbearing age	Providers must be updated/aware of the following contingencies (Massachusetts General Hospital):
	• Collaboration with obstetrician and essential early prenatal care
	• Birth control vs fertility consideration
	• Planned vs unplanned pregnancy/and risks associated
	• Consider psychotherapies plus low-risk medicines
	• No alcohol secondary to fetal birth defects
	• Risks vs benefits of pharmacologic treatment during pregnancy/postpartum time
	• Folate as precaution
	• Pregnancy/opioid issues: methadone/ buprenorphine (sole)
	• The new US FDA Pregnancy Labeling and Lactation Rule
	• Screening: evidence-informed screening lends to more accurate diagnosis and treatment, saving time and resources to recovery
	• Risk of neonatal symptoms, long-term effects, antidepressant risk, SSRI risks, persistent pulmonary hypertension of the newborn vs development of postpartum depression/psychosis[22]

Elderly	• Need for prescribing antidepressants for elderly to be evidence based • Start low, go slow • Avoid drug-drug interactions • Early screening/intervention for delirium onset • Screening Tool of Older People's Prescriptions (STOPP)[33] • BEERS Criteria[34]
Genetic pharmacologic testing	Genetic pharmacologic testing as a time savings for treatment efficacy. This area is promising but limited. Rosenblat and colleagues[35] completed a meta-analysis finding evidence to be limited and with methodological deficiencies. Still, the work provided evidence of faster, better response/remission rates when pharmacogenetics are used to provide treatment of depression

Data from Refs.[22,29–35]

and increasing frailty. In this age group, subthreshold symptoms can cause loss of functionality (see Fiske and colleagues).[28]

CLINICAL TREATMENT GOALS: REMISSION OF SYMPTOMS

Depression is treatable, with many paths to recovery, as outlined in **Box 1**. Unfortunately, true remission is generally unsought, with "less than" recovery generally received as an acceptable outcome, which differs from other somatic pathologic conditions. Depression begets depression: as a pathologic condition, depression is not held in high esteem by providers (see Grue and colleagues);[27] being stigmatized, depression ranks 30 of 38 disease categories in prestige globally: possessing less stature in terms of disability, rather than a "serious disability" such as myocardial infarction and HIV. The disease state itself is not taken seriously, given its pervasive incidence and prevalence. Therefore "less than" full remission of symptoms is unfortunately the norm, and too often accepted as an acceptable outcome compared with other pathologic conditions.

DISCUSSION

There are numerous barriers to effective management of depression in primary care that include the paucity of mental health providers, inadequately prepared providers, and the need for timely referrals to psychiatric providers when indicated. Current solutions include telemental health, measurement-based care, a Merit-Based Incentive Payment System, staff training, office-based consults/behavioral health provider(s), and integrative care model adoption.

The need for accurate differential diagnosis management pertinent to bipolar disorder includes lack of time for evidence-informed screens and thorough history taking because of varied presentations/co-morbidities. Differential diagnostics often result in diagnostic lateness of bipolarity and treatment of persons with bipolar affective disorders with antidepressant monotherapy leading to iatrogenic kindling mania risk. This can be addressed by appropriate screening and gathering of adequate history.

Other barriers include persistence of stigma related to mental health treatment, lack of psychoeducation for patients and providers, and time needed for a true cultural shift, which can take generations. However, the paradigm shift in primary delivery to

Table 2
New directions for mental health in primary care

Item/Definition	Current Status	Projected Impact
Measurement-based care (MBC)[36] MBC seeks: • Optimization, accuracy, and speed: patients receive most appropriate treatments and best possible results with least patient burden in a most economical way • To attain correct diagnosis and management as often and in as timely manner as possible • As compared with usual care, MBC more precisely defines problems through regular, targeted, assessment of key clinical outcomes informing an action plan	• Not standard clinical practice for mental health • Existing gap between research/practice outcomes • To implement MBC: establishment of clear expectations/guidelines • Foster practice-based implementation capacities • Change financial incentives • Assist providers adopting to MBC • Development/expansion of MBC science base • Engagement of consumers/families • Use of evidence-based screening/diagnostic instruments as a norm • Pharmacogenetic testing/assays	Measurement-based care adopted as standard of care could transform psychiatric practice, moving mental health into the health care mainstream, improving quality of care, access, enhancing recovery time, and lower economic burden for patients with mental illness • Examples: pharmacogenetic assays • Use of evidence-informed screens and treatments • Team approaches
Pharmacogenetic assays and updates[37]	Pharmacokinetic and/or pharmacodynamic assays determining individual genetic propensity for/against cytochrome P450 pathways, determining sense of particular medicine agent efficacy working optimally/sub-optimally/against genetic makeup. • Medicare reimbursed • Ease of use: Buccal swab • Accuracy continues to develop • Some firms update without added costs	• Savings of medication and indirect health care costs compared with those receiving treatment as usual • Projected increase in quality-adjusted life-years of 0.316 y • Evidence limited although used in practice

(continued on next page)

Table 2
(continued)

Item/Definition	Current Status	Projected Impact
Telehealth access[38]	Linking provider and patient through web-based means in an articulated agreement using agency to provide access for screen face-to-face encounters in which psychiatric mental health is provided. Rapid growth: • Driven by the increasing demand for mental health services • Shortage/distribution of mental health providers • Increasing technology availability • Third-party reimbursement	Telemental health limits/opportunities: • Access to care increased • Multiple logistical demands can lead to link interruptions • Some third-party payer limits • Organizational approach/support/technology are key on both side of encounter • Access increases care coordination • 24/7 coverage • Improve quality, equity, and affordability of depression management • Patients increasingly request patient centered access to care
Wellness-based reimbursement incentive payment strategies[39]	• Medicare access/Children's Health Insurance Program (CHIP) Reauthorization • Act of 2015 (Medicare Access and CHIP Reauthorization Act [MACRA]) a stepping stone for revised Part B Medicare payments • Core aspect of this legislation with permanent repealing of Sustainable Growth Rate • MACRA's Importance: key in development of new payment framework for health care delivery divided into the Merit-Based Incentive Payment System (MIPS)/advanced alternative payment methods • Introduced 2 y ago, in trial state to become mandatory at some point in near future	• Financial incentives for population wellness outcomes • Increased provider satisfaction • Confusion in the system relating to overhaul of payment system and the economic incentives based on the former/current system. • Encounter-based payments will be replaced by wellness, quality-based encounters, in time

(continued on next page)

Table 2 (continued)		
Item/Definition	Current Status	Projected Impact
	• Bonus incentive payments to be awarded to practices attaining wellness benchmarks • Private payers historically follow Medicare dynamics	
Integrative care model uptake[40,41]	• Integrative care, simply stated is where people can receive physical and mental wellness care in a setting/organization • Positive uptake for recipients of care for depression in integrative care settings reported by Cochrane Review meta-analysis[42] • Many levels of integrative care available • Provides coordination of care, payer, and transportation issues • Faces numerous challenges to fully fold into US health care services • Serves persons, communities, and mental wellness with regard to substance use issues • Both recipients of care and providers report increases in encounter satisfaction • Reduction of hospitalizations • Recovery and trauma • Centered framework adoption	• Uptake of model increased since Affordable Care Act and commensurate funding structures. • 70% of depression care is initiated and followed in primary care • Integrated electronic health records are essential, reducing service gaps/information gaps • Payer structuring is cumbersome but in progress

Data from Refs.[36–41]

wellness promoting Center for Medicare & Medicaid Services initiatives, rewarding wellness, rather than encounter volume, have initiated an industry disruption, but an essential culture shift among health care providers is needed. New treatment approaches for mental health in primary care are outlined in **Table 2**.

Depression is commonplace, most often recognized and treated in primary care[3] settings, by clinicians who may or may not be adequately prepared for its diverse presentations. Measurement-based practice promises assistance in more accurate diagnosis early on in presentations using treatment options based on evidence-informed practice. See **Box 2** for a review of current evidence-based clinical practice pearls.

> **Box 2**
> **Clinical pearls**
>
> Center for Medicare Systems in process of moving toward adoption of Merit-Based Incentive Payment System (MIPS)[36] and wellness initiatives
>
> Psychotherapy and psychopharmacology approaches combined yield; more robust results leading to recovery in insightful patients willing to participate[9]
>
> All patients with depression recommended to be screened for bipolar disorder/other differentials[43]
>
> Pediatric depression screening ages 12 to 17 years is recommended at every visit, can screen younger depending on development.[44] All adolescents to be screened for substance use at every encounter[42]
>
> Women of childbearing/lactation age should be treated pharmacologically with the least teratogenic and/or harmful approaches, with reliable birth control in place, if sexually active when not family planning[22,45]
>
> Screening of the elderly for depression at each encounter as a standard[46,47]
>
> Using measurement-based instruments for efficient screening/diagnostics/treatments[36,39]
>
> Where possible, use pharmacogenetic testing to reduce costs of time lost to efficacy[37]
>
> Access care/providers via telemental health, use of telehealth consults, and/or face–to–face care via telehealth when face–to–face mental health provider(s) not accessible[38]
>
> Integrative care models incorporate mental/physical wellness care within 1 organization, reducing service gaps due to relative accessibility[40–42]
>
> *Data from* Refs.[9,22,36–47]

SUMMARY

Pharmacogenetic assays may speed recovery through introduction of more accurately targeted medicines. Moving into the future, avenues such as integrative care, telehealth, and wellness-based reimbursement incentives promise a welcome change to a landscape needing dynamic restructure and the mental health encounter environment in primary care.

REFERENCES

1. World Health Organization. Depression and other common mental disorders: global health estimates. Geneva (Switzerland): World Health Organization; 2017. Available at: http://apps.who.int/iris/bitstream/handle/10665/254610/WHO-MSD-MER-2017.2-eng.pdf?sequence=1. Accessed November 11, 2018.
2. Pratt LA, Brody DJ. Depression in the U.S. household population, 2009-2012. NCHS Data Brief 2014;172:1–8. Available at: https://www.cdc.gov/nchs/data/databriefs/db172.htm. Accessed November 11, 2018.
3. Halverson J, Bienenfeld D, Bhalla R, et al. Depression clinical presentation: history, physical examination, major depressive disorder. 2018. Available at: Emedicine.medscape.com; https://emedicine.medscape.com/article/286759-clinical#showall. Accessed November, 24 2018.
4. World Health Organization. Depression. 2017. Available at: https://www.who.int/mental_health/management/depression/en/. Accessed November, 8 2018.
5. Mojtabai R, Olfson M, Han B. National trends in the prevalence and treatment of depression in adolescents and young adults. Pediatrics 2016;138(6):9.

6. World Health Organization. Adolescent mental health. 2018. Available at: http://www.who.int/mental_health/maternal-child/adolescent/en/. Accessed November, 15 2018.

7. Goldberg JS, Bell CE Jr, Pollard DA. Revisiting the monoamine hypothesis of depression: a new perspective. Perspect Medicin Chem 2014;6:1–8.

8. McEwen BS. Plasticity of the hippocampus: adaptation to chronic stress and allostatic load. Ann N Y Acad Sci 2001;933(1):265. Available at: https://libproxy.usouthal.edu/login?url=https://search.ebscohost.com/login.aspx?direct=true&db=edb&AN=91503744&site=eds-live.

9. Duman R. Pathophysiology of depression and innovative treatments: remodeling glutamatergic synaptic connections. Dialogues Clin Neurosci 2014;16(1):11–27. Available at: https://www-ncbi-nlm-nih-gov.libproxy.usouthal.edu/pubmed/24733968.

10. Sederer LI. The social determinants of mental health. Psychiatr Serv 2016;67(2):234–5.

11. Assari S. Social determinants of depression: the intersections of race, gender, and socioeconomic status. Brain Sci 2017;7(12). https://doi.org/10.3390/brainsci7120156.

12. Andermann A. Screening for social determinants of health in clinical care: moving from the margins to the mainstream. Public Health Rev 2018;39:19.

13. Rusner M, Berg M, Begley C. Bipolar disorder in pregnancy and childbirth: a systematic review of outcomes. BMC Pregnancy Childbirth 2016;16:331–72.

14. American Psychiatric Association. Diagnostic and statistical manual of mental disorders. 5th edition. Washington, DC: American Psychiatric Association; 2013.

15. SAMSHA-HRSA Center for Integrated Health Solutions. Screening tools. Available at: https://www.integration.samhsa.gov/clinical-practice/screening-tools. Accessed December 20, 2018.

16. US Preventive Services Task Force (nd.)PHQ-9. Available at: https://www.uspreventiveservicetaskforce.org/Home/GetFileByID218. Accessed November 30, 2018.

17. Prime MD. Prime-MD patient health questionnaire. Available at: http://www.oacbdd.org/clientuploads/Docs/2010/Spring%20Handouts/Session%20220j.pdf. Accessed November 30, 2018.

18. Bright futures (nd.) pediatric symptom checklist, instructions for use. Available at: https://wwwbrightfutures.org/mentalhealtyh/pdf/professionals/ped_symptom_chklst.pdf. Accessed November 30, 2018.

19. Posner K, Brent D, Lucas C, et al. Columbia-suicide severity rating scale. Columbia-suicide severity rating scale, pediatric-since last contact- communities and healthcare version 6/23/10. The Research Foundation for Mental Hygiene, Inc. Available at: https://cssrs.columbia.edu/wp-content/uploads/C-SSRS_Pediatric-SLC_11.14.16.pdf. Accessed November 30, 2018.

20. Megellan. Cage and Cage-AID introduction and scoring. Available at: https://docs.google.com/document/d/1_qwV9mb5BzHx1XZisGxCGTtOIuh68L3y24B-C58AYbI/edit. Accessed November 30, 2018.

21. American Psychological Association. Beck depression inventory. 2018. Available at: https://www.apa.org/pi/about/publications/caregivers/practice-settings/assessment/tools/beck-depression.aspx. Accessed November 30, 2018.

22. Massachusetts General Hospital Center for Women's Mental Health Reproductive Psychiatry Resource & Information Center. Psychiatric disorders during pregnancy, weighing the risks and benefits of pharmacologic treatment during

pregnancy. 2018. Available at: https://womensmentalhealth.org/specialty-clinics/psychiatric-disorders-during-pregnancy/. Accessed November 30, 2018.

23. Sage therapeutics. Using the edinburgh postnatal depression scale. 2018. Available at: https://www.knowppd.com/epds-ppd-screening/. Accessed November 30, 2018.

24. North American Menopause Society. Depression and menopause. 2018. Available at: https://www.menopause.org/for-women/menopauseflashes/mental-health-at-menopause/depression-menopause. Accessed November 30, 2018.

25. Greenberg S. The geriatric depression scale, revised 2012. Try this. Best practices in nursing care to older adults. 2019 Issue 4. Available at: https://consultgeri.org/try-this/general-assessment/issue-4.pdf. Accessed November 30, 2018.

26. Balsamo M, Cataldi F, Carlucci L, et al. Assessment of late-life depression via self-report measures: a review. Clin Interv Aging 2018;13:2021–44.

27. Grue J, Johannessen LE, Rasmussen EF. Prestige rankings of chronic diseases and disabilities. A survey among professionals in the disability field. Soc Sci Med 2015;124:180–6.

28. Fiske A, Wetherell JL, Gatz M. Depression in older adults. Annu Rev Clin Psychol 2009;5:363–89.

29. CDC. Suicide rates rising across the U.S. Comprehensive prevention goes beyond a focus on mental health concerns. CDC Newsroom. 2018. Available at: https://www.cdc.gov/media/releases/2018/p0607-suicide-prevention.html. Accessed November 30, 2018.

30. Zuckerbrot RA, Cheung A, Jensen PS, et al. Guidelines for Adolescent Depression in Primary Care (GLAD-PC): Part I. Practice preparation, identification, assessment, and initial management. Pediatrics 2018;141(3):1–21.

31. Moreland CS, Bonin L, Brent D, et al. Pediatric unipolar depression and pharmacotherapy: choosing a medication. UpToDate. The Netherlands: Wolters Kluwer; 2018. Available at: https://wwwuptodate-com.libproxy.usouthal.edu/contents/pediatric-unipolar-depression-andpharmacotherapy-choosing-a-medication?topicRef51231&source5see_link. Accessed November 26, 2018.

32. Tamburello AC, Kathpal A, Reeves R. Characteristics of inmates who misuse prescription medication. J Correct Health Care 2017;23(4):449–58.

33. Gers L, Petrovic M, Perkisas S, et al. Antidepressant use in older inpatients: current situation and application of the revised STOPP criteria. Ther Adv Drug Saf 2018;9(8):373–84.

34. By the American Geriatrics Society 2015 Beers Criteria Update Expert Panel. American Geriatrics Society 2015 updated beers criteria for potentially inappropriate medication use in older adults. J Am Geriatr Soc 2015;63(11):2227–46. Available at: https://www-ncbi-nlm-nih-gov.libproxy.usouthal.edu/pubmed/26446832.

35. Rosenblatt JD, Lee Y, McIntyre RS. The effect of pharmacogenomic testing on response and remission rates in the acute treatment of major depressive disorder: a meta-analysis. J Affect Disord 2018;241:484–91.

36. Harding KJ, Rush AJ, Arbuckle M, et al. Measurement-based care in psychiatric practice: a policy framework for implementation. J Clin Psychiatry 2011;72(8):1136–43.

37. Bousman CA, Hopwood M. Commercial pharmacogenetic-based decision-support tools in psychiatry. Lancet Psychiatry 2016;3(6):585–90.

38. Adams S, Rice MJ, Jones SL, et al. TeleMental health: standards, reimbursement, and interstate practice. J Am Psychiatr Nurses Assoc 2018;(4):295–305.

39. Hirsch JA, Rosenkrantz AB, Ansari SA, et al. Are you ready for MIPS? J Neurointerv Surg 2017;9:714–6.
40. SAMSHA-HRSA. Advancing behavioral health integration within NCQA recognized patient-centered homes. SAMSHA-HRSA Center for Integrated Health Services (online). Available at: https://www.integration.samhsa.gov/integrated-care-models. Accessed December 25, 2018.
41. SAMSHA-HRSA. Advancing behavioral health integration within NCQA recognized patient-centered homes. SAMSHA-HRSA national center for integrated health solutions. 2014. White Paper. Washington DC. Available at: https://docs.google.com/document/d/1IYmOBUsVDst_1zkcyglontUxfh47FQkkU9n9XbeYDJ4/edit#. Accessed Deccember 20, 2018.
42. Archer J, Bower P, Gilbody S, et al. Collaborative care for depression and anxiety problems. Cochrane Database Syst Rev 2012;(10):CD006525.
43. Tolliver BK, Anton RF. Assessment and treatment of mood disorders in the context of substance abuse. Dialogues Clin Neurosci 2015;17(2):181–90. Available at: https://www.ncbi.nlm.nih.gov/pubmed/26246792.
44. Knight J, Roberts T, Gabrielli J, et al. Adolescent alcohol and substance use and abuse. In: Tanski S, Garfunkel LC, Duncan PM, et al, editors. Performing preventative services: a bright futures handbook. 3rd edition. Cherry Hill (NJ): American Academy of Pediatrics; 2010. p. 103. Ch. 55.
45. Bonham A. Why are 50 percent of pregnancies in the U.S. unplanned? Special edition, A Woman's nation changes everything. The Shriver Report 10.21 2013. Available at: http://shriverreport.org/why-are-50-percent-of-pregnancies-in-the-us-unplanned-adrienne-d-bonham/. Accessed November 15, 2018.
46. Miller J, Johnson SL, Eisner L. Assessment tools for adult bipolar disorder. Clin Psychol 2009;16(2):188–201.
47. Bosanquet K, Adamson J, Atherton K, et al. Collaborative care for Screen-Positive Elders with major depression (CASPER plus): a multicentered randomized controlled trial of clinical effectiveness and cost-effectiveness. Health Technol Assess 2017;21(67):1–252.

The Physician's Physician
The Role of the Psychiatrist in Helping Other Physicians and Promoting Wellness

Keisuke Nakagawa, MD*, Peter M. Yellowlees, MBBS, MD

KEYWORDS

- Physician well-being • Wellness • Burnout • Suicide • Depression
- Physician health • Physician well-being committee • Physician health program

KEY POINTS

- Psychiatrists are strategically positioned to serve as leaders in their organizations' efforts to address physician health, including being experts at treating medical colleagues in distress.
- Psychiatrists can serve in several leadership roles at their organizations, including chief wellness officer, chair of the physician well-being committee, and in the state's physician health program.
- Culture change is needed to preserve the health of physicians. It is important to recognize the importance of physician wellness and self-care and adopt the "Quadruple Aim," which includes provider well-being as a core component of the health care system's priorities.
- Psychiatrists need to lead by example in implementing and innovating best practices for supporting physician health in their own practices and by spreading this knowledge to their colleagues.

INTRODUCTION

A recent survey found that nearly two-thirds of US physicians report feeling burnt out, depressed, or both, and it is estimated that approximately 300 to 400 physicians commit suicide every year.[1-3] Although the US health care system and medical culture have always put the patient first, the well-being of physicians has been largely ignored. Although studies have shown that physicians adopt better health care and physical lifestyle practices compared with the general population (regular exercise, less smoking, and less obesity), physicians are also noted to have high rates of mental health concerns.[4,5] At a time when the US health care system faces a critical physician

This article originally appeared in *Psychiatric Clinics*, Volume 42, Issue 3, September 2019.
Disclosure Statement: No disclosures.
Department of Psychiatry and Behavioral Sciences, UC Davis Health, 2230 Stockton Boulevard, Sacramento, CA 95817, USA
* Corresponding author.
E-mail address: drknakagawa@ucdavis.edu

shortage, improving physician health can help to maximize workforce productivity, increase quality of care, and derive more value out of every health care dollar spent.[6,7]

Many positive efforts are already underway by organizations such as the American Medical Association, the American Psychiatric Association, and the Accreditation Council for Graduate Medical Education (ACGME). These include offering online modules, creating toolkits, and mandating resident training on physician well-being, respectively.[8–10] However, significant work remains to adequately address these issues and the medical culture at large. Although physicians receive specialized medical training, their knowledge and expertise does not necessarily enable them to maintain their own personal wellness or model best practices for themselves.

THE PHYSICIAN'S PHYSICIAN: A PSYCHIATRIST'S ROLE
Psychiatrists Have Unique Skills to Treat Physicians

Psychiatrists are in a unique position to serve as the "physician's physician." Most physicians receive very limited training in psychiatry and do not have the skills and knowledge to detect early signs of burnout, depression, addictions, and suicidality in their colleagues or in themselves. This lack of formal training and experience makes it hard for many physicians to take proactive steps to speak to a colleague in distress. Other common causes of delays in addressing colleagues are fear of professional repercussions, damaging relationships, and negatively affecting team dynamics.

Psychiatrists receive substantial training in these skills during residency and throughout their careers. This places psychiatrists in prime position to help their organizations raise awareness and develop effective prevention, detection, and management programs. Historically, psychiatrists have not been proactive enough in promoting the relevance of their skills to help their colleagues and organizations tackle this hidden epidemic.

Psychiatrists Are Well Trained to Treat Very Important Person Physician Patients

Physicians may be challenging to treat. Overidentification, intimidation, and politics can play a significant role in negatively influencing care for the impaired physician who will likely be treated as a VIP. This may lead to deviations from the standard of care that other patients would have received.[11] One of the most common problematic tendencies is for the VIP (physician patient) to influence or dictate their own treatment plans. This leads to a tendency to deviate from standard treatment approaches that the treating physician would have typically made due to fear of upsetting the VIP.[11,12] Excluding physical examinations, delaying drug screens, and ignoring the role of the primary care physician are some common examples of deviations from the standard of care when treating VIPs.

Physicians may also have difficulty being completely honest with their physician patient, resorting to appeasing, or unnecessarily supporting their VIP's demands. This can lead to inappropriate or suboptimal treatments, as both parties lose clinical objectivity. It may be more appropriate and helpful to think of the "VIP" acronym as "Very Influential Patient" or "Very Intimidating Patient" instead of "Very Important Person."[12] This may bring more conscious awareness to the psychosocial traps and biases that can affect even the most cognizant physician.

Another major concern is protecting the privacy of the physician patient. Physician patients will be sensitive to being seen by other staff and colleagues while seeking care, and it is not uncommon for appointments to be scheduled outside of regular clinic hours. Physician patients often prefer to be referred outside of their practice network and pay cash to avoid having their employer or insurer having any record of their visits. Some physician patients also expect priority treatment such as being able to call their physician's cell phone directly.[11] It can be helpful to offer these, but it is critical to set clear limits.

Informal Consults: a Supportive Colleague Just One Phone Call Away

Within a health system or clinical network, psychiatrists can serve to help support and identify colleagues at risk for depression, burnout, and suicide. Physicians struggling with depression and burnout may try to hide their symptoms from colleagues for fear of professional repercussions, stigma, and judgment. Many will also be in self-denial and try to "power through" their struggle as other obstacles they have had to overcome in their life. Having a colleague who they can trust, talk to, and confide in can be one of the most effective first-line defenses. One of the most effective ways for organizations to identify struggling physicians is creating an informal referral network that includes a psychiatrist who is available to provide information and anonymous consultations.

BEST PRACTICES FOR ADDRESSING IMPAIRED PHYSICIANS AND PROMOTING WELLNESS

A large proportion of physicians report experiencing at least one symptom of burnout.[13] Many physicians have colleagues who are burnt out but are unaware of the fact and may hesitate to address such colleagues when they notice warning signs, because they receive little to no training on how to do so effectively. Having education on well-being for all physicians, and making self-care part of the culture of health care, are likely effective responses.

A Culture of Wellness as the First Defense

A clear message and acknowledgment of the impact of burnout from leadership such as the Chief Executive Officer and Chief Wellness Officer (CWO) are important first steps to promoting a culture of wellness across the organization, as long as this is done in a manner that does not blame physicians or make it seem that they are the problem. In reality, current evidence suggests that 80% of burnout is caused by administrative and systems issues, not by a lack of resilience from individual physicians. Creating open forums for staff to learn about wellness strategies and discuss burnout issues elevate the awareness of staff across the entire organization as a valuable first-line defense.[11] It is also important to create systems and processes such as anonymous hotlines, well-being committees, and reporting protocols that reduce the barrier to self-reporting or reporting a colleague (**Box 1**).

Addressing Impaired Physicians, Substance Abuse, and Addiction

Risk factors and warning signs for suicide are not different for physicians compared with the general public.[14] Educating staff on these warning signs is a critical first step to prevention, early identification, and management of burnt out physicians at risk for suicide.

It is important for colleagues to take immediate action if they notice changes in a colleague. Expressing concern for the individual, asking about their well-being, or suggesting that they speak to a mental health professional can be a critical first step to helping the individual.[11] Regularly reinforcing these points with the team at staff meetings, one-on-one sessions, and continuing medical education coursework can increase awareness and reduce the stigma that is one of the most common causes for delayed action by colleagues.

Box 1
Ten best practices for promoting wellness and addressing physician burnout

Leadership. Communicate a clear vision and plan for supporting wellness efforts. Acknowledge burnout issues and reinforce leadership's commitment to addressing them.

Well-Being Committee. Start a physician well-being committee and assign wellness champions across departments and employment levels.

Performance Metrics. Align staff performance metrics with wellness activities and objectives.

Quality Metrics. Incorporate wellness-oriented metrics as part of the organization's quality measures.

Annual Survey. Distribute an annual wellness survey to establish a concrete baseline and solicit feedback.

Interventions. Launch pilot programs based on feedback and ideas.

Data Collection. Use follow-up surveys and focus groups to measure progress and impact with quantitative and qualitative data.

Refinement. Use survey data and feedback to refine interventions and iterate on improvements. Scale successful interventions to increase impact and expand outreach.

Reinforcement. Meet regularly with leaders and staff to discuss progress, data, and interventions to promote wellness.

Systems. Establish processes to systematize key functions that reduce the barriers to getting help. Examples include anonymous self-reporting hotlines, processes for reporting colleagues, and well-being committees.

Data from American Medical Association (AMA), STEPS Forward™. Preventing Physician Burnout: improve patient satisfaction, quality outcomes and provider recruitment and retention; 2018; and Yellowlees PM. Physician suicide: cases and commentaries, 1st edition. Washington, DC: American Psychiatric Association Publishing; 2019.

It is vital to be educated on the difference between having a disorder, such as depression, and a disability or an impairment. The latter may cause work-related difficulties and require reporting through appropriate internal or external channels, potentially to a Physician Health Program, or occasionally directly to Medical Boards. Most physician patients with a psychiatric- or substance-related problem have an illness and are not impaired for work in any functional way, and they should be treated clinically and reassured that no reporting is necessary.

ORGANIZATIONAL LEADERSHIP ROLES FOR PSYCHIATRISTS TO CHAMPION PHYSICIAN WELL-BEING

Psychiatrists can play an instrumental role in driving a culture of physician well-being for their organizations. In 2017, the ACGME started requiring all accredited residency and fellowship programs "to address well-being more directly and comprehensively" (Section VI of Common Program Requirements).[10,15] This is an opportunity for psychiatrists to help craft policies, guidelines, and programs that fulfill these new requirements.

Psychiatrists can increasingly serve as valuable leaders and contributors to every organization by serving as CWO, chairing or being a member of a physician well-being committee, or working with a statewide physician health program (PHP). A description of each role is provided in more detail below summarizing key responsibilities, required skills, process for getting involved, and the kind of impact one can make in an organization by serving in such roles. These roles also offer opportunities for professional development and career enrichment for psychiatrists looking to expand the scope of their practice, engage in physician leadership, and leverage their clinical expertise to shape policies at the local and national levels.

Chair or Member of Physician Well-Being Committee

Physician well-being committees involve volunteer physicians at a hospital or health system and fulfill the 2001 mandate from the Joint Commission that requires accredited health care organizations to implement "a process to identify and manage matters of individual health for licensed independent practitioners which is separate from actions taken for disciplinary purposes." This has tended to comprise a physician well-being committee.[16,17]

The functions and practices of physician well-being committees vary significantly. Most committees focus on identification, assessment, and referral of impaired physicians to the State PHP, which takes care of the monitoring and management of the physician until they are deemed safe to return to practice. Both systems are meant to be nonpunitive and offer a safe, recovery process that does not involve the State Medical Board or de-licensing.

Physician well-being committees are good career entry points for physicians interested in getting more involved in physician health issues. Psychiatrists are well-positioned to chair these committees, given their expertise in mental health. Serving on these committees can offer a unique perspective on addiction and mental health issues, because the committee sits at the intersection of clinical practice, policy, and institutional leadership and management.

Chief Wellness Officer

CWOs are new executive level positions that often set the long-term vision, strategy, and implementation of wellness for the organization. Among the 168 LCME-accredited medical schools and 400 major teaching hospitals in North America, as of November 2018, 18 had appointed CWOs, only 2 of whom were psychiatrists.

CWOs require many different skillsets, although the addition of strong clinical expertise in mental health would seem to be most useful, making psychiatrists well positioned to fill these roles. A CWO typically manages a multidisciplinary team that spans the entire organization, has experience setting long-term vision and strategies, as well as developing shorter-term goals focused on implementation of organizational changes and well-being initiatives. CWOs have the potential to impact an organization's culture, productivity, and success. Workforce training and retention can be one of the most significant drivers of cost for any organization. Lost productivity due to physician burnout and depression is costly, leading to decreased patient volume, increased stress on other physicians who need to cover, and negative impact on quality of care as a consequence. One study calculated that the US health system incurs $3.4 billion in annual costs due to physician burnout, and a study conducted at Stanford University estimated the annual cost to their health system to be in the range of $8 million to $28 million.[6,18,19] Therefore, supporting a culture where physicians and staff can find more fulfillment, meaning, and joy in their work every day can have a significant impact on the long-term success of an organization.

State Physician Health Programs

PHPs are nonpunitive and nondisciplinary state-run programs that help physicians address their addictions and mental health conditions, recover, and create a safe, structured, and accountable plan to return to practice.

PHPs are composed of a medical director and a few full-time or part-time staff who are often psychiatrists or addiction specialists, and they are employed by the state running the PHP. It is important to note that their services are not generally free and have to be paid by physicians using them. This can cause a professional dilemma for impaired physicians, because complying with the PHPs' program may be a requirement to avoid being reported to the state medical board while they recover. However, the PHPs offer a valuable service for recovering physicians, and follow-up studies have shown that up to 80% of physicians with substance use disorders, including psychiatrists, return to practice within 5 years.[20,21]

TRAINING AND ORGANIZATIONAL CAPACITY BUILDING

There are 3 major training requirements: first, the need for self-care for all physicians; second, educational programs for physicians who wish to treat other physicians; third, institutional and departmental promotion and education of a culture of wellness. With new requirements set by ACGME for integrating physician health education in all residency programs starting in 2017, a more streamlined curriculum to assist physicians with their own self-care would be valuable to provide a standardized baseline of knowledge and skills for all physicians.[15,22]

Training in self-care and well-being is likely to be most effective when it is incorporated throughout the course of the physician's training starting in medical school. Most medical schools have resources available, including wellness counselors and academic advisors. This presents a great opportunity for psychiatry to play a more integral role in the medical school curriculum and throughout the training pipeline from medical school, to residency, to clinical practice. A comprehensive curriculum for self-care and well-being would cover a range of topics including resilience, regular participation in process-oriented reflective small groups, mindfulness training, and interpersonal skills development (**Box 2**).

Psychiatrists serving in organizational leadership capacities are strategically positioned to advocate for more exposure to their specialty during the critical period where students are assessing their careers and residency options.

No formal training program exists outside of psychiatry residency for physicians to be trained to manage physician health issues. Many physicians gain experience and knowledge by serving on committees or by treating physicians as patients. Although receiving "on-the-job" training such as this can be effective, there is wide variation in exposure and experience, and specialist training programs in this area are sorely needed.

EMBRACING CULTURAL EVOLUTION

In 2014, the Institute for Healthcare Improvement revised their original Triple Aim framework to include "Joy in Work" to make it the "Quadruple Aim."[23,24] Physicians and physicians-in-training need to be empowered to protect their health and well-being just as much as they are taught to put the patient's needs first. They both do not need to be at odds if the culture and practices evolve to protect both patients and physicians.

"It is unprofessional not to look after yourself," is a message that is rarely taught and needs to be emphasized more in the future. We need to teach a broad scope of professionalism beyond attire, appearance, timeliness, and bedside manners. The Hippocratic Oath is full of values that protect the patient's rights, but there is no mention of how physicians need to treat themselves. Many medical schools have final year

> **Box 2**
> **Key elements of comprehensive curriculum on physician self-care and well-being**
>
> *Small Groups.* Regular participation in process-oriented reflective small groups.
>
> *Networking and Relationships.* Teach ways to strengthen professional and social relationships and how to network widely and appropriately. Specific skill development in interpersonal professional relationships.
>
> *Simulations, Multimedia, and Experiential Training.* Media training, combined with experiential training using multiple communications technologies with patients and colleagues.
>
> *Mentorship.* Mentoring and mentee supervision opportunities throughout medical school and residency.
>
> *Self-Reflection.* Content and discussion of personal identity development and transformation, the interaction between burnout and physician health, empathy, compassion, and how to become reflective practitioners.
>
> *Mindfulness and Resilience Training.* Active participation and learning about resilience, mindfulness, exercise, nutrition, and relationships.
>
> *Psychiatry for Physicians.* Content on the specific psychiatric, substance abuse, and personality disorders that affect physicians and how to recognize and treat them in any physician, including the individual themselves.
>
> *Leadership and Skills Training.* Modules and discussion groups on leadership, financial, and business skills.
>
> *Systems Training.* Learning about organizational systems and the interactions that occur within them and an understanding of institutional awareness and resources that can be used to change institutions.
>
> *Adapting to Practice Changes.* Decision-making and clinical reasoning that takes into account future changes in medicine and technology such as the need for physicians to analyze large datasets and translate to patients.
>
> *Data from* Yellowlees PM. Physician suicide: cases and commentaries, 1st edition. Washington, DC: American Psychiatric Association Publishing; 2019.

students modify this oath annually and it is to be hoped that such modifications will increasingly include the importance of self-care as a professional attribute.

Psychiatrists Leading Health Care's Workforce into the Future

The country's health care workforce is rapidly changing with a new generation of physicians entering clinical practice and the baby boomer generation of physicians set to retire. Technologies such as telemedicine and smartphones are enabling more flexible and mobile work arrangements. Psychiatrists can lead a process in adapting to these new changes and evolve their practices accordingly. Today's culture and work environments need to change rapidly to support the values and work-life equilibria sought by the Millennial generation. The changes in residency applications to various specialties are indicators of the shift in workforce preferences with increasing applications to "lifestyle" specialties such as dermatology and emergency medicine. Although Millennials are often described as "high maintenance" or "entitled," they are also known to prioritize family, friends, and hobbies, making them more resilient to burnout and better at self-care than previous generations.[11,25,26] Millennials are responding to the pressures of modern medicine more effectively than previous generations of physicians, and the medical culture will have to change to take into account the needs of this upcoming generation of physicians.

Technology also plays an undeniable role in physician burnout. Electronic medical records, increased administrative workloads, and increasing emphasis on laboratories, evidence, and data analysis will inevitably affect the way physicians practice medicine and how much joy and meaning they can find in their daily practice.[27,28] How will physicians increase meaning and joy through patient care while integrating more data and technology into their clinical workflows? These are the difficult questions that need to be studied to guide the profession toward a more fulfilling practice in the future. Innovations in telemedicine, smartphones, and web-based technologies create new opportunities for physicians to adopt a more hybrid approach to their practice that integrates virtual care more into their daily practice. Psychiatrists have opportunities to shape the future practice of medicine, using their understanding of cognition and mental processes to improve workflows by designing innovative user experiences and products.

LEADING BY EXAMPLE: MODELING SELF-CARE

It is important to remember that psychiatrists are also vulnerable to burnout and depression although rates are low compared with other specialties.[28] Although we focus on opportunities to lead and support physician health in communities, we must lead by example as individuals and as a specialty. During residency, psychiatrists learn the professional demands of clinical practice, and this is a critical time to teach best practices on wellness and self-care to all psychiatric residents. Psychiatrists' everyday actions and behaviors can have the most impact on their colleagues and health systems.

From a research perspective, psychiatrists have the opportunity to advance their understanding of physician health and well-being through research, advocacy, and clinical excellence. Very few studies have evaluated the design, implementation, and effectiveness of physician health programs such as physician well-being committees or state PHPs, and self-care education programs need to be evaluated as they are introduced. Data are critical to understand what is working and what is not working and for the community to share best practices that lead to measurable outcomes. The growing physician health problem opens the door for new research opportunities and advocacy efforts that are well-suited for psychiatrists to lead.

SUMMARY

Increasing interest in physician health and well-being offers a unique opportunity for psychiatrists to elevate their profession's visibility and affect the organizational and national levels. The country's health care spending is on an unsustainable trajectory, while the physician shortage problem will only get worse as more physicians retire. Lost productivity due to physician burnout, depression, and addiction is no longer just a physician wellness issue, but it has become a national policy issue. For the health care system to gain more value out of every health care dollar, maintaining a healthy, productive physician workforce is absolutely critical.

Despite organized efforts to tackle this problem as state PHPs and the Joint Commission's mandate of implementing physician well-being committees, the culture and everyday practice of medicine still lags behind. There is an opportunity for psychiatrists to serve in numerous roles to help drive cultural change and become leaders at the organizational, regional, and national levels. Designing and implementing effective physician well-being programs requires experienced mental health professionals to provide guidance and expertise to maximize returns on these investments, while improving patient care and physician well-being.

REFERENCES

1. Peckham C. Medscape national physician burnout & depression report 2018 2018. Medscape. Available at: https://www.medscape.com/slideshow/2018-lifestyle-burnout-depression-6009235. Accessed August 22, 2018.
2. Center C, Davis M, Detre T, et al. Confronting depression and suicide in physicians: a consensus statement. JAMA 2003;289(23):3161-6.
3. Association of American Medical Colleges. Applicants and matriculants data - FACTS: applicants, matriculants, enrollment, graduates, MD/PhD, and residency applicants data - data and analysis - AAMC. Applicants and matriculants data. Available at: https://www.aamc.org/data/facts/applicantmatriculant/. Accessed August 23, 2018.
4. Helfand BKI, Mukamal KJ. Healthcare and lifestyle practices of healthcare workers: do healthcare workers practice what they preach? JAMA Intern Med 2013;173(3):242-4.
5. Compton MT, Frank E. Mental health concerns among Canadian physicians: results from the 2007-2008 Canadian Physician Health Study. ComprPsychiatry 2011;52(5):542-7.
6. Berg S. At Stanford, physician burnout costs at least $7.75 million a year. AMA Wire. 2017. Available at: https://wire.ama-assn.org/life-career/stanford-physician-burnout-costs-least-775-million-year. Accessed August 23, 2018.
7. Shanafelt T, Goh J, Sinsky C. The business case for investing in physician well-being. JAMA Intern Med 2017;177(12):1826-32.
8. Linzer M, Guzman-Corrales L, Poplau S. Preventing physician Burnout - STEPS forward.AMA | STEPS forward. Available at: https://www.stepsforward.org/modules/physician-burnout. Accessed August 23, 2018.
9. Goldman ML, Bernstein C, Chilton J, et al. Toolkit for well-being ambassadors: a manual - a guide for psychiatrists to improve physician well-being and reduce physician burnout at their institutions. 2017. Available at: https://www.psychiatry.org/psychiatrists/practice/well-being-and-burnout/well-being-resources. Accessed August 23, 2018.
10. Accreditation Council for Graduate Medical Education (ACGME). Improving physician well-being, restoring meaning in medicine. 2018. ACGME.Available at: https://www.acgme.org/What-We-Do/Initiatives/Physician-Well-Being. Accessed August 23, 2018.
11. Yellowlees PM. Physician suicide: cases and commentaries. 1st edition. Washington, DC: American Psychiatric Association Publishing; 2019.
12. Alfandre D, Clever S, Farber NJ, et al. Caring for 'very important patients'-ethical dilemmas and suggestions for practical management. Am J Med 2016;129(2):143-7.
13. Shanafelt TD, Hasan O, Dyrbye LN, et al. Changes in Burnout and satisfaction with work-life balance in physicians and the general US working population between 2011 and 2014. MayoClin Proc 2015;90(12):1600-13.
14. Preventing physician distress and suicide. Available at: https://edhub.ama-assn.org/steps-forward/module/2702599. Accessed December 28, 2018.
15. Accreditation Council for Graduate Medical Education (ACGME). ACGME common program requirements section VI with background and intent 2017. Available at: https://www.acgme.org/What-We-Do/Accreditation/Common-Program-Requirements. Accessed August 23, 2018.
16. CMA Legal Counsel and California Public, Protection and Physician Health. 5177 guidelines for physician well-being committees policies and procedures 2013.

Available at: https://www.csam-asam.org/sites/default/files/5177_oncall.pdf. Accessed August 8, 2013.

17. Joint commission requirement - MS.11.01.01. Available at: http://www.massmed.org/Physician_Health_Services/Joint_Commission/Joint_Commission_Requirement_-_MS_11_01_01/#.W375GugzpEY. Accessed August 23, 2018.

18. Goh J, Shasha Han MS, Shanafelt TD, et al. An economic evaluation of the cost of physician burnout in the United States. In: Abstract book. 2017. p. 102. San Francisco (CA): American Conference on Physician Health (ACPH); 2017. Available at: https://med.stanford.edu/content/dam/sm/CME/documents/brochures/2017/ACPH-Abstract-Book-FULL.pdf.

19. Hamidi MS, Bohman B, Sandborg C, et al. The economic cost of physician turnover attributable to burnout. In: Abstract book. 2017. p. 35. San Francisco (CA): American Conference on Physician Health (ACPH); 2017.

20. DuPont RL, McLellan AT, Carr G, et al. How are addicted physicians treated? A national survey of Physician Health Programs. J SubstAbuse Treat 2009; 37(1):1–7.

21. Yellowlees PM, Campbell MD, Rose JS, et al. Psychiatrists with substance use disorders: positive treatment outcomes from physician health programs. Psychiatr Serv 2014;65(12):1492–5.

22. White S. ACGME launches resources webpage for resident and faculty well-being. The DO 2018. Available at: https://thedo.osteopathic.org/2018/03/acgme-launches-resources-webpage-resident-faculty-well/. Accessed August 23, 2018.

23. Bodenheimer T, Sinsky C. From triple to quadruple aim: care of the patient requires care of the provider. Ann Fam Med 2014;12(6):573–6.

24. Feeley D. The triple aim or the quadruple aim? Four points to help set your strategy. IHIImprov Blog. 2017. Available at: http://www.ihi.org/communities/blogs/the-triple-aim-or-the-quadruple-aim-four-points-to-help-set-your-strategy. Accessed August 23, 2018.

25. Landrum S. Millennials to be the most high-maintenance in the workplace. Forbes 2018. Available at: https://www.forbes.com/sites/sarahlandrum/2018/01/12/millennials-to-be-the-most-high-maintenance-in-the-workplace/. Accessed August 23, 2018.

26. Hershatter A, Epstein M. Millennials and the world of work: an organization and management perspective. J Bus Psychol 2010;25(2):211–23.

27. Sinsky C, Colligan L, Li L, et al. Allocation of physician time in ambulatory practice: a time and motion study in 4 specialties. Ann Intern Med 2016;165(11): 753–60.

28. Arndt BG, Beasley JW, Watkinson MD, et al. Tethered to the EHR: primary care physician workload assessment using EHRevent log data and time-motion observations. Ann Fam Med 2017;15(5):419–26.

Mixed Features in Depression
The Unmet Needs of Diagnostic and Statistical Manual of Mental Disorders Fifth Edition

Isabella Pacchiarotti, MD, PhD[a], Giorgio D. Kotzalidis, MD, PhD[b],
Andrea Murru, MD, PhD[a], Lorenzo Mazzarini, MD, PhD[b],
Chiara Rapinesi, MD[b], Marc Valentí, MD, PhD[a],
Gerard Anmella, MD[a], Susana Gomes-da-Costa, MD[a],
Anna Gimenez, MD[a], Cristian Llach, MD[a], Giulio Perugi, MD[c],
Eduard Vieta, MD, PhD[a],*, Norma Verdolini, MD, PhD[a]

KEYWORDS

• Major depressive disorder • Bipolar disorder • DSM-5 • Mixed features specifier
• Nonoverlapping symptoms • Overlapping symptoms

KEY POINTS

- The identification of mixed features during a major depressive episode is important due to the worse course and treatment issues associated with this condition.
- Diagnostic and Statistical Manual of Mental Disorders Fifth Edition mixed features specifier criteria are controversial, because it includes typical manic symptoms, whereas it excludes overlapping excitatory symptoms that are frequently reported in mixed depression.
- Psychomotor agitation, mood lability, and aggressiveness are the new proposed criteria based on the results of the Bipolar Disorders: Improving Diagnosis, Guidance and Education-II-Mix study.
- Several clinical and course indicators of bipolarity were found to be associated with the presence of mixed characteristics, mainly overlapping excitatory symptoms, during a major depressive episode.

This article originally appeared in *Psychiatric Clinics*, Volume 43, Issue 1, March 2020.
^a Barcelona Bipolar and Depressive Disorders Program, Hospital Clinic, University of Barcelona, Institute of Neuroscience, IDIBAPS, CIBERSAM, 170 Villarroel st, 12-0, Barcelona, Catalonia 08036, Spain; ^b Neurosciences, Mental Health, and Sensory Organs (NESMOS) Department, Faculty of Medicine and Psychology, Sapienza University, Sant'Andrea University Hospital, UOC Psichiatria, Via di Grottarossa 1035-1039, Rome 00189, Italy; ^c Department of Clinical and Experimental Medicine, University of Pisa, Via Roma 67, Pisa 56100, Italy
* Corresponding author. Bipolar Disorders Unit, Institute of Neuroscience, IDIBAPS, CIBERSAM, Hospital Clínic de Barcelona, c/Villarroel, 170, 12-0, Barcelona 08036, Spain.
E-mail address: EVIETA@clinic.cat

Clinics Collections 11 (2021) 27–36
https://doi.org/10.1016/j.ccol.2020.12.027

INTRODUCTION

The identification of mixed features in bipolar disorder (BD) and major depressive disorder (MDD) is an open challenge in psychiatry, because an accurate diagnosis is a prerequisite for the initiation of adequate therapeutic approaches.[1–4] Although the importance of mixed states was increasingly recognized in the last decades, the Kraepelinian concept of a continuum between manic and depressive states was not incorporated into major psychiatric diagnostic systems such as the Diagnostic and Statistical Manual of Mental Disorders Third Edition (DSM-III), DSM-III-R, DSM-IV, DSM-IV-TR,[5–8] and the International Classification of Diseases, Tenth Edition.[9] Substantial changes to the diagnosis of BD mixed state were made in the DSM-5.

The DSM-IV–defined categorical approach of diagnosing mixed states (ie, a period of 1 week when the criteria are met for both a manic episode and a major depressive episode [MDE] nearly every day) has been replaced in DSM-5 by the dimensional mixed features specifier (MFS).[10] Despite the introduction of the MFS, substantial controversy still remains as to whether the definition proposed reflects the empirical evidence.[11,12]

MAJOR DEPRESSIVE EPISODE WITH MIXED FEATURES

The importance of promptly recognizing the presence of mixed characteristics during an MDE is mostly due to clinical variables associated with greater severity, namely the higher number of episodes[13]; the lower response or switch with antidepressants (ADs)[14]; the high prevalence of psychiatric comorbidities such as anxiety, substance use,[13] and borderline personality disorder[15]; the increased risk of suicide[16]; worse psychosocial functioning; and quality of life.[17]

In DSM-5, a depressive episode with MFS would apply if the criteria for an MDE are met along with 3 or more of the following nonoverlapping symptoms: elevated/expansive mood, inflated self-esteem, talkativeness, flight of ideas, increased energy, goal-directed activity, decreased need for sleep, and excessive involvement in activities that have high potential for adverse consequences.[10]

Major concerns still exist for the DSM-5 specifier particularly due to the exclusion of overlapping symptoms, such as distractibility, irritability, and psychomotor agitation. As a consequence, different classifications have been developed, such as the research-based diagnostic criteria for mixed depression (RBDC) that are defined by the presence of an MDE plus 3 out of 14 hypomanic symptoms. The included hypomanic symptoms differ between the 2 classifications: the DSM-5 includes the symptom "decreased need for sleep" that is not included in the RBDC. The RBDC includes overlapping symptoms between episodes of opposite poles and other symptoms such as aggression and affective lability that are not considered in the rubric of mixed symptoms in the DSM-5.

In 2015, a large multicenter study, the Bipolar Disorders: Improving Diagnosis, Guidance and Education (BRIDGE)-II-Mix study, was conducted in order to estimate the frequency of depressive mixed features during an MDE, considering not only the DSM-5 criteria but also the RBDC criteria. The latter identified 4 times more patients with MDE as having mixed features and yielded statistically more robust associations with several illness characteristics of BD than did DSM-5 criteria, such as family history of mania; lifetime suicide attempts; duration of the current episode greater than 1 month; atypical features; early onset history of AD-induced mania/hypomania; and lifetime comorbidity with anxiety, alcohol, and substance use disorders, attention-deficit/hyperactivity disorder, and borderline personality disorder.[18]

A recent cluster analysis of the same study identified an algorithm of predictive symptoms of mixed depression and supported the predominant role for overlapping "manic" symptoms in defining mixed depressive states, namely irritability, psychomotor agitation, and distractibility, together with other excitatory features shared with mania and atypical features, such as emotional lability, mood reactivity, absence of reduced appetite, and absence of psychomotor retardation, rather than by nonoverlapping manic symptoms.[19]

WHY DSM-5 DOES NOT FIT WITH REAL MIXED DEPRESSION?

Several aspects of the clinical presentation of MDE with MFS commonly seen in clinical practice unfortunately seem not to be reflected by the diagnostic DSM-5 criteria for mixed features. Particularly, it is quite infrequent to observe euphoria and grandiosity as mixed features in the context of an MDE both in bipolar and unipolar depression. Indeed, findings from the BRIDGE-II-Mix study highlighted that euphoria and grandiosity were rare mixed features (4.6% and 3.7%, respectively) among the entire sample.[18] Similarly, Sato and colleagues[20] found that in their sample euphoria and grandiosity ranged from 1% to 4% and stated that euphoria and grandiosity were too uncommon to be used for the selection of patients with depressive mixed states. Maj and colleagues[21] reported that no depressive patients, either agitated or nonagitated, presented elevated mood, inflated self-esteem, or grandiosity. Results from the Systematic Treatment Enhancement Program for Bipolar Disorder, including data of 1380 bipolar depressed patients, found that in those patients presenting subsyndromal mania or a full mixed episode the specific manic symptoms with the highest frequency did not include either elation or grandiosity.[22] These findings suggest that the "real-world" depressive patients with mixed features may have characteristics of hypo/manic behavior but they lack expansiveness typical of euphoria and grandiosity.[12]

With the aim of avoiding overdiagnosis, DSM-5 MFS has excluded the overlapping "manic" symptoms, leaving many patients with mixed depression undiagnosed.[12] Many investigators have claimed how overlapping symptoms, such as anxiety, psychomotor agitation, mood lability, irritability, and distractibility, are the most frequently observed in mixed patients and may actually represent the core features of mixed depression.[12,23,24] In the BRIDGE-II-Mix study including 2811 unipolar or bipolar depressed patients, the most frequent manic/hypomanic symptoms according to the RBDC mixed criteria were irritable mood (32.6%), emotional/mood lability (29.8%), distractibility (24.4%), psychomotor agitation (16.1%), impulsivity (14.5%), aggression (14.2%), racing thoughts (11.8%), and pressure to keep talking (11.4%).[18] Interestingly, in a recent cluster analysis of the BRIDGE-II-Mix study, although nonoverlapping DSM-5 mixed symptoms were more represented among the group of depressive patients with mixed features, the symptoms that better predicted the mixed cluster were irritable mood, emotional/mood lability, psychomotor agitation, distractibility mood reactivity, absence of reduced appetite, and absence of psychomotor retardation, pointing out that none of these correspond to DSM-5 MFS criteria.[19]

Noteworthy, most of the overlapping symptoms have been found to be associated with clinical and course variables related to a bipolar diathesis such as BD diagnosis, family history of hypomania, atypical features, early age of onset, history of switch with ADs, suicide attempts, comorbidity with alcohol and substances disorders, attention deficit hyperactivity disorder (ADHD) and borderline personality disorder, probably indicating a better "affinity" of these features to the bipolar spectrum.[18] Similarly, Malhi and colleagues[23] found that the so-called DIP symptoms, including distractibility, irritability, and psychomotor agitation, were fundamental to define mixed depression and all 3 were key features in indicating a clinical course that suggests a bipolar spectrum disorder.

This leads to another important issue: the capability of the DSM-5 to capture the real accurate diagnosis of mixed presentations. In fact, overlapping criteria have been excluded by DSM-5 because they were thought to be nonspecific.[23] As a consequence, the choice of a more "specific" approach has been made at the expenses of the "sensitivity" of the classification.[25,26] In fact, DSM-5 MFS presented a 100% specificity but only 5.1% sensitivity,[27] as also highlighted in the recent cluster analysis of the BRIDGE-II-Mix group.[19] This means that up to 95% of patients presenting with mixed features according to the DSM-5 are wrongly diagnosed as having "pure" affective episodes with huge clinical and therapeutic implications.[25,27]

The speculative wish to avoid "overlapping" symptoms, such as psychomotor agitation, irritability, and mood lability, the most common features of mixed depression across the literature, is very restrictive, allowing the diagnosis of mixed depression only in 1 out of 4 cases.[18] Certainly, these symptoms may be nonspecific but to exclude them entirely may be not justified, in the absence of any evidence that the remaining criteria are sufficiently sensitive.[28]

THE CLINICAL RELEVANCE OF MIXED SYMPTOMS NOT INCLUDED IN DSM-5 CRITERIA: RESULTS FROM BRIDGE-II-MIX STUDY
Psychomotor Agitation

DSM-5 criteria for MFS currently exclude psychomotor agitation, making it diagnostically irrelevant because it represents one of the symptoms defining the B criterion of an MDE in DSM-5. Conversely, the concept of agitation and psychomotor excitement has been consistently proposed as the key point of mixed depression across the literature. Actually, Koukopoulos and colleagues,[12,16] based on their clinical experience, considered the classic "agitated depression" the most dramatic clinical picture of depressive mixed states, being psychomotor agitation, when present, a fairly distinctive symptom to make the diagnosis of mixed depression. Moreover, in a pooled post hoc analysis of both the BRIDGE and the BRIDGE-II-Mix studies, psychomotor agitation was closely related to bipolarity and was found to characterize an especially difficult-to-treat subgroup of patients, requiring a more complex regimen of pharmacologic treatment.[29]

Affective Lability

The psychopathologic construct of affective lability assumed a central role both as a traitlike clinical feature in mixed episodes[30] and as one of the 3 most frequent state features in mixed depression, together with agitation and irritability.[12] Traditionally, affective lability in a depressive mixed episode was considered as a risk factor of shifting between MDD and BD[31,32] and was found to be strongly associated with atypical depression, in which the core symptom is mood reactivity,[10] that has been typically related to bipolar depression.[32]

In a post hoc analysis of the BRIDGE-II-Mix study,[33] more than a half of the patients reporting affective lability were diagnosed with a DSM-5 MDE with mixed features. Several findings from this study seem to support that the presence of affective lability during an MDE was associated with mixicity, particularly with a more severe clinical condition, such as the severity of cooccurring hypo/manic symptoms during an MDE. Furthermore, mood reactivity was the variable most significantly associated with affective lability, and vice versa, leading the investigators to review their results in the light of a unique continuum between mood states, concluding that the intertwined association between affective lability and mood reactivity might bridge the gap between mixed and atypical depression.[33] Consistently, affective lability and mood reactivity are 2 of the 7 clinical features proved to be the best predictors of membership of the mixed cluster in the cluster analysis of the BRIDGE-II-Mix study.[19]

Aggressiveness

Aggressiveness is not currently considered as a DSM diagnostic criterion of MFS in either bipolar or unipolar depressive episodes despite its prevalence being around 15% in an MDE, according to RBDC mixed criteria.[18] In a post hoc analysis of the BRIDGE-II-Mix study[34] focused on this behavioral construct, the most relevant clinical variable associated with aggressiveness was the presence of a DSM-5 MDE with mixed features. Several findings from this study supported its association with bipolarity per se, independently from comorbid disorders such as borderline personality disorder and substance abuse, for example, the higher frequency of BD diagnosis in depressed patients with aggressiveness, whereas a diagnosis of unipolar depression was negatively correlated with aggressive behaviors. Moreover, MDE patients with aggressiveness showed higher rates of family history for BD as well as younger age at the first depressive episode. Taken together, these results might have important implications in terms of the reconsideration of aggressiveness for diagnostic criteria for the MFS.

The proposed mixed features are shown in **Fig. 1**.

CLINICAL INDICATORS OF "MIXICITY" THAT SUGGEST A BIPOLAR DIATHESIS

Interestingly, the RBDC criteria, but not DSM-5 criteria, for MFS were found to be associated with several indicators of bipolarity, as mentioned earlier.[18]

Since the publication of the BRIDGE-II-Mix study, several post hoc analyses found that different clinical variables related to a bipolar diathesis were more likely associated with the presence of mixed features during a bipolar or unipolar MDE (**Fig. 2**).

Suicidality

The presence of suicidality was the focus of a post hoc analysis by Popovic and colleagues,[35] which found that depressed patients with a previous history of suicide attempts presented distinct clinical features that suggest a bipolar diathesis, such as a first-degree family history of BD, psychotic and atypical features, more (hypo)manic switches with AD, and higher rates of treatment resistance. Moreover, suicidal behavior was associated with RBDC mixed features, particularly risky behavior, psychomotor agitation, and impulsivity.

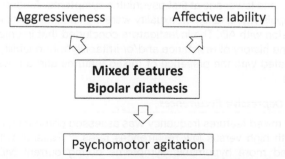

Fig. 1. New proposed mixed features: results from BRIDGE-II-Mix study.

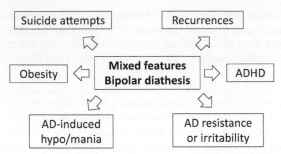

Fig. 2. Clinical and course features that suggest BD: results from BRIDGE-II-Mix study.

Antidepressant-Induced Hypomania

The emergence of new hypo/manialike responses to AD treatment in patients diagnosed as having a major depressive disorder (MDD-AIHM) has been assessed by Barbuti and colleagues.[36] The investigators compared patients in the MDD-AIHM group with those suffering from MDD or BD without a history of AD-induced hypo/mania and found that in the MDD-AIHM group, familiarity for BD and rates of atypical features and comorbid psychiatric disorders were similar to that of patients with BD and significantly more frequent compared with the MDD group. MDD-AIHM patients presented clinical course variables associated with BD, such as more than 3 affective episodes and higher rates of treatment resistance. The frequency of MDE with MFS was similar in patients of the MDD-AIHM and BD groups and significantly higher in both groups than in the MDD group. This led the investigators to claim the need for the DSM-5 inclusion of patients with MDD with AIHM within the rubric of BD.

Treatment Resistance or Worsening of Depression Associated with Antidepressant

Another recent analysis from the BRIDGE-II-Mix group was aimed at exploring the possible association between different inadequate patterns of response to ADs and bipolarity in unipolar depressive patients.[37]

Patients with or without a history of resistance to AD treatment and with or without a previous AD-induced irritability and mood lability have been compared. Those with AD treatment resistance showed higher rates of psychotic features, history of suicide attempts, emotional lability and impulsivity as mixed features, comorbid borderline personality disorder, and polypharmacologic treatment.

Patients presenting previous affective lability and irritability following AD treatment showed significantly higher rates of first-degree family history for BD, previous treatment-resistant depression, atypical features, psychiatric comorbidities, lifetime suicide attempts, and lower age at first psychiatric symptoms. Among mixed features, distractibility, impulsivity, and hypersexuality were significantly associated with worsening of depression with AD. The investigators concluded that in unipolar depressed patients, a lifetime history of resistance and/or irritability/mood lability in response to ADs was associated with the presence of mixed features and a possible underlying bipolar diathesis.

Higher Rates of Depressive Recurrences

The presence of mixed features frequency was assessed comparing unipolar depressive patients with high versus low recurrences rates.[38] Patients with higher recurrences presented more hypomanic symptoms during current MDE, resulting in higher rates of mixed depression according to both DSM-5 and RBDC criteria.

Moreover, they presented clinical indicators of bipolarity such as earlier depressive onset, more family history of BD, more atypical features, suicide attempts, treatment resistance, (hypo)manic switches when treated with AD, and higher psychiatric comorbidities.

Obesity

A comparison of patients with or without obesity (body mass index >30) presenting an MDE was conducted in a subanalysis of the BRIDGE-II-Mix study.[39] Obese depressed patients showed higher rates of history of (hypo)manic switches during AD treatment, atypical depressive features, comorbid eating disorders, and anxiety disorders. Psychomotor agitation, distractibility, increased energy, and risky behaviors were the mixed features more frequently presented among obese patients. When hypersomnia was studied with the metabolic aspects in the same sample, the cooccurrence of hypersomnia and overweight/obesity represented a more extreme clinical phenotype of bipolarity complicated by treatment-related adverse effects and mixed features.[40]

Psychiatric Comorbidities

The presence of psychiatric comorbidities, particularly those sharing an important underpinning impulsive component, has been related in a sample of depressed patients with mixed features and bipolarity. The presence of mixed features during an MDE in comorbidity with borderline personality disorder was associated with a more complex course of illness associated with bipolarity, reduced treatment response, and worse outcomes.[41] Similarly, in those patients presenting a comorbid ADHD, mixed features and bipolar clinical course indicators were more represented.[42]

SUMMARY

A proper identification of an MDE with mixed features is of huge importance not only for the diagnostic implications but also for clinical practice due to the worse course and treatment issues associated with this condition.

The DSM-5 made an important step in this sense by introducing the specifier "with mixed features," thus recognizing for the first time that symptoms of opposite polarity may co-occur during an MDE of either BD-I, BD-II, or unipolar MDD and are diagnostically different from pure episodes within these 3 clinical entities. Conversely, the DSM-5 criteria for MFS during an MDE are based on the putative construct of avoiding overdiagnosis due to overlapping symptoms. The definition of MDE with MFS according to DSM-5 is controversial because it includes typical manic symptoms, such as elevated mood and grandiosity, that were found to be rare among patients with mixed depression, whereas it excludes overlapping excitatory symptoms that are frequently reported in mixed depression. Leaving out these 3 symptoms means that only 25% of patients with mixed depression will actually meet DSM-5 criteria. In this sense, the authors agree with Koukopoulos and Sani's position that is to rename the clinical identity of these symptoms as "excitatory" instead of "manic," in order to underline the different nature of this excitatory component from the pure manic symptom presentation in defining mixed features during an MDE.

Indeed, the BRIDGE-II-Mix group claimed at including in the rubric of MFS symptoms, such as psychomotor agitation, mood lability, and aggressiveness, which are not currently considered as mixed features in the DSM-5.

Furthermore, despite the DSM-5 MFS may characterize also a unipolar mixed depression, we argue that the presence of excitatory overlapping symptoms may describe more specifically a subgroup of depressed patients uncovering a bipolar diathesis. This is in line with the findings of the studies mentioned earlier, in which several clinical and course indicators of bipolarity, such as suicidality, AD-induced hypo(mania), treatment resistance or worsening of depression associated with AD, higher rates of depressive recurrences, metabolic issues such as overweight or obesity, and the presence of specific psychiatric comorbidities, ADHD, and borderline personality disorder in particular were found to be associated with the presence of mixed characteristics, mainly overlapping excitatory symptoms, during an MDE.

The aforementioned considerations suggest the need of a deep revision of the MFS in depression for the planned DSM-5 text revision.

DISCLOSURE

Dr I. Pacchiarotti has received CME-related honoraria or consulting fees from ADAMED, Janssen-Cilag, and Lundbeck. Dr A. Murru has received grants, honoraria, or consulting fees from, Janssen, Lundbeck, and Otsuka. Prof. G. Perugi has acted as consultant of Lundbeck, Angelini, FB-Health. He received grant/research support from Lundbeck and Angelini. He is on the speaker/advisory board of Sanofi-Aventis, Lundbeck, FB-Health, and Angelini. Pr E. Vieta has received grants and served as consultant, advisor, or CME speaker for the following entities: AB-Biotics, Abbott, Allergan, Angelini, AstraZeneca, Bristol-Myers Squibb, Dainippon Sumitomo Pharma, Farmindustria, Ferrer, Forest Research Institute, Gedeon Richter, GlaxoSmithKline, Janssen, Lundbeck, Otsuka, Pfizer, Roche, SAGE, sanofi-aventis, Servier, Shire, Sunovion, Takeda, the Brain and Behaviour Foundation, the Spanish Ministry of Science and Innovation (CIBERSAM), the EU Horizon 2020, and the Stanley Medical Research Institute. Dr G.D. Kotzalidis, Dr L. Mazzarini, Dr C. Rapinesi, Dr M. Valentí, Dr G. Anmella, Dr S. Gomes-da-Costa, Dr A. Gimenez, Dr C. Llach, and Dr N. Verdolini has been supported by a BITRECS. BITRECS project has received funding from the European Union's Horizon 2020 research and innovation programme under the Marie Skłodowska-Curie grant agreement No 754550 and from "La Caixa" Foundation.

REFERENCES

1. Grande I, Berk M, Birmaher B, et al. Bipolar disorder. Lancet 2016;387(10027): 1561–72.

2. Solé E, Garriga M, Valentí M, et al. Mixed features in bipolar disorder. CNS Spectr 2017;1–7. https://doi.org/10.1017/S1092852916000869.

3. Vieta E, Berk M, Schulze TG, et al. Bipolar disorders. Nat Rev Dis Prim 2018;4: 18008.

4. Vieta E, Salagre E, Grande I, et al. Early intervention in bipolar disorder. Am J Psychiatry 2018;175(5):411–26.

5. American Psychiatric Association. Diagnostic and statistical manual of mental disorders 3rd edition. Washington, DC; 1980.

6. American Psychiatric Association. Diagnostic and statistical manual of mental disorders. 3rd edition, Rev. Washington, DC: Author.; 1987.

7. American Psychiatric Association. Diagnostic and statistical Manual of mental disorders. 4th edition. Washington, DC: Author.; 1994.

8. American Psychiatric Association. Diagnostic and statistical manual of mental disorders. 4th edition, text revision. Washington, DC: Author.; 2000.

9. World Health Organization. International statistical classification of diseases and related health problems, 10th Revision (ICD-10). Geneva (Switzerland): Author.; 1992.

10. American Psychiatric Association. Diagnostic and statistical manual of mental disorders. 5th edition. Washington, DC: American Psychiatric Association; 2013.
11. Takeshima M, Oka T. DSM-5-defined 'mixed features' and Benazzi's mixed depression: Which is practically useful to discriminate bipolar disorder from unipolar depression in patients with depression? Psychiatry Clin Neurosci 2015; 69(2):109–16.
12. Koukopoulos A, Sani G. DSM-5 criteria for depression with mixed features: a farewell to mixed depression. Acta Psychiatr Scand 2014;129(1):4–16.
13. Angst J, Cui L, Swendsen J, et al. Major depressive disorder with subthreshold bipolarity in the national comorbidity survey replication. Am J Psychiatry 2010; 167(10):1194–201.
14. Smith DJ, Forty L, Russell E, et al. Sub-threshold manic symptoms in recurrent major depressive disorder are a marker for poor outcome. Acta Psychiatr Scand 2009;119(4):325–9.
15. Zimmermann P, Brückl T, Nocon A, et al. Heterogeneity of DSM-IV major depressive disorder as a consequence of subthreshold bipolarity. Arch Gen Psychiatry 2009;66(12):1341.
16. Koukopoulos A, Sani G, Koukopoulos AE, et al. Melancholia agitata and mixed depression. Acta Psychiatr Scand Suppl 2007;115(433):50–7.
17. McIntyre RS, Soczynska JK, Cha D, et al. The prevalence and illness characteristics of DSM-5-defined "mixed feature specifier" in adults with major depressive disorder and bipolar disorder: results from the International Mood Disorders Collaborative Project. J Affect Disord 2015;172:259–64.
18. Perugi G, Angst J, Azorin J-M, et al. Mixed features in patients with a major depressive episode: the BRIDGE-II-MIX study. J Clin Psychiatry 2015;76(3): e351–8.
19. Brancati GE, Vieta E, Azorin J-M, et al. The role of overlapping excitatory symptoms in major depression: are they relevant for the diagnosis of mixed state? J Psychiatr Res 2019;115:151–7.
20. Sato T, Bottlender R, Schröter A, et al. Frequency of manic symptoms during a depressive episode and unipolar "depressive mixed state" as bipolar spectrum. Acta Psychiatr Scand 2003;107(4):268–74. Available at: http://www.ncbi.nlm.nih. gov/pubmed/12662249. Accessed July 11, 2018.
21. Maj M, Pirozzi R, Magliano L, et al. Agitated "unipolar" major depression: prevalence, phenomenology, and outcome. J Clin Psychiatry 2006;67(5):712–9. Available at: http://www.ncbi.nlm.nih.gov/pubmed/16841620. Accessed July 21, 2019.
22. Goldberg JF, Perlis RH, Bowden CL, et al. Manic symptoms during depressive episodes in 1,380 patients with bipolar disorder: findings from the STEP-BD. Am J Psychiatry 2009;166(2):173–81.
23. Malhi GS, Byrow Y, Outhred T, et al. Exclusion of overlapping symptoms in DSM-5 mixed features specifier: heuristic diagnostic and treatment implications. CNS Spectr 2017;22(2):126–33.
24. Perugi G, Quaranta G, Dell'Osso L. The significance of mixed states in depression and mania. Curr Psychiatry Rep 2014;16(10):486.
25. McIntyre RS, Lee Y, Mansur RB. A pragmatic approach to the diagnosis and treatment of mixed features in adults with mood disorders. CNS Spectr 2016; 21(S1):25–33.
26. Vieta E, Valentí M. Mixed states in DSM-5: Implications for clinical care, education, and research. J Affect Disord 2013;148(1):28–36.

27. Stahl SM. Mixed-up about how to diagnose and treat mixed features in major depressive episodes. CNS Spectr 2017;22(02):111–5.
28. Perugi G. ICD-11 mixed episode: nothing new despite the evidence. Bipolar Disord 2019;21(4):376–7.
29. Barbuti M, Mainardi C, Pacchiarotti I, et al. The role of different patterns of psychomotor symptoms in major depressive episode: pooled analysis of the BRIDGE and BRIDGE-II-MIX cohorts. Bipolar Disord 2019. [Epub ahead of print].
30. Mackinnon DF, Pies R. Affective instability as rapid cycling: theoretical and clinical implications for borderline personality and bipolar spectrum disorders. Bipolar Disord 2006;8(1):1–14.
31. Akiskal HS, Maser JD, Zeller PJ, et al. Switching from "unipolar" to bipolar II. An 11-year prospective study of clinical and temperamental predictors in 559 patients. Arch Gen Psychiatry 1995;52(2):114–23.
32. Benazzi F. The relationship of major depressive disorder to bipolar disorder: continuous or discontinuous? Curr Psychiatry Rep 2005;7(6):462–70. Available at: http://www.ncbi.nlm.nih.gov/pubmed/16318825. Accessed July 21, 2019.
33. Verdolini N, Menculini G, Perugi G, et al. Sultans of swing: a reappraisal of the intertwined association between affective lability and mood reactivity in a post hoc analysis of the BRIDGE-II-MIX study. J Clin Psychiatry 2019;80(2). https://doi.org/10.4088/JCP.17m12082.
34. Verdolini N, Perugi G, Samalin L, et al. Aggressiveness in depression: a neglected symptom possibly associated with bipolarity and mixed features. Acta Psychiatr Scand 2017. https://doi.org/10.1111/acps.12777.
35. Popovic D, Vieta E, Azorin J-M, et al. Suicide attempts in major depressive episode: evidence from the BRIDGE-II-Mix study. Bipolar Disord 2015;17(7):795–803.
36. Barbuti M, Pacchiarotti I, Vieta E, et al. Antidepressant-induced hypomania/mania in patients with major depression: evidence from the BRIDGE-II-MIX study. J Affect Disord 2017;219:187–92.
37. Perugi G, Pacchiarotti I, Mainardi C, et al. Patterns of response to antidepressants in major depressive disorder: drug resistance or worsening of depression are associated with a bipolar diathesis. Eur Neuropsychopharmacol 2019;29(7):825–34.
38. Mazzarini L, Kotzalidis GD, Piacentino D, et al. Is recurrence in major depressive disorder related to bipolarity and mixed features? Results from the BRIDGE-II-Mix study. J Affect Disord 2018;229:164–70.
39. Petri E, Bacci O, Barbuti M, et al. Obesity in patients with major depression is related to bipolarity and mixed features: evidence from the BRIDGE-II-Mix study. Bipolar Disord 2017;19(6):458–64.
40. Murru A, Guiso G, Barbuti M, et al. The implications of hypersomnia in the context of major depression: results from a large, international, observational study. Eur Neuropsychopharmacol 2019;29(4):471–81.
41. Perugi G, Angst J, Azorin J-M, et al. Relationships between mixed features and borderline personality disorder in 2811 patients with major depressive episode. Acta Psychiatr Scand 2016;133(2):133–43.
42. Vannucchi G, Medda P, Pallucchini A, et al. The relationship between attention deficit hyperactivity disorder, bipolarity and mixed features in major depressive patients: Evidence from the BRIDGE-II-Mix Study. J Affect Disord 2019;246:346–54.

Psychotherapy for Mixed Depression and Mixed Mania

Brittany O'Brien, PhD[a,b,1], Delphine Lee, LCSW[b],
Alan C. Swann, MD[a,b], Sanjay J. Mathew, MD[a,b],
Marijn Lijffijt, PhD[a,b,*,1]

KEYWORDS

- Psychotherapy • Mixed features • Patient-centered approach
- Evidence-based treatment • Suicide • Anxiety • Hypomania

KEY POINTS

- Treatment guidelines for mixed depression and for mixed (hypo)mania focus generally on pharmacologic intervention.
- In individuals with major depressive disorder, psychotherapy in conjunction with psychopharmacology has treatment effects almost twice as large compared with single intervention.
- Because of the clinical profile, mixed depression defined as (past) major depressive episode with 2 or more manic symptoms could benefit from psychotherapies for bipolar disorder.
- Psychotherapies for mixed states should incorporate modules for reducing suicide risk and anxiety, characteristics of mixed states, and adapt a person-centered rather than manualized approach.

INTRODUCTION

Worldwide, 11% to 13% of adults have a lifetime history of major depressive disorder (MDD),[1,2] and 1% of adults worldwide have a lifetime history of bipolar disorder (BD)[2]; 23.8% of individuals with MDD and 35.2% of individuals with BD experience at least 3 (hypo)manic symptoms during a major depressive episode (MDE), and 35.1% of individuals with BD experience at least 3 MDE symptoms during a (hypo)manic episode.[3] Irrespective of primary episode, the presence of at least 2 symptoms of the opposite

This article originally appeared in *Psychiatric Clinics*, Volume 43, Issue 1, March 2020.
[a] Michael E. DeBakey VA Medical Center, Houston, TX 77030, USA; [b] Menninger Department of Psychiatry and Behavioral Sciences, Baylor College of Medicine, 1977 Butler Boulevard, Houston, TX 77030, USA
[1] Both authors contributed equally to this work.
* Corresponding author. Menninger Department of Psychiatry and Behavioral Sciences, Baylor College of Medicine, 1977 Butler Boulevard, Houston, TX 77030.
E-mail address: marijn.lijffijt@bcm.edu

Abbreviations

BD	Bipolar disorder
CBT	Cognitive-behavioral therapy
DBT	Dialectical behavior therapy
MDD	Major depressive disorder
MDE	Major depressive episode

pole is associated with an earlier age onset, rapid cycling, a higher risk of psychosis, a higher risk of a substance use disorder, enhanced anxiety, a higher risk of a suicide attempt,[4–7] and increased treatment resistance.[7,8] In BD, MDE with irritability is associated with delayed recovery.[9]

Treatment guidelines for mixed states focus almost exclusively on pharmacologic interventions and electroconvulsive therapy.[10] Guidance about psychological interventions is absent, despite evidence of the efficacy and extended benefits of psychological interventions across psychiatric disorders, in particular when combined with pharmacotherapy.[11,12] To our knowledge there is no evidence-based psychotherapy for mixed depression or mixed (hypo)mania.

The presence of mixed states present several challenges for treatment, including:

1. A higher likelihood of a severe illness course, with early onset and frequent and/or prolonged periods of affective and behavioral instability.
2. Increased susceptibility to comorbid addiction, trauma-related disorders, and suicide.
3. Treatment targets that shift, in various combinations, over time.

The approach for any psychotherapy treatment plan for mixed states will benefit from being tailored to the patient given his or her specific clinical profile. The treatment plan needs also to be flexible, accounting for the changing and varying needs of a patient at different stages of the illness course. In this article, we (i) describe the clinical characteristics of mixed depression and/or (hypo)mania, (ii) present evidence-based methods and techniques that we believe should be considered for patients with mixed states, and (iii) present a case report to illustrate a tailored, adaptive psychotherapy treatment plan for a patient with MDD with mixed features.

CLINICAL CHARACTERISTICS OF MIXED STATES

To meet criteria for mixed states, an individual must meet (or have met) clinical criteria for MDE and/or a (hypo)manic episode with at least some symptoms of the opposite pole. The *Diagnostic and Statistical Manual of Mental Disorders*, 5th edition, defines the mixed features specifier as having at least 3 symptoms of the opposite pole excluding irritability and psychomotor agitation.[13] However, these diagnostic criteria will likely misdiagnose a proportion of individuals as having pure MDE or pure (hypo)mania, even though they would benefit from treatment for mixed states. Research has shown a more severe clinical illness course for individual who have MDE or (hypo)mania with at least 2 symptoms of the opposite pole, including irritability and agitation. MDE with at least 2 (hypo)manic symptoms in the context of MDD overlap with clinical characteristics of BD rather than MDD.[14] Mixed MDE in the context of MDD or BD is associated with symptoms of overactivation (irritability, psychic and psychomotor agitation, talkativeness, flight of ideas, or racing thoughts); other symptoms of mania, including expansive mood, rarely occur during mixed depression.[5,15–18] In addition to mania-associated overactivation, mixed MDE is also characterized by mood lability, including anger.[17] Worry and negative self-evaluation cuts across mixed depression and (hypo)mania.[5] Depression and (hypo)mania with at least 2 symptoms of the opposite pole have been associated with increased anxiety. Depression and (hypo)mania with at least 3 symptoms of the opposite pole have been associated with increased suicide risk.[5] These findings suggest 3 things:

1. Individuals with MDE or (hypo)mania are at higher risk of a more severe illness course and premature mortality when at least 2 symptoms of the opposite pole are present, including the presence of irritability and agitation.
2. Mixed MDE in the context of MDD resembles the clinical characteristics of MDE in the context of BD, suggesting that individuals with mixed MDE in the context of MDD may more optimally benefit from treatments designed for BD than for MDD.
3. Interventions of mixed states must address the increased risk of suicide and enhanced anxiety.

CONSIDERATIONS FOR PSYCHOTHERAPY OF MIXED STATES

A literature search in PubMed, Google Scholar, WorldCat, and the Cochrane Library revealed no psychotherapy studies specifically for mixed depression or (hypo)mania. This finding suggests that there are few resources for psychosocial treatments specifically designed to meet the needs of patients with mixed depression or (hypo)mania.

Fortunately, a rich array of psychotherapies already exist for MDD and BD from which interventions can be drawn to create an integrated, evidence-based treatment plan tailored to each patient's clinical profile. Because the clinical characteristics of mixed depression in MDD overlap with the clinical characteristics of BD,[14] clinicians are encouraged to consult evidence-based therapies for BD that address the range of symptoms that may occur in a manic, depressive, or mixed episode of the illness. Given the usual severity of illness for patients with mixed states, psychological interventions have to be adjunctive and complementary to pharmacologic intervention rather than used as a stand-alone treatment.

Evidence-based treatment for BD include cognitive-behavioral therapy (CBT), family-focused therapy, and interpersonal and social rhythms therapy.[19] CBT is based on the premise that mood disturbance is the consequence of maladaptive, dysfunctional thinking and that problematic cognitions can be modified.[19–21] Family-focused therapy is based on the premise that caregiver criticism and hostility contribute to and increase relapse risk, which can be modified by changing communication among family members and increasing problem-solving skills.[19] Interpersonal and social rhythms therapy attributes BD-associated mood episodes as a disturbance to circadian rhythms, which can be modified by regulating daily routines and sleep–wake rhythms.[19]

CBT, family-focused therapy, and interpersonal and social rhythms therapy consist of interventions aimed at teaching of coping skills, social and communication skills, symptom recognition, capitalizing on personal strength and resources, functional thinking, adaptive thinking, relaxation, problem solving, sleep–wake cycles, and mindfulness. Although each therapy is unique in terms of structure and emphasis, all include psychoeducation. Controlled clinical trials have shown immediate and sustained effects of these therapies to attenuate symptoms of depression and of mania, lengthen time to relapse, diminish time ill, improve sleep, and improve medication adherence.[19,22–26] CBT is effective in decreasing suicidal behaviors[27] as well as symptoms of anxiety in the context of anxiety disorders.[28]

Interventions for mixed states should also address suicide risk and anxiety. Dialectical behavior therapy (DBT), developed originally for borderline personality disorder (which clinically resembles mixed states) and suicidality,[29] proposes that overt and covert actions are learned behaviors and are amendable through cognitive modification, training of new skills, exposure, and dealing with unexpected situations. DBT reduces self-directed violent behaviors[30,31] by increasing mindfulness, emotion regulation, and distress tolerance.[25]

In this article, we propose a person-centered treatment approach that integrates evidence-based psychological interventions to address common challenges and symptoms that present in episodes of MDD or BD with mixed states. Treatment addresses (i) illness-related safety, (ii) therapy participation, (iii) current symptoms and difficulties, and (iv) relapse prevention. Many of the techniques that we refer to have been used in psychotherapy trials for BD. **Fig. 1** and **Table 1** display the breakdown and the proposed interventions for psychotherapy for a patient with mixed states. We conclude with a case example of Laura to illustrate a tailored, adaptive psychotherapy treatment plan for a patient with MDD with mixed features.

PHARMACOLOGIC TREATMENT

Treatment guidelines of mixed states recommend pharmacologic interventions and/or electroconvulsive therapy.[10] Communication between the health care providers providing medication management and providing psychotherapy is vital to align treatment goals and manage issues related to potential noncompliance.

Assessment of Mixed States and Symptoms

The Schedule for Affective Disorders and Schizophrenia (SADS) is a clinical interview that assesses severity of symptoms of depression, mania, suicidality, anxiety, and psychosis associated with mixed states that would otherwise require various separate forms;[32–34] the SADS has a change version, which can be used at follow-up. Treatment providers can also assess each disorder and problem area independently (see **Table 1**).

ILLNESS-RELATED SAFETY ISSUES AND TREATMENT PARTICIPATION
Suicide Risk Management

Development of a safety plan, approached in a collaborative and constructive fashion, can provide an early opportunity in therapy for alliance building between patient and

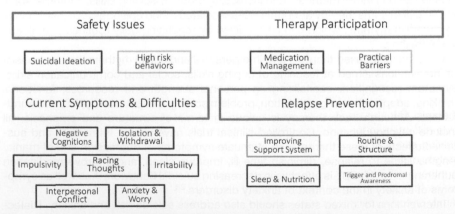

Fig. 1. Diagram of interventions for mixed depression or mixed (hypo)mania.

Table 1
Symptoms of mixed states and interventions

Symptom	Assessment Tool	Interventions
Suicide risk	Collaborative Assessment and Management of Suicidality (CAMS) Beck Scale for Suicide Ideation (BSSI) Sheehan Suicide Tracking Scale (S-STS) Concise Health Risk Tracking Scales (CHRT-SR; CHRT-C)	Collaborative assessment and management of suicidality Crisis response plan (CRP) Distress tolerance skills (DBT) Cognitive-behavioral therapy (CBT)
Impulsivity	Barratt Impulsiveness Scale (BIS-11) UPPS Impulsivity Behavior Scale (UPPS)	Mindfulness (DBT) Emotional regulation skills (DBT) Distress tolerance skills (DBT) Coping ahead (DBT)
Irritability/agitation	Irritability, Depression, Anxiety (IDA) Scale	Emotion regulation skills (DBT) Interpersonal and social rhythms therapy (IPSRT)
Low mood	Beck Depression Inventory (BDI)	Accumulating positives (DBT)
Worry and anxiety	Penn State Worry Questionnaire (PSWQ) Generalized Anxiety Disorder 7-item screening (GAD-7)	Cognitive Restructuring (CBT) Mindfulness (DBT) Worry time Relaxation skills
Negative cognitions	Beck Depression Inventory (BDI)	Cognitive restructuring (CBT) Mindfulness (DBT) Cognitive Defusion (ACT)
Sleep	Pittsburg Sleep Quality Index (PSQI)	Cognitive-behavioral therapy for insomnia (CBT-I) Interpersonal and social rhythm therapy (IPSRT)
Racing thoughts	Focussed clinical interview	Reducing internal and external overstimulation (CBT) Organization strategies (PST; CBT)
Interpersonal conflict/strained relationships	Focused clinical interview	Interpersonal Effectiveness (DBT)
Isolation and withdrawal	UCLA Loneliness Scale	Increasing social support and interactions with family/friends (IPT)

therapist.[35] It also creates a model for adaptive, active, and collaborative coping. Suicide risk interventions commonly teach cognitive reframing techniques and problem-solving skills. Stress reframing can be especially valuable for patients with mixed states, many of whom will have developed an enhanced reactivity to stressors.[36,37] Another helpful technique is to identify specific reasons to live, which orients patients to the future. Helping patients to identify or reconnect with social supports, whether family or community groups, is recommended to increase the number of people a patient can rely on for support during times of crisis.

High-Risk Behaviors

Patients who experience increased activation are often at risk of engaging in behaviors endangering themselves and possibly others. High-risk sexual behaviors, excessive spending, and making investments in ventures that are seemingly too good to be true are common behaviors that signal to others a patient is unwell and in need of treatment. Oftentimes, insight is limited regarding the negative consequences of these behaviors in the moment, but may be improved after the fact. A discussion about the short-term versus long-term consequences of the behaviors should be had, emphasizing the benefit of establishing concrete, practical barriers to safeguard the patient from painful and potentially irreversible long-term consequences. Implementation of these boundaries and safeguards should be discussed with relevant family members and legal or financial representatives.

THERAPY PARTICIPATION
Treatment Adherence

Patients and their support network benefit from being educated on the complexities and challenges that come specifically with mixed states. The goal is to move from compliance and adherence to responsible participation.

Practical Barriers

Patients could face significant practical barriers. Challenges to accessing care because of financial, transportation, and scheduling limitations should be addressed to minimize their impact on treatment.

SYMPTOMS AND DIFFICULTIES

A careful assessment of a patient's current symptoms and concerns will inform the selection of evidence-based interventions to improve: coping skills, social and communication skills, symptom recognition, personal strength and resource recognition, functional and adaptive thinking, problem solving skills, sleep–wake cycles, relaxation, and mindfulness skills. As noted, treatment targets may shift. For example, therapy may initially address a combination of depression and overactivation and the associated risk of suicidal behavior. At a later point, interactions between affect or action control and interpersonal communication may be the appropriate focus of treatment and require different interventions. Controlled clinical trials have shown immediate and sustained effects of those modules to improve depression and mania, improve sleep, improve medication adherence,[19,22–26] and to diminish suicidal behaviors[27] and anxiety.[28] Specific interventions should be selected to best suit a patient's clinical profile, his or her circumstances, and a provider's training in delivering the interventions. **Table 1** displays commonly observed symptoms with mixed states, and displays a variety of evidence-based treatments as examples of interventions for those symptoms.

RELAPSE PREVENTION

In BD, the use of behavioral coping mechanisms during a prodromal phase reduced risk of relapse and was associated with fewer mood episodes.[38] Mood charts are used across a variety of disorders. Several good templates are available online. The mood chart should not be too complex, but should be customized based on episode prodromes that the patient and therapist have identified. Mood charts are a vehicle to increase a sense of control, and to facilitate alliance and communication with the therapist.

CASE STUDY

Laura was a 27-year-old, married, accountant who was referred for psychotherapy by her psychiatrist. She began experiencing a lot of "ups and downs" in college. In her senior year, close friends called Laura's parents because she had stopped attending class, was up most of the night, and had expressed a wish to no longer live. She took a medical leave of absence from school, sought treatment, and was diagnosed with MDD with mixed features. Since then, she had been "off and on" prescribed mood stabilizers, more recently "off" since meeting and marrying her husband 1 year ago. She started feeling more irritable and anxious 6 months after they were married. She also started having difficulty focusing at work. About 3 months ago, conflict with coworkers regarding her increasing unreliability resulted in a confrontation with her boss and his suggestion that she resign. Laura's husband and parents were understanding of Laura's difficulties and tried their best to be supportive. However, they were also growing tired and increasingly frustrated by her moodiness, seeming lack of effort to get herself back on track, and not knowing how to help her.

Laura arrived to her first psychotherapy appointment with her husband and mother, wearing wrinkled, casual attire. She appeared tired and ungroomed. She stated that the past few months had been "awful" since losing her job, and that she experienced significant difficulty maintaining basic self-care habits and keeping up with household chores. She described low mood, irritability, racing thoughts, and chronic worry about her marriage and finances. She also noted binge eating, insomnia, and suicidal ideation in the past month. She spent most of the day in bed watching television while her husband was at work. At night, she paced around her house. Her marriage was especially strained since her husband discovered several thousand dollars of credit card debt from online shopping sprees and a withdrawal from her 401K to purchase a lavish all-inclusive vacation for their anniversary. Laura reported abstaining from alcohol and denied engaging in illicit substance use. During the initial phase of treatment, the provider conducted an assessment of safety concerns, factors that posed barriers to engaging in treatment, and current symptoms associated with presenting concerns. **Fig. 1** illustrates the organization of the treatment planning as well as the focal points and interventions used.

Psychoeducation

Psychoeducation was provided to Laura and her family on the expected course, recurrence, and prognosis of MDD with mixed features. Family members were also provided with information regarding the evidence of effectiveness and benefits of psychotherapy. Expectations for therapy were addressed, particularly the recommendation that Laura's family be involved in her treatment. This process included her family helping to establish structure and provide support during periods of greater illness severity, as well as learning to spot emerging prodromal symptoms and helping her to access appropriate levels of care. Laura's reported history of noncompliance with prescribed medications was addressed by providing psychoeducation on the effectiveness of medication. This information was shared with Laura's husband and parents to support compliance during periods when Laura was feeling better and might feel less motivated to take her medication.

Safety Concerns

A safety plan was developed using the crisis response plan model to address suicidal ideation. Laura was guided in a narrative assessment of the most recent crisis and identified thoughts, emotions, behaviors, and bodily sensations to outline possible warning signs of increased risk. Contacts she could reach out to when feeling at increased risk of self-harm were also identified. These people included Laura's husband, parents, and a cousin. Distracting and pleasant activities that were familiar, relaxing, and did not pose risk for overspending were identified, including taking her dog for walk, working on a puzzle, and baking. Laura expressed often feeling overwhelmed by the intensity of her suicidal thoughts. For this reason, distress tolerance skills taken from DBT were introduced and included into her safety plan. Finally, cognitive restructuring techniques were applied to challenge and modify suicidal thoughts.

Targeted Symptom Interventions

The following treatment interventions were applied to target Laura's symptoms and to improve her general coping skills. A variety of evidence based interventions may have been used for these symptoms and were selected based on Laura's receptiveness to the CBT and DBT models:

- *Irritability*: In addition to relaxation skills to decrease irritability, mindfulness skills were introduced to increase emotion awareness, bodily sensations, and the presence of primary and secondary emotions. Emotion regulation skills from DBT were also introduced to address emotional reactivity.
- *Racing thoughts*: To combat Laura's racing thoughts, factors contributing to overstimulation in the environment (noise, clutter, and being in crowds) were identified and removed where possible. She was also educated on the importance of being adherent to medication to manage this symptom. Finally, Laura was taught organizational and time management strategies.
- *Anxiety and worry*: Laura learned cognitive restructuring skills to address thoughts that perpetuated her anxiety and worry. Relaxation techniques such as progressive muscle relaxation and paced breathing were also practiced during and between sessions.
- *Negative cognitions*: Laura engaged in chronic negative thoughts about unemployment, hygiene, and perceived burden on her spouse. Cognitive restructuring techniques were used to identify and modify maladaptive thinking patterns.
- *Isolation and withdrawal*: Since she became ill, Laura significantly decreased time spent outside of her home and with other people. Small goals were made each week to engage in pleasurable, easy-going activities with a friend or a family member outside of the house. It was important when selecting these activities that they felt manageable and were familiar, so as not to induce anxiety.
- *Interpersonal conflict*: Laura's symptoms and history of illness contributed to significant strain on her marriage. They had also made it difficult for Laura to maintain friendships and get along with others. Interpersonal effectiveness skills taken from DBT were introduced to increase her comfort in communicating emotions and needs that increased responsiveness from spouse, parents, and friends.
- *Impulsivity*: Emotional regulation strategies such as (i) chain analysis of the presenting problem and distress tolerance skills taken from DBT were incorporated to increase awareness of impulsive urges, and (ii) mindfulness of possible consequences and alternative behaviors. These coping skills helped Laura to problem solve and identify practical steps to manage her urges to shop online.

Relapse Prevention Interventions

After mapping out Laura's patterns associated with the described symptoms, Laura became more aware of the contributing factors and warning signs that her symptoms were emerging and worsening. **Fig. 2**—drawn from the CBT model—was completed

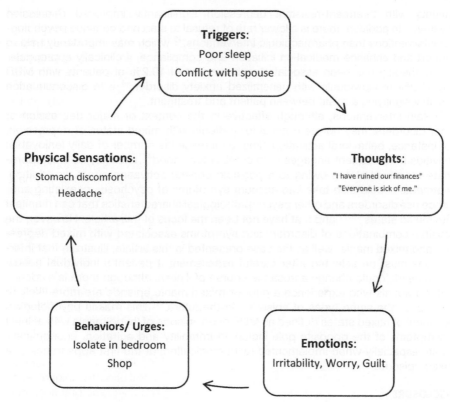

Fig. 2. Laura's personalized illness cycle.

to personalize the relationship between Laura's specific triggers, thoughts, emotions, behaviors, and physical sensations. The figure was shared with her family members to educate them on early warning signs as well. A copy was kept on Laura's phone and posted at home for reference. To decrease risk of relapse, Laura's sleep habits and daily routines were evaluated. Sleep interventions from CBT for insomnia (sleep restriction is contraindicated for Laura), including stimulus control, were applied. Laura was also recommended to regularly exercise. Laura and her provider developed regular daily routines that helped her to plan ahead and balance tasks, chores, and leisure activities to support her mood and relationships. As her symptoms remitted, Laura felt well enough to return to work. She and her provider prepared for changes to her routines and modified daily schedule to ensure she had adequate time to complete scheduled activities during the day and maintain good sleep habits.

SUMMARY

Current treatment guidelines for patients with mixed depression or (hypo)mania focus almost exclusively on psychopharmacological and electroconvulsive therapy interventions,[10] foregoing evidence-based psychosocial treatments. Psychosocial interventions have been proven effective for MDD,[39–41] BD,[19,24] suicidal behaviors,[27] and anxiety.[28] In MDD, psychological and pharmacologic interventions have both similar efficacy, with combined treatment having effects that could be twice as large compared with single interventions.[11,12,39] Adding CBT to treatment as usual in patients with treatment-resistant depression significantly improved depression severity.[42] In addition, there is a lower rate of refusal to start and continue psychological interventions than pharmacologic interventions,[43] which may importantly help to support and enhance medication initiation and compliance, if clinically appropriate. Psychotherapy has been associated with dropout of 19.2% of patients with MDD and 15.2% of individuals with generalized anxiety disorder,[44] with discontinuation possibly signifying a misfit between patient and treatment.

Certain interventions, although effective in the context of major depression or other disorders, may not be optimal for patients with mixed states of depression. For instance, behavioral activation aims to increase the number of daily (enjoyable) activities that a patient engages in to combat low mood[41] and may be less appropriate for mixed states owing to a possible general activating effect. In addition, treatments should also take into account symptoms of psychosis, coexisting substance use disorders and other psychopathological characteristics that can manifest with mixed states[4,5,45] and that have not been the focus of this article. However, the possible combinations of disorders and symptoms associated with mixed depression and mixed mania, well as the case presented in this article, illustrate that interventions must be selected after careful assessment a patient's individual needs. These needs could change across the course of illness, although there is evidence that individuals who experience a pure or mixed manic episode are more likely to experience the same types of episodes in the future.[46] This makes psychological treatment of mixed states defined as MDE or an episode of (hypo)mania with at least 2 symptoms of the opposite pole including irritability and agitation, economically viable, especially when implemented (with medication) at the first appearance of a mixed episode.

DISCLOSURE

The authors have nothing to disclose related to this work. Drs B. O'Brien, A.C. Swann, S.J. Mathew and M. Lijffijt are supported by the use of resources and facilities at the Michael E. Debakey VA Medical Center, Houston, Texas.

REFERENCES

1. Kessler RC, Sampson NA, Berglund P, et al. Anxious and non-anxious major depressive disorder in the World Health Organization World Mental Health Surveys. Epidemiol Psychiatr Sci 2015;24:210–26.
2. Merikangas KR, Jin R, He J-P, et al. Prevalence and correlates of bipolar spectrum disorder in the world mental health survey initiative. Arch Gen Psychiatry 2011;68:241–51.
3. Vázquez GH, Lolich M, Cabrera C, et al. Mixed symptoms in major depressive and bipolar disorders: a systematic review. J Affect Disord 2018;225:756–60.
4. Swann AC, Janicak PL, Calabrese JR, et al. Structure of mania: depressive, irritable, and psychotic clusters with different retrospectively-assessed course patterns of illness in randomized clinical trial participants. J Affect Disord 2001;67:123–32.
5. Swann AC, Steinberg JL, Lijffijt M, et al. Continuum of depressive and manic mixed states in patients with bipolar disorder: quantitative measurement and clinical features. World Psychiatry 2009;8:166–72.
6. Balázs J, Benazzi F, Rihmer Z, et al. The close link between suicide attempts and mixed (bipolar) depression: implications for suicide prevention. J Affect Disord 2006;91:133–8.

7. Azorin J-M, Aubrun E, Bertsch J, et al. Mixed states vs. pure mania in the French sample of the EMBLEM study: results at baseline and 24 months–European mania in bipolar longitudinal evaluation of medication. BMC Psychiatry 2009; 9:33.

8. Jha MK, Malchow AL, Grannemann BD, et al. Do baseline sub-threshold hypomanic symptoms affect acute-phase antidepressant outcome in outpatients with major depressive disorder? Preliminary findings from the randomized CO-MED trial. Neuropsychopharmacology 2018;43:2197–203.

9. Yuen LD, Shah S, Do D, et al. Current irritability associated with hastened depressive recurrence and delayed depressive recovery in bipolar disorder. Int J Bipolar Disord 2016;4(1):15.

10. Verdolini N, Hidalgo-Mazzei D, Murru A, et al. Mixed states in bipolar and major depressive disorders: systematic review and quality appraisal of guidelines. Acta Psychiatr Scand 2018;138:196–222.

11. Cuijpers P, Sijbrandij M, Koole SL, et al. Adding psychotherapy to antidepressant medication in depression and anxiety disorders: a meta-analysis. World Psychiatry 2014;13:56–67.

12. Cuijpers P, Dekker J, Hollon SD, et al. Adding psychotherapy to pharmacotherapy in the treatment of depressive disorders in adults: a meta-analysis. J Clin Psychiatry 2009;70(9):1219–29.

13. APA. Diagnostic and statistical manual of mental disorders. 5th edition. Arlington (VA): American Psychiatric Association; 2013.

14. Sato T, Bottlender R, Schröter A, et al. Frequency of manic symptoms during a depressive episode and unipolar "depressive mixed state" as bipolar spectrum. Acta Psychiatr Scand 2003;107:268–74.

15. Malhi GS, Byrow Y, Outhred T, et al. Exclusion of overlapping symptoms in DSM-5 mixed features specifier: heuristic diagnostic and treatment implications. CNS Spectr 2017;22:126–33.

16. Koukopoulos A, Sani G, Ghaemi SN. Mixed features of depression: why DSM-5 is wrong (and so was DSM-IV). Br J Psychiatry 2013;203:3–5.

17. Sani G, Vöhringer PA, Napoletano F, et al. Koukopoulos' diagnostic criteria for mixed depression: a validation study. J Affect Disord 2014;164:14–8.

18. Akiskal HS, Benazzi F, Perugi G, et al. Agitated "unipolar" depression reconceptualized as a depressive mixed state: implications for the antidepressant-suicide controversy. J Affect Disord 2005;85(3):245–58.

19. Geddes JR, Miklowitz DJ. Treatment of bipolar disorder. Lancet 2013;381: 1672–82.

20. Hofmann SG, Asnaani A, Vonk IJJ, et al. The efficacy of cognitive behavioral therapy: a review of meta-analyses. Cognit Ther Res 2012;36:427–40.

21. Leichsenring F, Hiller W, Weissberg M, et al. Cognitive-behavioral therapy and psychodynamic psychotherapy: techniques, efficacy, and indications. Am J Psychother 2006;60:233–59.

22. Chu C-S, Stubbs B, Chen T-Y, et al. The effectiveness of adjunct mindfulness-based intervention in treatment of bipolar disorder: a systematic review and meta-analysis. J Affect Disord 2018;225:234–45.

23. Hofmann SG, Sawyer AT, Witt AA, et al. The effect of mindfulness-based therapy on anxiety and depression: a meta-analytic review. J Consult Clin Psychol 2010; 78:169–83.

24. Vallarino M, Henry C, Etain B, et al. An evidence map of psychosocial interventions for the earliest stages of bipolar disorder. Lancet Psychiatry 2015;2:548–63.

25. Eisner L, Eddie D, Harley R, et al. Dialectical behavior therapy group skills training for bipolar disorder. Behav Ther 2017;48:557–66.
26. Lukens EP, McFarlane WR. Psychoeducation as evidence-based practice: considerations for practice, research, and policy. Brief Treat Crisis Interv 2004;4: 205–25.
27. Tarrier N, Taylor K, Gooding P. Cognitive-behavioral interventions to reduce suicide behavior: a systematic review and meta-analysis. Behav Modif 2008;32: 77–108.
28. Carpenter JK, Andrews LA, Witcraft SM, et al. Cognitive behavioral therapy for anxiety and related disorders: a meta-analysis of randomized placebo-controlled trials. Depress Anxiety 2018;35:502–14.
29. Swales MA. Dialectical behaviour therapy: description, research and future directions. Int J Behav Consult Ther 2009;5(2):164–77.
30. DeCou CR, Comtois KA, Landes SJ. Dialectical behavior therapy is effective for the treatment of suicidal behavior: a meta-analysis. Behav Ther 2019;50:60–72.
31. Panos PT, Jackson JW, Hasan O, et al. Meta-analysis and systematic review assessing the efficacy of Dialectical Behavior Therapy (DBT). Res Soc Work Pract 2014;24:213–23.
32. Endicott J, Spitzer RL. Use of the research diagnostic criteria and the schedule for affective disorders and schizophrenia to study affective disorders. Am J Psychiatry 1979;136:52–6.
33. Endicott J, Spitzer RL. A diagnostic interview: the schedule for affective disorders and schizophrenia. Arch Gen Psychiatry 1978;35:837–44.
34. Endicott J, Cohen J, Nee J, et al. Hamilton depression rating scale. Extracted from regular and change versions of the schedule for affective disorders and schizophrenia. Arch Gen Psychiatry 1981;38(1):98–103.
35. Ellis TE, Green KL, Allen JG, et al. Collaborative assessment and management of suicidality in an inpatient setting: results of a pilot study. Psychotherapy 2012. https://doi.org/10.1037/a0026746.
36. Lijffijt M, Hu K, Swann AC. Stress modulates illness-course of substance use disorders: a translational review. Front Psychiatry 2014;5:83.
37. Lijffijt M. Stress and addiction. In: Swann AC, Moeller FG, Lijffijt M, editors. Neurobiology of addiction. 1st edition. New York: Oxford University Press; 2016. p. 153–75.
38. Lam D, Wong G, Sham P. Prodromes, coping strategies and course of illness in bipolar affective disorder–a naturalistic study. Psychol Med 2001;31:1397–402.
39. Cuijpers P, Berking M, Andersson G, et al. A meta-analysis of cognitive-behavioural therapy for adult depression, alone and in comparison with other treatments. Can J Psychiatry 2013;58:376–85.
40. Barth J, Munder T, Gerger H, et al. Comparative efficacy of seven psychotherapeutic interventions for patients with depression: a network meta-analysis. PLoS Med 2013;10:e1001454.
41. Ekers D, Webster L, Van Straten A, et al. Behavioural activation for depression; an update of meta-analysis of effectiveness and sub group analysis. PLoS One 2014;9(6):e100100.
42. Ijaz S, Davies P, Williams CJ, et al. Psychological therapies for treatment-resistant depression in adults. Cochrane common mental disorders group. Cochrane Database Syst Rev 2018. https://doi.org/10.1002/14651858.CD010558.pub2.
43. Swift JK, Greenberg RP, Tompkins KA, et al. Treatment refusal and premature termination in psychotherapy, pharmacotherapy, and their combination: a meta-analysis of head-to-head comparisons. Psychotherapy 2017;54:47–57.

44. Swift JK, Greenberg RP. A treatment by disorder meta-analysis of dropout from psychotherapy. J Psychother Integr 2014;24:193–207.
45. Swann AC. The strong relationship between bipolar and substance-use disorder. Ann N Y Acad Sci 2010;1187:276–93.
46. Baldessarini RJ, Salvatore P, Khalsa H-MK, et al. Dissimilar morbidity following initial mania versus mixed-states in type-I bipolar disorder. J Affect Disord 2010;126(1–2):299–302.

Diagnosis, Clinical Features, and Therapeutic Implications of Agitated Depression

Gaia Sampogna, MD*, Valeria Del Vecchio, MD, PhD,
Vincenzo Giallonardo, MD, Mario Luciano, MD, PhD,
Andrea Fiorillo, MD, PhD

KEYWORDS

- Agitated "unipolar" depression • Mixed states • Suicide • Psychomotor agitation
- Treatments

KEY POINTS

- Depression is a complex disorder with multiple symptomatic clusters, including affective, cognitive, and physical dimensions, with a heterogeneous clinical presentation.
- Agitated "unipolar" depression is a distinct affective syndrome conceptualized as lying on the continuum of the bipolar disorder spectrum or as a distinct unipolar depression. This difference has obvious therapeutic and prognostic implications.
- The clinical picture of agitated "unipolar" depression is characterized by low mood, diminished interest in activities, and psychomotor excitation, whereas melancholic depression is characterized by retarded psychomotor functioning and anhedonia.
- Agitated "unipolar" depression requires a personalized management and treatment plan, which should include mood stabilizers, atypical antipsychotics, and benzodiazepines. The use of antidepressants is controversial.

INTRODUCTION

Depression is a complex, severe mental disorder with multiple symptomatologic dimensions, including affective, cognitive, and physical symptoms.[1,2] In the last decade, a significant increase in the incidence of the disorder of almost 20% has been observed.[3,4] In 2015, depressive disorders were the greatest contributor to nonfatal health loss. The average lifetime prevalence of major depressive disorder (MDD) is estimated to be 14.6% in high-income countries.[5] Moreover, MDD represents the leading cause of disability worldwide,[6] accounting for 2.5% of global Disability Adjusted Life Years lost, especially in women. Depression has been traditionally

This article originally appeared in *Psychiatric Clinics*, Volume 43, Issue 1, March 2020.
Department of Psychiatry, University of Campania "Luigi Vanvitelli", Largo Madonna delle Grazie, Naples 80138, Italy
* Corresponding author.
E-mail address: gaia.sampogna@gmail.com

described as a clinical state characterized by low mood, reduced levels of energy, and reduction in motor and physic activity, with disturbances in motivation, reward, and arousal.[7] Some patients with major depression present activation as a product of inner tension and anxiety, which is defined as "psychic pain," a type of activation completely different from the goal-oriented one present during a manic episode. Therefore, the clinical presentation of major depressive disorder can be very heterogeneous, with some patients presenting features of psychomotor excitation together with sad mood and diminished interest in activities. Patients with agitated depression are characterized by a depressed and anxious mood with inner, psychic agitation, whereas psychomotor agitation could even not be present.[8] This clinical condition has been neglected in recent years, and it does not appear as a full clinical diagnosis in modern classification systems. However, more recently, there has been a renewed clinical and research interest toward this syndrome, which is a "difficult to treat" subtype of depression, often refractory to antidepressant treatments.

Along the years, agitated "unipolar" depression has been conceptualized as a mixed affective state[9] or as a type of major depressive episode associated with subsyndromal symptoms of mania.[10] Historically, Kraepelin[11] and Weygandt[12] defined "excited depression," in which symptoms of excitement and inhibition were present in the same episode, which was developed from the concept of *melancholia agitata*. More recently, Akiskal and colleagues[13] underlined that agitated depression is a distinct affective syndrome characterized by intraepisode noneuphoric hypomanic symptoms and a family history of bipolar disorder, lying on a continuum of the bipolar disorder spectrum.

THE PROBLEM OF CLASSIFICATION OF AGITATED "UNIPOLAR" DEPRESSION

In the modern classification systems, the diagnosis of agitated depression is unclear and misleading. In 1978, with the approval of Research Diagnostic Criteria, agitated depression was considered a subtype of depressive episode, which could be present either during a major depressive disorder or during a bipolar disorder.[10] In the third edition of the Diagnostic and Statistical Manual for Mental Disorders (DSM-III),[14] the category of MDD included several depressive states, such as melancholic depression (with psychomotor retardation and anhedonia) and agitated depression. However, this categorization has not been acknowledged in the subsequent versions of the DSM and in the International Classification of Diseases (ICD). In the DSM-IV, a diagnosis of mixed episode could be formulated as a combination of a full manic episode with a major depressive episode at the same time in the course of bipolar disorders. However, this condition was very rare in ordinary clinical practice,[15] and it has not been used routinely by clinicians worldwide. The DSM-5 has included the specifier "with mixed features" in both the chapters on depressive and bipolar disorders.[16] The main advantage of the introduction of this specifier is that it can be applied to both groups of patients, increasing the clinical utility of those diagnoses. In fact, this change has given to clinicians the possibility to capture the most common subthreshold presentations of mixed states; however, some limitations still persist.[17,18] The "mixed features" specifier is defined by the presence of at least 3 hypomanic signs or symptoms during a depressive episode in the context of major depressive disorder or bipolar disorder or by more than 3 depressive features present during a (hypo)manic episode in bipolar disorder. According to the DSM-5, in order to reach the symptoms' criteria threshold for mixed features, agitation, distractibility, impulsivity, and sleep-loss should not be considered, because these symptoms are nonspecific and already listed among the symptoms of both depressive and (hypo)manic episodes.[19,20]

More in detail, the definition provided in the DSM-5 focuses on the presence of nonoverlapping manic symptoms during a major depressive episode. However, the exclusion of these features has been highly criticized, because it limits the identification of many mixed affective states.[21–23] Other investigators have argued that nonspecific and common symptoms shall not be excluded if robust scientific evidence confirm that they have enough sensitivity for making the diagnosis.[24–26] This controversy underlines the limitations of the current categorial diagnostic systems, in which the identification of clear boundaries between pure mania and pure depression, as well as between unipolar and bipolar disorders, is not possible.[27–30] These clinical conditions lay on a continuum and probably a prototypical approach, as described in the seminal works by Kraepelin[11] and Weygandt,[31] is needed, considering the clinical presentation of the syndrome as a whole and not just its individual symptoms.[32–34]

In contrast to the DSM-5, the 11th revision of the International Classification of Disorders released by the World Health Organization[35,36] categorizes mixed episodes as characterized by the presence of persistent, prominent, and rapidly alternating manic/hypomanic and depressive symptoms in a single episode lasting for at least 2 weeks. Moreover, the ICD-11 provides additional details on the contrapolar symptoms and episode-qualifiers.[37–39] The decision to keep the definition of mixed episodes similar to that of the ICD-10 is due to the fact that this approach was validated by several studies. Guidance is provided regarding the typical contrapolar symptoms observed when manic or depressive symptoms predominate.

Recently, using the criteria developed by Koukopoulos and colleagues,[9] an alternative model for classifying depressive mixed states has been proposed, focusing on the presence of psychic agitation, marked irritability, and marked mood lability, with or without other excitatory symptoms.[24,40] Koukopoulos' perspective is broad, including not only DSM-based manic symptoms but also psychic excitation.[9,41] Sani and colleagues[8] have provided a definition of mixed depression using diagnostic validators such as the presence of psychic agitation, marked irritability, and mood reactivity, with an absence of psychomotor retardation, thus further confirming the validity of these criteria. This concept of mixed depression is in line with the Kraepelinian nosology, in which a central role is given to psychic agitation, accompanied or not by motor agitation. According to this model, psychic pain, suicidal ideas, anxiety, agitation, and other symptoms, which are the core features of mixed depression, are due to an excitatory process.[9]

WHAT IS AGITATED "UNIPOLAR" DEPRESSION?

The original definitions of agitated "unipolar" depression described an affective state in which mood and ideation were in the negative polarity and activity in the opposite polarity.[11] It has also been called "excited depression" or "depression with excitatory symptoms," pointing out the presence of symptoms of excitement (ie, restlessness, talkativeness, flight of ideas, irritability) together with a depressed mood within the same affective episode.

Koukopoulos and Koukopoulos[9] proposed that agitated depression should be considered as a mixed affective state, laying on the bipolar disorder spectrum. Akiskal and colleagues[13] in a clinical sample of 254 "unipolar" patients found a strong association between agitated depression and depressive mixed state, as regards the presence of distractibility, racing/crowded thoughts, irritable mood, talkativeness, and risky behaviors in both definitions. They concluded that bipolar features can be found also in "unipolar" depressed patients and that agitated major depression can be considered as part of the bipolar spectrum, defining what we call a depressive mixed state.[42]

This conceptualization is in line with the classical definitions proposed by German psychopathologists, who included agitated depression among mixed states. "Activated depression," "agitated depression," and "depression with mixed features" would represent three overlapping clinical categories.[13] Compared with nonagitated depressed patients, during a depressive episode, patients with agitated depression present several bipolar features, including distractibility, racing/crowded thoughts, irritability, talkativeness, and risky behaviors (all classified as hypomanic symptoms).[13]

Several clinical studies have been conducted in order to describe the clinical features of agitated "unipolar" depression. In a sample of day-care patients, Perugi and colleagues[43] found that patients with agitated depression have irritable mood, pressured speech, flight of ideas, psychotic symptoms, and psychomotor agitation. Other studies[44,45] carried out in clinical samples confirmed that agitated depression is a more severe variant of bipolar depression, whose most common manic symptoms are irritability, greater talkativeness, distractibility, and racing thoughts.

Agitated depression is quite common in outpatient settings,[13] but patients with these clinical characteristics can be found also in other settings, such as primary care, tertiary care, outpatient, and inpatient units, further supporting the idea that agitated depression is a common clinical presentation.

In agitated depression, psychomotor agitation is not a sufficient symptom for characterizing this subtype of affective disorder,[13] whereas the main feature is the combination of low mood with many hypomanic symptoms.

Two subtypes of mixed depression have been proposed recently[46]: the classic agitated depression, characterized by anxiety and restlessness with motor agitation, and a second type, mainly characterized by inner psychic tension, racing and crowded thoughts, mood lability, and talkativeness, without motor agitation.[9,46] Koukopoulos identified several independent predictors of the mixed depressive state, such as premorbid temperament, course of illness, family history, worsening of the clinical status with antidepressants, and improvement with sedatives.[46] In both forms, patients can present suicidal ideation and psychotic features. Many sociodemographic and lifetime clinical features are associated with the presence of agitated depression, such as female gender,[47] more lifetime mixed episodes,[22] and the presence of suicide attempts.[48] Also, some characteristics of the index episode are associated with a higher risk of developing agitated features, such as distractibility, increased talkativeness, longer duration of the episode,[49] suicidal ideation,[50] and suicidal behavior[51] (**Box 1**).

Box 1
Main clinical features of agitated depression

- Dysphoric mood
- Emotional lability
- Psychic and/or motor agitation
- Talkativeness, crowded and/or racing thoughts
- Rumination
- Initial or middle insomnia
- Impulsive suicidal attempts
- Verbal outbursts

Agitated depression occurs in 7% to 60% of patients with major depressive disorder. In a recent study by Serra and colleagues,[51] agitated depression was present in 32% of patients, with a slightly higher prevalence in patients with bipolar II disorder (BD-II) (36.8%) compared with patients with BD-I (30.3%). However, in this study the lifetime diagnosis was not a significant predictor of the presence of agitated depression, even after controlling for other clinical and sociodemographic characteristics. The investigators argued that the different prevalence rates found between the two disorders could be due to the heterogeneity of the definition of depression with mixed features.[50] Patients with agitated depression have a poorer prognosis compared with patients with a nonagitated depression, given the inadequate response to antidepressants in the former group.[13,52]

The mixed depressive syndrome is not a transitory condition, but it can persist for several weeks or months. The clinical picture is characterized by dysphoric mood, emotional lability, psychic and/or motor agitation, talkativeness, crowded and/or racing thoughts, rumination, and initial or middle insomnia. Impulsive suicidal attempts are also frequent. The most frequently reported complaints by family members include patients' irritability, verbal outbursts, physical aggression, and hypersexuality.[46]

However, according to Swann,[7] agitation can be considered a dimensional part of the core depressive syndrome. Therefore, agitated depression should not necessarily be considered a mixed state, laying on the bipolar spectrum disorder. In particular, agitation can be considered a cross-cutting symptom of both bipolar and depressive disorders, with two different types of agitation: the former characterized by inner tension, which is most typical of depressive states, corresponding to "psychic pain"; and the latter characterized by disinhibited goal-oriented behavior, which is more frequent in manic episodes.

SUICIDALITY IN AGITATED DEPRESSION

Suicidal behaviors are due to the interaction between biological, psychosocial, and sociocultural factors. People suffering from agitated depression are at high risk of suicide, especially for the presence of racing thoughts and general restlessness. Because of flight of ideas and high levels of impulsivity, patients can take life-threatening decisions and risky behaviors. Other elements concurring to the high suicidal risk include the rapid cycling course, the predominant depressive polarity, the high levels of anxiety, the use of substances, and the presence of hopelessness and insomnia.[53–57]

Akiskal and colleagues[13] identified the presence of suicidal ideation as an independent predictive factor of having agitated depression, whereas other previous studies found a robust association between psychomotor agitation and suicidal ideation.[58–61]

More recently, Popovic and colleagues[62] found that depressed patients with impulsivity, risky behaviors, reckless driving or promiscuity, psychomotor agitation (such as pacing around a room, wringing one's hands or pulling off clothing and putting it back on, and other similar actions) have a 50% higher risk of attempting suicide compared with depressed patients without these behaviors. Therefore, the early identification of risky behaviors, psychomotor agitation, and impulsivity in patients with a major depressive episode may be crucial to reduce the risk of suicide and to develop appropriate suicide prevention plans.

Another important issue in suicidal patients with agitated depression is the role of antidepressant medications.[62] Patients taking antidepressants who become suicidal are usually in an activated state, characterized by increased energy before mood improvement. This phase, which has been defined as "activation syndrome," is characterized by agitation, irritability, impulsivity, and hostility. These symptoms represent the most common (hypo)manic symptoms occurring during a major depressive episode.[51,63] Therefore, it may be that those "unipolar" depressed patients treated with antidepressants have a paradoxic (or poor) response to antidepressants, resulting in increased suicidal behaviors.

THERAPEUTIC IMPLICATIONS

Agitated depression is a severe clinical condition that requires a specific management and treatment plan. The main challenge is represented by its adequate identification and appropriate diagnosis.[50,64] In case of patients with treatment-resistant depression, who failed to respond to treatment with 4 or 5 sequential trials of antidepressants over a period of years, a diagnosis of agitated depression should always be considered.[65] Moreover, many patients with this disorder—even if they are on a long-term pharmacologic management—do not remit and report a worsening of symptoms, mainly an exacerbation of irritability, sleep disturbances, restlessness, anxiety, or dysphoric mood for a year or more. Moreover, when psychomotor symptoms are present during a depressive episode and are misdiagnosed, there is the risk to prescribe inappropriate pharmacologic or psychological treatments. The concept of agitated depression proposes that the origin of psychic pain, suicidal ideas, anxiety, agitation, and other symptoms is an excitatory process, instead of a depressive one.

An accurate description of the clinical features of agitated "unipolar" depression is essential for successful treatment, because these patients need different treatments compared with those with a nonagitated depression.

One of the main challenges for psychiatrists in managing agitated depression is the lack of specific clinical guidelines.[66] In fact, available guidelines provide clinical recommendations for the treatment of unipolar depression, bipolar depression, and bipolar mania, whereas the authors found only one guideline specifically focusing on patients with a major depressive episode with mixed features.[67] Therefore, clinicians manage agitated depression following the guidelines for the treatment of major depressive disorder or bipolar disorder. The authors believe that this approach should be revised, because agitated depression represents a clinical condition with specific features and different prognostic implications compared with nonagitated depression.

In fact, the use of antidepressants in this condition is still controversial, because many studies found that these drugs can induce hypomanic symptoms.[68] In particular, patients with bipolar I disorder with a current mixed depression episode have a higher risk of mood switching when they take antidepressants compared with patients with BD-I without a mixed depression.[12,69] Therefore, an antidepressant monotherapy is not recommended in patients with mixed depression of any type (unipolar, BP II, or BP I), given the potential role of these drugs to increase psychomotor agitation,[70] whereas mood stabilizers or antipsychotics may reduce agitation and associated hypomanic symptoms.[9,65,68]

Although no drugs are currently approved by the Food and Drug Administration and European Medicines Agency for the treatment of agitated depression, antipsychotics and benzodiazepines have been used successfully for the treatment of this clinical condition. In particular, second-generation antipsychotics, such as asenapine, lurasidone, olanzapine, quetiapine and ziprasidone, have been tested for the treatment of depression with mixed features. Also, aripiprazole and cariprazine have shown some efficacy in improving both manic and depressive symptoms.[64]

Mood stabilizers can be used in patients with agitated depression in order to prevent mood swings and angry outbursts. However, except lamotrigine, no other mood stabilizer is approved for use in any kind of depression (unipolar, mixed, bipolar). As regards lithium, it is well known that it has antisuicidal, antiaggression, anticycling, and antimanic effects, and therefore it should be considered, whenever possible, as an effective augmentation strategy in these patients.[71,72] Benzodiazepines may be used as additional short-term medications and their beneficial effects confirm the excitatory nature of agitated depression.[73]

SUMMARY

Agitated "unipolar" depression represents a potentially dangerous clinical entity, given the high associated risk of suicide. It is extremely relevant for clinicians, mental health professionals, patients, carers, and all mental health stakeholders to adequately identify, diagnose, and treat it. This clinical condition has been neglected for many years, and therefore, there is still an open and ongoing debate about the correct classification of this disorder. In particular, it should be clarified whether this condition belongs to the group of depressive disorders or to the group of bipolar disorders. However, although already Kraepelin identified this state more than a century ago, during the evolution of modern psychiatry, the importance of mixed states has been inconstantly recognized by psychiatrists. Infact, the concept of a continuum between manic and depressive states has not been incorporated into the modern psychiatric diagnostic systems. With the approval of the DSM-5, the introduction of the specifier "with mixed features" has broadened the diagnosis of major depression, although this definition is still not adequate to capture the complexity of this clinical syndrome.

In conclusion, agitated "unipolar" depression is a severe psychiatric condition, too often misdiagnosed, which needs to be adequately addressed by researchers and identified and treated by clinicians.[74,75] In particular, considering the high levels of suicidal ideation and suicidal behaviors in these patients, it is also a public health priority to promote a correct identification and clinical management of these patients.

ACKNOWLEDGMENTS

The authors would like to acknowledge Carmela Palummo, Benedetta Pocai, Luca Steardo Jr, Arcangelo Di Cerbo, and Francesca Zinno, all from the Department of Psychiatry of the University of Campania "L. Vanvitelli", Naples, Italy.

DISCLOSURE

The authors have nothing to disclose.

REFERENCES

1. Fiorillo A, Carpiniello B, De Giorgi S, et al. Assessment and management of cognitive and psychosocial dysfunctions in patients with major depressive disorder: a clinical review. Front Psychiatry 2018;9:493.
2. McIntyre RS, Cha DS, Soczynska JK, et al. Cognitive deficits and functional outcomes in major depressive disorder: determinants, substrates, and treatment interventions. Depress Anxiety 2013;30:515–27.
3. Reynolds CF RD, Patel V. Screening for depression: the global mental health context. World Psychiatry 2017;16:316–7.
4. Ormel J, Cuijpers P, Jorm AF, et al. Prevention of depression will only succeed when it is structurally embedded and targets big determinants. World Psychiatry 2019;18:111–2.

5. Kessler RC, Bromet EJ. The epidemiology of depression across cultures. Annu Rev Public Health 2013;34:119–38.

6. World Health Organization. Depression and other common mental disorders: global health estimates. 2017. Available at: http://apps.who.int/iris/bitstream/10665/254610/1/WHO-MSD-MER-2017.2-eng.pdf. Accessed November 25, 2019.

7. Swann AC. Activated depression: mixed bipolar disorder or agitated unipolar depression? Curr Psychiatry Rep 2013;15(8):376.

8. Sani G, Vöhringer PA, Napoletano F, et al. Koukopoulos' diagnostic criteria for mixed depression: a validation study. J Affect Disord 2014;164:14–8.

9. Koukopoulos A, Koukopoulos A. Agitated depression as a mixed state and the problem of melancholia. Psychiatr Clin North Am 1999;22:547–64.

10. Spitzer RL, Endicott J, Robins E. Research diagnostic criteria for a selected group of functional disorders. 3rd edition. New York: New York State Psychiatric Institute Biometrics Inst; 1978.

11. Kraepelin E. Manic-depressive insanity and paranoia. Edinburgh (Scotland): E & S Livingstone; 1921.

12. Benazzi F. Agitated depression: a valid depression subtype? Prog Neuropsychopharmacol Biol Psychiatry 2004;28:1279–85.

13. Akiskal HS, Benazzi F, Perugi G, et al. Agitated "unipolar" depression reconceptualized as a depressive mixed state: implications for the antidepressant-suicide controversy. J Affect Disord 2005;85:245–58.

14. American Psychiatric Association. Diagnostical and statistical manual of mental disorders (DSM-III). DSM–III. 3rd edition. Washington, DC: American Psychiatric Association; 1980.

15. First MB, Rebello TJ, Keeley JW, et al. Do mental health professionals use diagnostic classifications the way we think they do? A global survey. World Psychiatry 2018;17:187–95.

16. Benazzi F. Depressive mixed states: unipolar and bipolar II. Eur Arch Psychiatry Clin Neurosci 2000;250:249–53.

17. American Psychiatric Association. Diagnostic and statistical manual of mental disorders. 5th edition. Washington, DC: American Psychiatric Association; 2013.

18. Luciano M, Sampogna G, Del Vecchio V, et al. Critical evaluation of current diagnostic classification systems in psychiatry: the case of DSM-5. Riv Psichiatr 2016;51:116–21.

19. Pingani L, Luciano M, Sampogna G, et al. The crisis in psychiatry: a public health perspective. Int Rev Psychiatry 2014;26:530–4.

20. Malhi GS, Byrow Y, Outhred T, et al. Exclusion of overlapping symptoms in DSM-5 mixed features specifier: heuristic diagnostic and treatment implications. CNS Spectr 2017;22:126–33.

21. Zimmerman M. Measures of the DSM-5 mixed-features specifier of major depressive disorder. CNS Spectr 2017;22:196–202.

22. Perugi G, Angst J, Azorin J-M, et al. Mixed features in patients with a major depressive episode: the BRIDGE-IIMIX study. J Clin Psychiatry 2015;76:e351–8.

23. Tondo L, Vázquez GH, Pinna M, et al. Characteristics of depressive and bipolar disorder patients with mixed features. Acta Psychiatr Scand 2018;138:243–52.

24. Brancati GE, Vieta E, Azorin JM, et al. The role of overlapping excitatory symptoms in major depression: are they relevant for the diagnosis of mixed state? J Psychiatr Res 2019;115:151–7.

25. Koukopoulos A, Sani G, Ghaemi SN. Why DSM-5 is wrong (and so was DSM-IV). Br J Psychiatry 2013;203:3–5.

26. Malhi GS, Lampe L, Coulston CM, et al. Mixed state discrimination: a DSM problem that won't go away? J Affect Disord 2014;158:8–10.
27. Lahey BB, Krueger RF, Rathouz PJ, et al. Validity and utility of the general factor of psychopathology. World Psychiatry 2017;16:142–4.
28. Maj M. Why the clinical utility of diagnostic categories in psychiatry is intrinsically limited and how we can use new approaches to complement them. World Psychiatry 2018;17:121–2.
29. Fulford KWM, Handa A. Categorical and/or continuous? Learning from vascular surgery. World Psychiatry 2018;17:304–5.
30. Jablensky A. The dialectic of quantity and quality in psychopathology. World Psychiatry 2018;17:300–1.
31. Ghaemi SN. After the failure of DSM: clinical research on psychiatric diagnosis. World Psychiatry 2018;17:301–2.
32. Weygandt W. Uber die mischzustande des manisch-depressiven irreseins. Munchen (Germany): Verlag von S.F. Lechmann; 1899.
33. Borsboom D, Robinaugh DJ, Rhemtulla M, et al, Psychosystems Group. Robustness and replicability of psychopathology networks. World Psychiatry 2018;17:143–4.
34. Kendler KS. Classification of psychopathology: conceptual and historical background. World Psychiatry 2018;17:241–2.
35. Schultze-Lutter F, Theodoridou A. The concept of basic symptoms: its scientific and clinical relevance. World Psychiatry 2017;16:104–5.
36. Reed GM, Keeley JW, Rebello TJ, et al. Clinical utility of ICD-11 diagnostic guidelines for high-burden mental disorders: results from mental health settings in 13 countries. World Psychiatry 2018;17:306–31.
37. Luciano M, Sampogna G, Del Vecchio V, et al. The Italian ICD-11 field trial: interrater reliability in the use of diagnostic guidelines for schizophrenia and related disorders. Riv Psichiatr 2019;54:109–14.
38. Chakrabarti S. Mood disorders in the international classification of Diseases-11: Similarities and differences with the diagnostic and statistical manual of mental Disorders 5 and the international classification of Diseases-10. Indian J Social Psychiatry 2018;34:17–22.
39. Perugi G. ICD-11 mixed episode: nothing new despite the evidence. Bipolar Disord 2019;21:376–7.
40. Koukopoulos A, Sani G, Koukopoulos AE, et al. Melancholia agitata and mixed depression. Acta Psychiatr Scand 2007;115:50–7.
41. Koukopoulos A, Sani G. DSM-5 criteria for depression with mixed features: a farewell to mixed depression. Acta Psychiatr Scand 2014;129:4–16.
42. Koukopoulos A, Sani G, Koukopoulos AE, et al. Endogenous and exogenous cyclicity and temperament in bipolar disorder: review, new data and hypotheses. J Affect Disord 2006;96:165–75.
43. Akiskal HS, Benazzi F. Family history validation of the bipolar nature of depressive mixed states. J Affect Disord 2003;73:113–22.
44. Perugi G, Akiskal HS, Micheli C, et al. Clinical characterization of depressive mixed state in bipolar-I patients: Pisa-San Diego collaboration. J Affect Disord 2001;67:105–14.
45. Maj M, Pirozzi R, Magliano L, et al. Agitated depression in bipolar I disorder: prevalence, phenomenology, and outcome. Am J Psychiatry 2003;160:2134–40.
46. Maj M, Pirozzi R, Magliano L, et al. Agitated "unipolar" major depression: prevalence, phenomenology, and outcome. J Clin Psychiatry 2006;67:712–9.

47. Faedda GL, Marangoni C, Reginaldi D. Depressive mixed states: a reappraisal of Koukopoulos' criteria. J Affect Disord 2015;176:18–23.
48. Benazzi F, Helmi S, Bland L. Agitated depression: Unipolar? Bipolar? or Both? Ann Clin Psychiatry 2002;14:97-104.
49. Rihmer A, Gonda X, Balazs J, et al. The importance of depressive mixed states in suicidal behaviour. Neuropsychopharmacol Hung 2008;10:45–9.
50. Vázquez GH, Lolich M, Cabrera C, et al. Mixed symptoms in major depressive and bipolar disorders: A systematic review. J Affect Disord 2018;225:756–60.
51. Serra F, Gordon-Smith K, Perry A, et al. Agitated depression in bipolar disorder. Bipolar Disord 2019;21(6):547–55.
52. Takeshima M, Oka T. Association between the so-called "activation syndrome" and bipolar II disorder, a related disorder, and bipolar suggestive features in out-patients with depression. J Affect Disord 2013;151:196–202.
53. Maj M. "Mixed" depression: drawbacks of DSM-5 (and other) polythetic diagnostic criteria. J Clin Psychiatry 2015;76:e381–2.
54. Batty GD, Gale CR, Tanji F, et al. Personality traits and risk of suicide mortality: findings from a multi-cohort study in the general population. World Psychiatry 2018;17:371–2.
55. Oquendo MA, Bernanke JA. Suicide risk assessment: tools and challenges. World Psychiatry 2017;16:28–9.
56. Pietrzak RH, Pitts BL, Harpaz-Rotem I, et al. Factors protecting against the development of suicidal ideation in military veterans. World Psychiatry 2017;16:326–7.
57. Erbuto D, Innamorati M, Lamis DA, et al. Mediators in the association between affective temperaments and suicide risk among psychiatric inpatients. Psychiatry 2018;81:240–57.
58. Fico G, Caivano V, Zinno F, et al. Affective temperaments and clinical course of bipolar disorder: an exploratory study of differences among patients with and without a history of violent suicide attempts. Medicina 2019;55:390.
59. Sato T, Bottlender R, Schröter A, et al. Frequency of manic symptoms during a depressive episode and unipolar 'depressive mixed state' as bipolar spectrum. Acta Psychiatr Scand 2003;107:268–74.
60. Fisher K, Houtsma C, Assavedo BL, et al. Agitation as a moderator of the relationship between insomnia and current suicidal ideation in the military. Arch Suicide Res 2017;21:531–43.
61. Stange JP, Kleiman EM, Sylvia LG, et al. Specific mood symptoms confer risk for subsequent suicidal ideation in bipolar disorder with and without suicide attempt history: multi-wave data from STEP-BD. Depress Anxiety 2016;33:464–72.
62. Popovic D, Vieta E, Azorin JM, et al. Suicide attempts in major depressive episode: evidence from the BRIDGE-II-Mix study. Bipolar Disord 2015;17:795–803.
63. Courtet P, Lopez-Castroman J. Antidepressants and suicide risk in depression. World Psychiatry 2017;16:317–8.
64. Caligiuri MP, Gentili V, Eberson S, et al. A quantitative neuromotor predictor of antidepressant non-response in patients with major depression. J Affect Disord 2003;77:135–41.
65. Stahl SM, Morrissette DA, Faedda G, et al. Guidelines for the recognition and management of mixed depression. CNS Spectr 2017;22:203–19.
66. Steinert T. Chance of response to an antidepressant: what should we say to the patient? World Psychiatry 2018;17:114–5.

67. Bak M, Weltens I, Bervoets C, et al. The pharmacological management of agitated and aggressive behaviour: a systematic review and meta-analysis. Eur Psychiatry 2019;57:78–100.
68. University of South Florida, College of Behavioural & Community Sciences. Florida best practice psychotherapeutic medication guidelines for adults. Florida Medicaid Drug Therapy Management Program for Behavioral Health. University of South Florida; 2015.
69. Ghaemi SN, Hsu DJ, Soldani F, et al. Antidepressants in bipolar disorder: the case for caution. Bipolar Disord 2003;5:421–33.
70. Bottlender R, Sato T, Kleindienst N, et al. Mixed depressive features predict maniform switch during treatment of depression in bipolar I disorder. J Affect Disord 2004;78:149–52.
71. Akiskal HS, Pinto O. The evolving bipolar spectrum. Prototypes I, II, III, and IV. Psychiatr Clin North Am 1999;22:517–34.
72. Alda M. Who are excellent lithium responders and why do they matter? World Psychiatry 2017;16:319–20.
73. Sani G, Fiorillo A. The use of lithium in mixed states. CNS Spectr 2019;28:1–3.
74. Dell'Osso B, Albert U, Atti AR, et al. Bridging the gap between education and appropriate use of benzodiazepines in psychiatric clinical practice. Neuropsychiatr Dis Treat 2015;11:1885–909.
75. Kessing LV, Bukh JD. The clinical relevance of qualitatively distinct subtypes of depression. World Psychiatry 2017;16:318–9.

Telepsychiatry
A New Treatment Venue for Pediatric Depression

David E. Roth, MD[a],*, Ujjwal Ramtekkar, MD, MPE, MBA[b],
Sofija Zeković-Roth, LAc, DOM[a]

KEYWORDS

- Telepsychiatry • Telehealth • Telemedicine • Depression • Child psychiatry
- Adolescent psychiatry

KEY POINTS

- Telepsychiatry is being deployed to treat pediatric depression in several different models of care. The benefits of using it to provide direct care in homes, schools, primary care offices, juvenile correction centers, and residential facilities are well established.
- Telepsychiatry has the potential to improve prevention, early identification, and treatment of pediatric depression. Telepsychiatry removes the geographic barrier between patients and providers, which lowers the cost of providing treatment and decreases the time, effort, and lost income usually associated with transporting either patients/families or providers to rural and underserved communities.
- Telepsychiatry outcomes and patient satisfaction ratings are sometimes superior to sessions held in traditional face-to-face venues.
- Engaging, building relationships, and communicating with telepsychiatry patients are significantly different from traditional medical settings.
- Effective use of telepsychiatry requires Webside manners and the intentional shaping of both an authentic treatment experience and provider-patient relationships. When telepsychiatry staging and nonverbal and verbal communication skills are properly used, telepsychiatry sessions feel authentic to both patients and providers, and treatment outcomes meet or exceed traditional face-to-face venues.

 Video content accompanies this article at www.childpsych.theclinics.com.

This article originally appeared in *Child and Adolescent Psychiatric Clinics*, Volume 28, Issue 3, July 2019.
Disclosure Statement: None of the authors has any relationship with a commercial company that has a direct financial interest in subject matter or materials discussed in article or with a company making a competing product.
^a Mind & Body Works, Inc., 3340 Wauke Street, Honolulu, HI 96815-4452, USA; ^b Partners for Kids, Nationwide Children's Hospital, 700 Children's Way, Columbus, OH 43215, USA
* Corresponding author.
E-mail address: drroth@mind-bodyworks.com

INTRODUCTION

Contemporary children and adolescents are immersed in interactive media, including social media, online videos, video chat, and video games. It is estimated that more than 70% of teenagers are interacting on 1 or more social media sites on the Internet and approximately 25% of teenagers are constantly connected to Internet.[1] Although caution has been advised against such excessive media use, it reflects the exposure and comfort level youth have with technology. Because they are already using video technology to socialize and play, telepsychiatry is a good fit and appropriate treatment venue with most youth.

TELEPSYCHIATRY
Definition

The Centers for Medicaid & Medicare Services defines telehealth as the use of telecommunications and information technology to provide access to health assessment, diagnosis, intervention, consultation, supervision, and information across distance that seeks to seeks to improve a patient's health by permitting 2-way, real-time, interactive communication between a patient and a physician or practitioner at a distant site. This electronic communication means the use of interactive telecommunications equipment that includes, at minimum, audio and video equipment.[2] The term, *telepsychiatry*, refers to behavioral and mental health services that are provided via synchronous telecommunications technologies, including discipline-specific applications, such as telepsychiatry and telepsychology. Telepsychiatry refers to the use of secure, Health Insurance Portability and Accountability Act (HIPAA)–compliant videoconferencing to connect the psychiatric provider at the destination site with youth and/or their families at the origination site. If the videoconference is live, it is called synchronous telepsychiatry or simply telepsychiatry. If the interaction involves the exchanging of information at different times over a period of time, it is considered asynchronous telepsychiatry.

Laws

The prescription of medications by a telepsychiatrist is impacted by clinical and legal requirements. The clinical monitoring responsibility can be shared with a physician extender or clinician at the origination site or the youth's primary care provider. Standard tools, however, such as the Abnormal Involuntary Movement Scale and other neuropsychiatric assessments, can be used reliably over videoconferencing[3] to monitor for neurologic side effects. When depressed youth have comorbid conditions, such as attention-deficit/hyperactivity disorder or anxiety, the telepsychiatrist has to comply with federal regulations when prescribing Schedule II controlled substances, including stimulant medications and benzodiazepines. These federal regulations began in 2008 with the Ryan Haight Online Pharmacy Consumer Protection Act and were updated in late 2018. The current regulations include specific situations that require special registration with the Drug Enforcement Administration and a requirement that at least 1 in-person visit occurs before prescription of the controlled substances.[2] The federal government update to this act in 2018 provides a special registration for telepsychiatry. This allows a provider to prescribe controlled substances without an in-person visit in 7 categories of clinical practice. These include public health emergencies, working with the Indian Health Service, collaboration with another practitioner at the patient site, and during medical emergencies. A good summary of this special registration is available online from the Congressional Research Service. Telepsychiatrists must maintain active medical licenses for the state(s) in which the patient and provider are located at the time of treatment. Similar restrictions often apply to hospital credentialing and malpractice insurance. Several states have additional requirements and regulations, so the authors recommend telepsychiatrists regularly consult with agencies that track these changes. These include the Center for Connected Health Policy (www.cchpca.org), the American Telemedicine Association (www.americantelemed.org), and the Center for Telehealth and e-Health Law (www.ctel.org).

USING TELEPSYCHIATY TO TREAT DEPRESSION
Proved Efficacy

Landmark studies of the efficacy, feasibility, and acceptability of telepsychiatry service for children living in nonmetropolitan communities found high satisfaction rates in pediatric providers as well as youth. The service was shown to be feasible with good utilization rates in primary care settings.[4,5] Treating youth via telepsychiatry is well accepted by families and they report high satisfaction with the care delivered.[6] Telepsychiatry actually has several advantages over traditional face-to-face sessions. Youth treated with telepsychiatry feel a greater sense of safety and control when dealing with an unfamiliar adults (psychiatrists and other mental health professionals) and greater sense of personal space. They miss less school for sessions, and coordination of care with their other providers and teachers is improved.

Child and adolescent mental health studies of diagnostic accuracy and effectiveness of telepsychiatry treatment demonstrated positive outcomes for children in different settings.[7,8] The growing body of pediatric telepsychiatry literature also includes clinical guidelines for practicing telepsychiatry. The American Academy of Child and Adolescent Psychiatry has published clinical guidelines based on the systematic review and recommendations of the telepsychiatry committee.[2] The American Telemedicine Association published "Practice Guidelines for Telemental Health With Children and Adolescents" in 2017.[9]

Decrease Barriers to Care

Pediatric depression is associated with significant morbidity, including suicide. Despite the potential safety risks of this condition, only a small proportion of youth with depression receive adequate treatment in a timely manner due to barriers (discussed previously). The gap between the high need for care and limited access to care can be mitigated by telepsychiatry. Telepsychiatry has the potential to improve prevention, early identification, and treatment of pediatric depression. Telepsychiatry removes the geographic barrier between patients and providers, which lowers the cost of providing treatment and decreases the time, effort, and lost income usually associated with transporting either patients or providers to rural and underserved communities.[10–12]

Better Collaboration

Telepsychiatry potentially facilitates collaboration between child and adolescent mental health providers and other professionals. Schools and primary care providers can obtain consultations and collaborate with these providers through telehealth with a frequency and intensity usually unobtainable because of logistical barriers.[13] This makes telepsychiatry less expensive and more cost effective than other medical specialties that require additional technological devices necessary for physical examinations and testing. Cost savings have been demonstrated most clearly with newer programs that do not rely on expensive equipment and use the recently available array of secure technology.[14]

Cost Benefits

Mental health disorders affect approximately 15 million children and adolescents in the United States and are a national public health concern. Pediatric depression not only clinically impairs children but also disrupts family systems, often reducing children's adult functioning when it persists into adulthood. Pediatric depression is a clinical burden to the patients and their families, and it is also a financial burden to our society. Although the cost of pediatric depression alone has not been definitively determined, because the total annual cost of adult depression is estimated to be more than $83 billion, pediatric depression is likely a substantial portion of the total annual cost of all pediatric mental health disorders, which is at least $247 billion.[15,16] The overall impact and cost of this mental health burden are expected to rise due to several barriers in providing timely and adequate treatment. These include a critical shortage of child and adolescent psychiatrists, inadequate access to mental health providers with specialized training in treating children, significant geographic distances to reach rural communities, and socioeconomic/resource disparities in rural areas where primary medical care facilities are less concentrated and specialty care access is often suboptimal.[17] These access issues pose overall disadvantages with regard to social determinants of health, such as financial burden to afford transportation, lost wages from attending sessions, specialist copays, affordability of medications, lack of health insurance, poverty, unstable housing, and decreasing income due to worsening economies in those areas.[18] The social determinants related to finances and access often result in the delay of early identification and intervention for childhood mental illness, nonadherence to treatment, inadequate frequency of therapeutic interventions, and overall poor long-term functional outcomes.

MODELS OF TELEPSYCHIATRIC CARE
Direct Care and Collaborative Care/Consultation

Telepsychiatry is being deployed to treat pediatric depression in several different models of care. The benefits of using it to provide direct care in homes, schools, primary care offices, emergency departments, juvenile correction centers, and residential facilities are well established.[19–21] Rapid adoption is being facilitated by the falling cost of telemedicine hardware and the ubiquity of Internet-connected personal devices capable of running telemedicine apps. Recently, collaborative care telepsychiatry consultation models have been adopted because Medicare is reimbursing these consultations. In this model of care, the treatment plan is devised collaboratively with the consulting psychiatrist, but the primary care provider is responsible for implementation of the treatment plan, including medication management, care coordination, monitoring, and follow-up. This collaborative relationship supports the primary care provider and improves patient access to quality care.[22]

Project Extension for Community Healthcare Outcomes

Another model of telepsychiatry consultation is Project Extension for Community Healthcare Outcomes (ECHO). This hub-and-spoke model aims to improve primary care providers' abilities to confidently screen and provide care for children with mild to moderate psychiatric disorders. Project ECHO model outcomes indicate that it is an effective and potentially cost-saving model that increases participant knowledge and patient access to health care in remote locations.[23]

ENGAGING PATIENTS, BUILDING RAPPORT, AND DEVELOPING GOOD WEBSIDE MANNERS

Engaging, building relationships, and communicating with patients in the telepsychiatry venue are significantly different from traditional medical settings. Cameras, microphones, and speakers alter voices, change how participants are seen, and flatten emotional expressions. In order to appear as genuine, trustworthy, and empathic as they normally do in traditional clinical settings, telepsychiatrists need to adjust their communication patterns. Many of these adjustments are techniques used by newscasters, actors, and television studios to engage viewers and ensure clear and emotionally congruent communication with the audience.

Like an actor stepping onto the stage, telepsychiatrists must immediately engage a patient's attention and convince the patient that they are trustworthy, competent, empathic, and responsive to their needs.[24] Providers who seem naturally empathic and create good rapport are instinctually communicating well both verbally and nonverbally with their patients.[25] Adolescent depression treatment outcomes are better when the alliance is strong.[26]

The importance of using and observing congruent nonverbal communication cannot be overstated. More than two-thirds of communicated meaning comes from nonverbal messages, not the actual words spoken.[27] If a provider's nonverbal communication does not reinforce and support the verbal communication, the provider seems odd or insincere.[28] Insufficient, unobserved, or incongruent nonverbal communication weakens the provider-patient relationship.[29] It is often not what is said, but how it is said, that matters most to patients.[25,30]

A provider's bedside manner is the unique mixture of verbal and nonverbal communication used when communicating in a professional role with different patients in different settings.[31] During medical training, providers learned how to modify their bedside manner (consciously or unconsciously) to fit the clinical setting (hospital, emergency department, clinic, nursing home, or nursery). These modifications promote good communication that are appropriately nuanced to engage patients of different ages, genders, maturity, and cultures. It is the authors' opinion that telepsychiatry is not a technology but rather a new clinical setting in which providers must adjust how they communicate to engage patients and maintain therapeutic relationships. Telepsychiatrists must adapt their bedside manners to this venue, a communication style often called Webside manners.

This unspoken need to operate differently in a new clinical venue may be a contributing factor to the pervasive but gradually decreasing resistance to telepsychiatry among established providers. A better understanding of nonverbal communication and mastery of the conscious adjustments providers can make, however, give novice telepsychiatrists more confidence and help them overcome the limitations of this technology. This article reviews the categories of nonverbal communication and how telepsychiatrists can intentionally use and monitor nonverbal communication to successfully engage, diagnose, and treat children and adolescents suffering from depression. This article also reviews the nonverbal impact of the physical setting, including room selection, participant arrangement, and camera framing, on engagement and rapport.

ADOPTING GOOD WEBSIDE MANNERS

A provider's physical appearance, grooming, uniform/dress, and interactions become a more significant part of how patients make a first impression and how they judge a provider as trustworthy, competent, and empathic.[25,32] The provider's physical appearance is restricted by the camera frame, which limits patients' ability to see the provider and surroundings. Patients have less visual information about the provider and where the provider is working to inform and influence their perception and acceptance of the provider (**Box 1**).

Erect and open body posture (**Fig. 1**) communicates to patients that a provider is a confident, nonjudgmental, and trustworthy authority figure who is paying attention to their needs.[33,34] Moving toward or away from the camera approximates the effect of interpersonal space during in-person sessions. For example, moving slightly closer to the camera communicates more interest or attention. If a depressed patient seems defensive, moving slightly away from the camera conveys the perception of giving the patient more space. The picture-in-picture function on the monitor helps providers to monitor how their image is projected and stay within the frame.

Because patients can see only the facial expressions, gestures, movements, and activities that fall within the camera frame, providers must replace large gestures with smaller ones that are seen more easily.[35] Common gestures, like outstretched arms, can be replaced with hand gestures or emotionally congruent facial expressions.[36] Hand gestures, like waving and the thumbs-up sign, also can replace engaging physical contacts like handshakes and fist bumps. Children especially seem to enjoy these hand gestures (**Fig. 2**).

A provider's tone of voice affects the relationship.[37] The provider must sound honest, compassionate, and intelligent while speaking slowly, loudly, and clearly enough to be easily heard and understood through the microphone but without sounding robotic. Many novice providers speak robotically due to performance anxiety or distractions by the electronics, for example, a medical record that is simultaneously projected onto a monitor during the session. Smiling while speaking makes a provider sound warm and approachable. Placing a smiley face sticker next to the camera is a good reminder for those who often look or sound too serious.

There is a transmission delay during synchronous telepsychiatry sessions that, although brief, affects communication. Therefore, pauses and turn-taking are more important for providers to manage. Giving the patient an extra moment to reply in conversation may seem like a long pause but replicates a normal pause during in-person conversation. If there is a significant lag between 1 or more parties in a multicenter session, the provider may need to allow for even longer pauses. When patients feel they are encouraged to speak, they are more likely to feel their needs were fulfilled.[38]

Due to the slight audio transmission delay, verbal encouragers, like "yes," "tell me more," and "go on," are harder to use during telepsychiatry. If participants

---

Box 1
Limitations of telepsychiatry technology on the provider

- See the patient
- Be seen by the patient
- Be heard and understood
- Make gestures
- Maintain eye contact
- Touch
- Smell
- Demonstrate usual good bedside manner

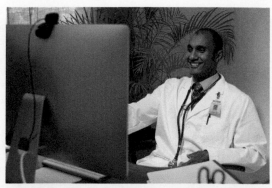

Fig. 1. Good posture suggests to others that you are healthy, confident, and deserving of their respect. (*Courtesy of* D. Roth, MD, FAAP, FAPA, Honolulu, HI.)

have already resumed speaking, they stop speaking to listen to the encourager, thereby interfering with communication. Therefore, experienced providers frequently use gestures, such as the thumbs-up gesture, to facilitate the reciprocal exchange of information while maintaining engagement and without interrupting the speaker (**Fig. 3**). The other approach is to nod and smile. After thousands of telepsychiatry sessions, the authors suggest the most important nonverbal rapport-building strategy is to periodically nod and smile while a patient is talking. Nodding and smiling reassure patients that a provider is listening and encourages them to continue.[25] Consider placing a sticky note that says "Nod and Smile!" on the monitor until these become natural.

OPTIMIZING THE AUTHENTICITY OF THE EXPERIENCE
Room Selection

Optimizing the telepsychiatry experience begins with appropriate room selection (**Box 2**). In telepsychiatry, the camera is turned on and—boom!—the provider is suddenly meeting with the patient. There are no grand hospital architecture, professional decor, and staff interactions to mentally prepare a patient for the clinical encounter. To make matters worse, a patient's site may be a home, school, or another provider's

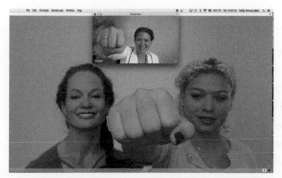

Fig. 2. A fist bump or hand waving gesture can help open and close a session. This gesture replaces the physical contact like handshakes normally used as part of greeting patients. (*Courtesy of* D. Roth, MD, FAAP, FAPA, Honolulu, HI.)

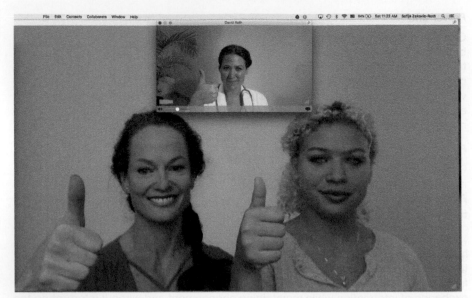

Fig. 3. Using the thumbs-up and other meaningful gestures can signal agreement or other thoughts without interrupting the speaker. Audio transmission delays make it difficult to rapidly state an affirmative verbally without talking over the other speaker. These gestures also are helpful when many participants want to signal agreement or vote on an idea at the same time. (*Courtesy of* D. Roth, MD, FAAP, FAPA, Honolulu, HI.)

office—all settings the provider cannot control. It is entirely up to the provider to make it feel like an authentic medical experience.

Good room selection begins with thoughtful selection, arrangement, and appearance of the rooms at both patient and provider sites. Telepsychiatrists often have to work with a wide range of rooms, but with the right setup, sessions can be conducted successfully in classrooms, conference rooms, treatment rooms, offices, living rooms, and bedrooms. After the room at the patient's site is selected, it should be tailored to support videoconferences, accommodate the routine number of participants, and maximize participants' focus during the session. If a child's motor skills, play, exploration, and movements are being assessed, the room should be large enough for these activities to fit within the camera frame (**Fig. 4**).

Box 2
Room selection in telepsychiatry

Room selection should ensure that

- Everyone feels comfortable
- Distractions are minimized
- Everyone is able to see each other
- Everyone is able to hear each other
- The room maintains visual and auditory privacy
- Room size accommodates the clinical encounter
- Décor minimizes camera distortions

Power and Network

One of the most important considerations in room selection for sites using consumer-based equipment or cloud videoconferencing is proximity to the Wi-Fi router to maintain a strong Internet connection. If connecting through a computer, it should be plugged into the router with an ethernet cable to provide the strongest and most stable video and auditory signals. Plugging the router, modem, computer, and monitor(s) into a combination surge protector and battery backup ensures that the connection does not drop if there is a momentary electrical surge or loss of power.

Privacy

Commercial telepsychiatry vendors advertise whether they meet HIPAA standards, including software encryption, and if they would sign a HIPAA Business Associate Agreement. Many popular video chat programs like FaceTime and Viber are not HIPAA-compliant.

Both sites must ensure that they can restrict access to the session. Family sessions may be best accommodated in a kitchen or family room, but these are high-traffic areas. Individual sessions, and some parent-child sessions, may be conducted away from other family in a bedroom, office, or porch. Many depressed teenagers prefer the privacy of a bedroom. If the telepsychiatrist routinely wants a parent's input during the session, it should be set up to occur at the beginning and/or end of the session. This helps with consent for treatment changes and getting parental input about home and school functioning. It gives the telepsychiatrist a chance to assess the parent's feelings about the youth and treatment efficacy while preserving the youth's privacy, as appropriate. It may be helpful to tell the parent when to join the session. This decreases parent and youth anxiety about who should be in the room and who has input into the session, and the provider can avoid being carried around the home as the youth looks for the parent.

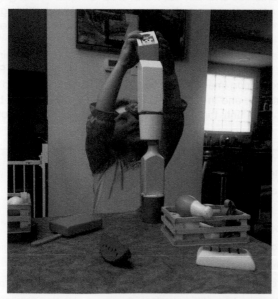

Fig. 4. When working with children, it is necessary to widen the camera's field of view to appreciate the task given to the child or to observe the child's behavior. (*Courtesy of* D. Roth, MD, FAAP, FAPA, Honolulu, HI.)

Audio privacy may be the largest obstacle to privacy (**Box 3**). The privacy of the patient site is held to the same HIPAA standards as a traditional clinic, nursing home, school, or hospital. Like any other clinical setting, the provider's voice and the patient's voice should be difficult or impossible to hear outside of the videoconferencing room.

Another privacy concern is whether to include a clinical staff member as a coordinator/presenter at the patient site during the session. Coordinators can provide valuable assistance with the telepsychiatry technology, emotionally support the patient, and provide immediate help in a clinical crisis. Additionally, they can provide educational material to patients' families, assist with follow-through on recommendations, and help ensure continuity of care. The presence of a coordinator in the session, however, may negatively affect the therapeutic relationship with a depressed patient. An uncomfortable patient may withhold disclosing critical information to a provider, and shy patients may not ask the coordinator to leave the room. Technical, confidentiality, and ethics trainings for the coordinator are highly encouraged.

Room Setup

Selecting a room with a camera-friendly color scheme makes it easier a the camera to focus on the participant instead of the background. The camera should be focused on a wall that is painted a soft neutral shade to help the participant's image stand out from the wall. Decorations in the provider's room should be minimal and professional, reflecting the services delivered.

Camera Framing and Positioning

The telepsychiatry provider has to overcome the visual field deficit created by the camera. Cameras have a limited field of view, whereas the human eye has both central and peripheral vision. How the provider positions and zooms the camera determines what the participants see and can have a profound impact on engagement with the participant. It is a compromise between being too close, which greatly limits the viewing of gestures, and too far, which makes the provider harder to see and harder to hear and may include distracting background objects.

The telepsychiatry provider should sit approximately 2 ft to 4 ft directly back from the camera. This usually put the image in the middle of the frame. Providers should check this self-monitoring image at the beginning of each session to ensure their image is large, centered, and in focus. Telepsychiatry providers can then adjust their chair height or camera until the eyes are approximately one-third down from the top

---

Box 3
Audio privacy in telepsychiatry

Ways to improve audio privacy

- Close windows

- Block gaps below doors

- Place a white noise machine outside and beside the door to the telepsychiatry room.

- Put carpet or an area rug on the floor.

- Add pillows to couches, curtains on windows, and/or tapestries on walls to absorb sound

- When remodeling, use decoupling soundproofing construction techniques.

- Consider using a headset microphone

of the self-monitor image (**Fig. 5**). This creates the natural-looking framing commonly used to make television newscasters appear attentive and engaging. Encourage the patient to similarly adjust positioning and camera framing at the beginning of the session.

Thoughtful camera placement improves the mental status examination. A participant's camera should be positioned at a sufficient distance to allow visualization of a child's motor abilities and play as well as dysmorphic facial features, facial expressions, hygiene, clothing, tics, and gestures.

Provider eye contact is significantly related patients' perceptions of a provider's connectedness and empathy.[39] The camera may not be located above the monitor, however, causing participants to make eye contact in the wrong direction. Therefore, the provider's camera should be directly in front of the provider, positioned at eye level, and immediately above or below the participant's image (**Fig. 6**). If a separate Web camera is available, place it on top of the computer or on a shelf so that it is positioned directly over the patient's image on the screen.

When using a portable device for a telepsychiatry session, place it on a desk or table so it does not move around. Handheld devices should be propped up at shoulder height and at arm's length from the user's body to make the eye contact feel more natural. This also prevents excessive camera movement, which causes the camera to lose focus, degrades image quality, and can make the other participants feel seasick (Video 1). If a single participant is using a phone or tablet, it should be positioned in vertical/portrait orientation. This improves the eye contact between participants because the other participant's eyes are closer to the camera. If the device needs to capture 2 or more people in the frame, turning the device to the horizontal/landscape position often creates a larger frame that encompasses more of the room, but eye contact may be misaligned.

If an electronic medical record (EMR) is used during the session and can be projected onto the screen, place it in a window below the participants' images. This causes the provider to constantly nod up and down in a positive and affirmative manner when glancing at the EMR (**Fig. 7**). By contrast, if the EMR window is placed lateral to the participant images, the provider is constantly making negative, head-shaking gestures during the session. Medical providers spend 30% of the visit length gazing at the EMR.[39] Telepsychiatrists should minimize the time spent looking at the EMR to maintain eye contact and rapport with the patient, even if this means charting very little during the session.

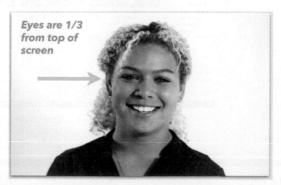

Fig. 5. Follow this rule used in television studios: when framing a person for a videoconference, have the person's eyes approximately one-third below the top of the frame and in the center of the frame. (*Courtesy of* D. Roth, MD, FAAP, FAPA, Honolulu, HI.)

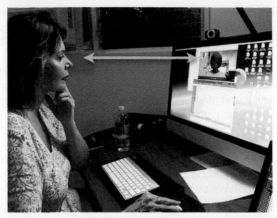

Fig. 6. Virtual eye contact is created when you appear to be looking at the person because you have juxtaposed the participant's image and your camera. When juxtaposed, you are looking at the camera when you are looking at the participant's image on your screen. This is much easier than trying to look at a camera lens. (*Courtesy of* D. Roth, MD, FAAP, FAPA, Honolulu, HI.)

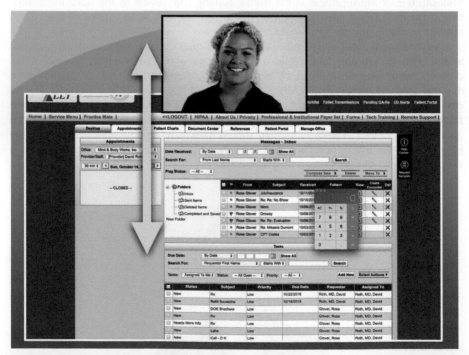

Fig. 7. By stacking a patient's image above or below the EMR, your head is moving up and down in a "yes" movement every time you reference the EMR. When arranged side-by-side, your head repeatedly makes a "no" movement. (*Courtesy of* D. Roth, MD, FAAP, FAPA, Honolulu, HI.)

Staying Within the Camera Frame

Drifting out of the camera frame is a common problem, because people move around in their chairs and often slouch (**Fig. 8**). Most software displays the provider's picture as a smaller self-monitor image on the screen. Even if providers are uncomfortable watching themselves on camera, they need to monitor their image. If they do not, they run the danger of disappearing from the other participants' screens, diminishing their ability to perceive the provider and distracting them. When the provider moves out of the frame the participants are reminded they are not face-to-face and this detracts from the authenticity of the experience.

Providers should ensure their hand and arm gestures are visible within the frame. Exclude moving objects like fans from the frame because they are distracting and degrade the picture. Digitally rendering these movements uses up valuable bandwidth and computer processing power, causing the participant's image and voice clarity to degrade.

Youth and Family Seating Arrangement

If there is only 1 participant at the remote site, the participant should sit 2 ft to 4 ft away from the camera and screen (**Fig. 9**). Each additional participant should be moved another 2 ft back from the camera (**Fig. 10**). If 2 people to 3 people want to sit within 3 ft of the camera, they have to sit shoulder to shoulder to fit in the frame (**Fig. 11**). Although armchairs are comfortable, chairs with straight backs and without armrests accommodate 2 people to 3 people closer to the camera. This often is necessary when the microphone or speakers are marginally adequate to the task.

When working with families, have them position the camera far enough away to see most of the room and keep all the participants within the frame so they do not have to adjust it during the session. Many seating arrangements can work for children. Children can sit next to a parent, between parents, on a parent's lap, or in front of parents in either their own chair or on the floor (**Fig. 12**). When focusing on a single youth who can remain in a chair, have the youth sit close to the camera. The chairs should be stationary to keep children from rolling them out of the frame and light enough for the

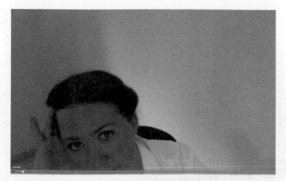

Fig. 8. Drifting out of the frame reminds the patient that you are on a screen and takes away from immersion in the experience. This often happens when telehealth providers turn off or hide their self-monitoring image. The way self-consciousness novice providers feel when seeing themselves on camera commonly fades with practice. (*Courtesy of* D. Roth, MD, FAAP, FAPA, Honolulu, HI.)

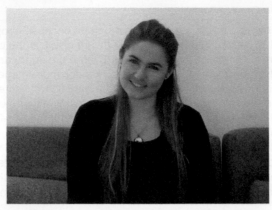

Fig. 9. If there is only 1 participant at the remote site, the participant should sit 2 ft to 4 ft feet away from the camera and screen. (*Courtesy of* D. Roth, MD, FAAP, FAPA, Honolulu, HI.)

parent to reposition them. Sometimes a hyperactive or agitated youth cannot remain in the camera frame. Consider keeping the parent(s) in the frame and call the child back to the camera when needed to answer a question (Video 2). Occasionally anxious, depressed, and defiant youth refuse to sit within the camera frame. If behavior management strategies fail to move the youth, then prior to the next session instruct the parent or session facilitator to turn off the self-monitor image and sit the youth farther away from the camera. This makes it more likely that the youth is at least partially within the camera frame.

Lighting

Lighting affects quality of the videoconferencing session.[35] Cameras need more light than human eyes to produce a clear image with accurate colors. An insufficiently illuminated room prevents participants from seeing each other clearly, detecting nonverbal communication, and identifying physical signs and symptoms and detracts from the authenticity of the experience.[32] Backlighting should be avoided. This occurs

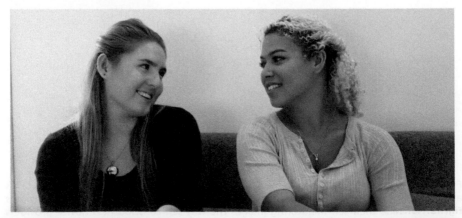

Fig. 10. Move each additional participant 2 ft or more back from the camera. (*Courtesy of* D. Roth, MD, FAAP, FAPA, Honolulu, HI.)

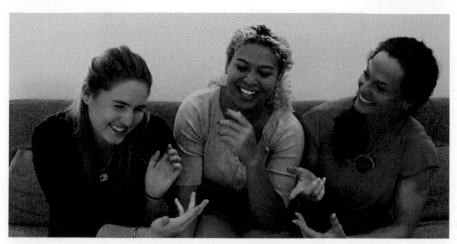

Fig. 11. If 2 people or 3 people want to sit within 3 ft of the camera, they have to sit shoulder-to-shoulder to fit in the frame. (*Courtesy of* D. Roth, MD, FAAP, FAPA, Honolulu, HI.)

when a bright light comes from behind the person, such as when participants are seated with their backs to a window or bright light (**Fig. 13**).

Room lighting should be considered early in room selection and when the position of the camera is determined. Copious indirect lighting, such as floor lamps that bounce light off the ceiling, is key to a good lighting plan (**Fig. 14**). It looks natural and softer and does not cause glare or shadows. Removing or covering reflective surfaces that cause glare also helps optimize the video image.

Audio Quality

Rooms should be selected to minimize common interfering sounds, including printers, air conditioners, fans, intercoms, animals, lawn equipment, and outside traffic. Most rooms are not perfectly quiet, however, and the provider should work with staff at

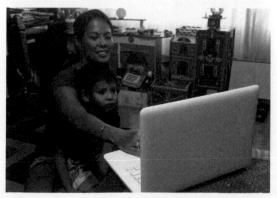

Fig. 12. When working with small children, having children sit on a parent's lap is a good way to keep them within the camera frame and engaged in the session. (*Courtesy of* D. Roth, MD, FAAP, FAPA, Honolulu, HI.)

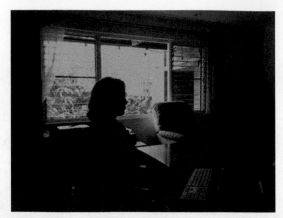

Fig. 13. Backlighting is a common problem in telehealth sessions. Cameras need more light in front of the subject rather than behind or to the side. When the light is misplaced, the camera is unable to properly render colors and light balance and keep the people brighter than the background. (*Courtesy of* D. Roth, MD, FAAP, FAPA, Honolulu, HI.)

the patient site to implement strategies to decrease background noise. If the provider is the only person in the room, the provider could use a headset microphone that eliminates most background sounds, minimizes keyboard clicks, and also ensures that participants' voices are not overheard.

Telepsychiatry providers must have a backup plan in case the audio connection fails. Usually, a conference speakerphone or smartphone can provide an adequate duplex connection, allowing the session to continue with suboptimal but sufficient video.

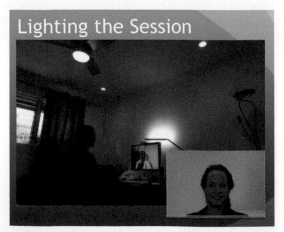

Fig. 14. Telehealth sessions need to be lit more brightly than other rooms to appear as they normally do to the human eye. Cameras need more light to correctly render the image details including color, contrast, and depth of field. A simple rule to follow is have 1 additional light in front of the subject or indirectly (and off camera) lighting the whole room to make the room seem as bright on camera as it does in face-to-face sessions. (*Courtesy of* D. Roth, MD, FAAP, FAPA, Honolulu, HI.)

SUMMARY

Telepsychiatry is rapidly becoming an established medical venue for treating depressed children and adolescents. Effective use of telepsychiatry requires Webside manners and the intentional shaping of both an authentic treatment experience and provider-patient relationships. When these staging and nonverbal and verbal communication skills are properly used, telepsychiatry sessions feel authentic to both patients and providers, and treatment outcomes meet or exceed traditional face-to-face venues and improve access to care. With sufficient practice, providers can become as effective and comfortable treating depressed pediatric patients via telepsychiatry as they are in other clinical venues. Additional resources for optimizing the telepsychiatry session are available at www.telepsychiatryguide.org, www.telepsychiatryresourcecenter.org, and www.americantelemed.org.

SUPPLEMENTARY DATA

Supplementary data to this article can be found online at https://doi.org/10.1016/j.chc.2019.02.007.

REFERENCES

1. Council on Communications and Media. Media use in school-aged children and adolescents. Pediatrics 2016. https://doi.org/10.1542/peds.2016-2592.
2. American Academy of Child and Adolescent Psychiatry (AACAP) Committee on Telepsychiatry and AACAP Committee on Quality Issues. Clinical update: telepsychiatry with children and adolescents. J Am Acad Child Adolesc Psychiatry 2017. https://doi.org/10.1016/j.jaac.2017.07.008.
3. Amarendran V, George A, Gersappe V, et al. The reliability of telepsychiatry for a neuropsychiatric assessment. Telemed J E Health 2011. https://doi.org/10.1089/tmj.2010.0144.
4. Myers KM, Valentine JM, Melzer SM. Feasibility, acceptability, and sustainability of telepsychiatry for children and adolescents. Psychiatr Serv 2007. https://doi.org/10.1176/ps.2007.58.11.1493.
5. Myers KM, Valentine JM, Melzer SM. Child and adolescent telepsychiatry: utilization and satisfaction. Telemed J E Health 2008. https://doi.org/10.1089/tmj.2007.0035.
6. Gloff NE, Lenoue SR, Novins DK, et al. Telemental health for children and adolescents. Int Rev Psychiatry 2015. https://doi.org/10.3109/09540261.2015.1086322.
7. Elford R, White H, Bowering R, et al. A randomized, controlled trial of child psychiatric assessments conducted using videoconferencing. J Telemed Telecare 2000. https://doi.org/10.1258/1357633001935086.
8. Nelson E-L, Barnard M, Cain S. Treating childhood depression over videoconferencing. Telemed J E Health 2003. https://doi.org/10.1089/153056203763317648.
9. Myers K, Nelson E-L, Rabinowitz T, et al. American telemedicine association practice guidelines for telemental health with children and adolescents. Telemed J E Health 2017;23(10):779–804.
10. Yilmaz SK, Horn BP, Fore C, et al. An economic cost analysis of an expanding, multi-state behavioural telehealth intervention. J Telemed Telecare 2018. https://doi.org/10.1177/1357633X18774181.
11. Russo JE, McCool RR, Davies L. VA telemedicine: an analysis of cost and time savings. Telemed J E Health 2016;22(3):209–15.

12. Bashshur RL, Shannon GW, Bashshur N, et al. The empirical evidence for telemedicine interventions in mental disorders. Telemed J E Health 2016;22(2):87–113.
13. Scott Kruse C, Karem P, Shifflett K, et al. Evaluating barriers to adopting telemedicine worldwide: a systematic review. J Telemed Telecare 2018;24(1):4–12.
14. Behere PB, Mansharamani HD, Kumar K. Telepsychiatry: reaching the unreached. Indian J Med Res 2017;146(2):150–2.
15. Nelson EL, Cain S, Sharp S. Considerations for conducting telemental health with children and adolescents. Child Adolesc Psychiatr Clin N Am 2017;26(1):77–91.
16. Greenberg PE, Kessler RC, Birnbaum HG, et al. The economic burden of depression in the United States: how did it change between 1990 and 2000? J Clin Psychiatry 2003. https://doi.org/10.4088/JCP.v64n1211.
17. Merikangas KR, He JP, Burstein M, et al. Service utilization for lifetime mental disorders in U.S. adolescents: results of the national comorbidity surveyAdolescent supplement (NCS-A). J Am Acad Child Adolesc Psychiatry 2011. https://doi.org/10.1016/j.jaac.2010.10.006.
18. Allen J, Balfour R, Bell R, et al. Social determinants of mental health. Int Rev Psychiatry 2014. https://doi.org/10.3109/09540261.2014.928270.
19. Butterfield A. Telepsychiatric evaluation and consultation in emergency care settings. Child Adolesc Psychiatr Clin N Am 2018;27(3):467–78.
20. Nelson E-L, Barnard M, Cain S. Feasibility of telemedicine intervention for childhood depression. Couns Psychother Res 2006. https://doi.org/10.1080/14733140600862303.
21. Thomas JF, Novins DK, Hosokawa PW, et al. The use of telepsychiatry to provide cost-efficient care during pediatric mental health emergencies. Psychiatr Serv 2018;69(2):161–8.
22. Martínez V, Rojas G, Martínez P, et al. Remote collaborative depression care program for adolescents in araucanía region, Chile: randomized controlled trial. J Med Internet Res 2018;20(1):e38.
23. Zhou C, Crawford A, Serhal E, et al. The impact of project ECHO on participant and patient outcomes: a systematic review. Acad Med 2016. https://doi.org/10.1097/ACM.0000000000001328.
24. Feldman RS. Applications of nonverbal behavioral theories and Research 1992. Available at: https://www.taylorfrancis.com/books/9781317782667. Accessed September 15, 2018.
25. Riess H, Kraft-Todd G. E. M. P. A. T. H. Y.: A tool to enhance nonverbal communication between clinicians and their patients. Acad Med 2014;89(8):8–10.
26. Shirk SR, Gudmundsen G, Kaplinski HC, et al. Alliance and outcome in cognitive-behavioral therapy for adolescent depression. J Clin Child Adolesc Psychol 2008;37(3):631–9.
27. Leathers D. Successful nonverbal communication: principles and applications. 3rd edition 1997. Available at: https://www.taylorfrancis.com/books/9781315542317. Accessed September 15, 2018.
28. Knapp ML, Hall JA, Horgan TG. Nonverbal communication in human interaction, eighth edition, international edition 2007. Available at: https://books.google.com/books?hl=en&lr=&id=rWoWAAAAQBAJ&oi=fnd&pg=PP1&dq=6.%09Knapp+M,+Hall+J,+Horgan+T:+Nonverbal+Communication+in+Human+Interaction,+8th+Ed.+Wadsworth,+Boston,+2014.&ots=4RqBTSsXcC&sig=Bq_1D2B9m KHi7NNemn5HfNS6abs. Accessed September 15, 2018.
29. Henry SG, Fuhrel-forbis A, Rogers MAM, et al. Patient Education and Counseling Association between nonverbal communication during clinical interactions and

outcomes : a systematic review and meta-analysis86. Elsevier; 2012. p. 297–315. https://doi.org/10.1016/j.pec.2011.07.006.
30. Burgoon J, Guerrero L, Floyd K. Nonverbal communication, vol. 201, 2015. p. 1–6. Available at: https://content.taylorfrancis.com/books/download?dac=C2015-0-61479-2&isbn=9781317346074&format=googlePreviewPdf. Accessed September 15, 2018.
31. Patel RA, Hartzler A, Pratt W, et al. Visual feedback on nonverbal communication : a design exploration with healthcare professionals. Pervasive Heal 2013. https://doi.org/10.4108/icst.pervasivehealth.2013.252024.
32. Glueck D. Establishing therapeutic rapport in telemental health. In: Myers K, Turvey C, editors. Telemental health. Waltham (MA): Elsevier; 2013. p. 29–46. https://doi.org/10.1016/B978-0-12-416048-4.00003-8.
33. Brugel S, Postma-nilsenová M, Tates K. The link between perception of clinical empathy and nonverbal behavior : the effect of a doctor' s gaze and body orientation. Patient Educ Couns 2015;98(10):1260–5.
34. Ebner N, Thompson J. @ Face value? Nonverbal communication & trust development in online video-based mediation. Int J Online Disput Resolut 2016;1–7. https://doi.org/10.1089/1050725027610164 94.
35. Onor ML, Misan S. The clinical interview and the doctor–patient relationship in telemedicine. Telemed J E Health 2005;11(1):102–5.
36. Savin D, Glueck DA, Chardavoyne J, et al. Bridging cultures: child psychiatry via videoconferencing. Child Adolesc Psychiatr Clin N Am 2011;20(1):125–34.
37. McHenry M, Parker PA, Baile WF, et al. Voice analysis during bad news discussion in oncology: reduced pitch, decreased speaking rate, and nonverbal communication of empathy. Support Care Cancer 2012;20(5):1073–8.
38. Dijkstra H, Albada A, Klöckner Cronauer C, et al. Nonverbal communication and conversational contribution in breast cancer genetic counseling. Patient Educ Couns 2013;93(2):216–23.
39. Montague E, Asan O. Dynamic modeling of patient and physician eye gaze to understand the effects of electronic health records on doctor – patient communication and attention. Int J Med Inform 2013;83(3):225–34.

Depression in Youth with Autism Spectrum Disorder

Florencia Pezzimenti, MEd[a], Gloria T. Han, MA[b],
Roma A. Vasa, MD[c], Katherine Gotham, PhD[d],*

KEYWORDS

- Depression • Mood • Dysthymia • Autism • ASD • Psychiatric comorbidity
- Assessment • Treatment

KEY POINTS

- Depression is a commonly cooccurring disorder in individuals with autism spectrum disorder (ASD), with lifetime rates approximately 4 times greater than the general population when pooled across age ranges (7.7% in child ASD samples; 40.2% in adults with ASD).

- Depression in ASD compromises adaptive functioning and quality of life and is associated with increased risk of medication and service use, suicidality, other forms of self-injury, and caregiver burden.

- Assessment and diagnosis of depression in young people with ASD are challenging because of symptom overlap between the disorders and lack of validated psychometric instruments for assessing depressive symptoms in ASD.

- Evidence for effective treatment of depression in youth with ASD is limited, but adapted psychotherapies show some promise.

This article originally appeared in *Child and Adolescent Psychiatric Clinics*, Volume 28, Issue 3, July 2019.

Disclosure Statement: Sources of support included the National Institute of Mental Health R01-MH113576, K01-MH103500, T32-MH18921. Content is solely the responsibility of the authors and does not necessarily represent the official views of the NIH. No funding body or source of support had a role in the study design, data collection, analysis, or interpretation, or writing of this manuscript.

[a] Department of Psychiatry and Behavioral Sciences, Vanderbilt University Medical Center, 1500 21st Avenue South, Village at Vanderbilt, Room 2246, Nashville, TN 37212, USA; [b] Department of Psychology, Vanderbilt University, 111 21st Avenue South, Wilson Hall, Room 205, Nashville, TN 37240, USA; [c] Department of Psychiatry and Behavioral Sciences, Johns Hopkins University School of Medicine, Kennedy Krieger Institute, 3901 Greenspring Avenue, Baltimore, MD 21211, USA; [d] Department of Psychiatry and Behavioral Sciences, Vanderbilt University Medical Center, 1500 21st Avenue South, Village at Vanderbilt, Room 2252, Nashville, TN 37212, USA
* Corresponding author.
E-mail address: katherine.gotham@vanderbilt.edu

Clinics Collections 11 (2021) 83–95
https://doi.org/10.1016/j.ccol.2020.12.031
2352-7986/21/© 2020 Elsevier Inc. All rights reserved.

INTRODUCTION

For several decades, the focus on understanding autism spectrum disorder (ASD) seemed to leave little room for research on cooccurring affective disorders. In addition, diagnostic overshadowing, or the tendency for clinicians to overlook or dismiss depressive symptoms or behaviors as attributes of ASD, largely obscured clinical awareness of depression in youth with ASD. Pioneering work[1,2] raised awareness of the syndrome of depression in ASD, and over the past decade, there has been a sharp increase in the number of research publications on this topic. The number of youth presenting with cooccurring ASD and depression often exceeds the clinical capacity to intervene in many (possibly most) regions throughout North America as well as globally. Stakeholders and funding agencies are swiftly coming to realize the importance and urgency of research on depression in ASD. Here, the authors provide an overview of the prevalence, impact, presentation, and risk factors associated with cooccurring depression in children and adolescents with ASD. Clinical guidelines for the assessment and treatment of depression in the ASD population are also provided, with the caveat that these are emerging fields in which research is ongoing.

PREVALENCE AND IMPACT OF DEPRESSION IN AUTISM SPECTRUM DISORDER

Establishing accurate and reliable prevalence rates of depression in ASD is challenging due to method variance (eg, population-based vs convenience sample estimates; self-report vs caregiver report of depressive symptoms). However, the literature suggests that depression commonly cooccurs with ASD, with prevalence estimates that exceed estimates from the general population and comparable subpopulations, such as those with intellectual disability.[3] In samples of children and adolescents with ASD, current rates of depression generally fall in the range of 1% to 10% as diagnosed by parent report; these same studies tend to report elevated subsyndromal depression rates for an additional 10% to 15% of their samples.[4,5] In a convenience sample of 1272 youth with ASD enrolled in the Autism Speaks Autism Treatment Network, parents reported depression diagnoses for 20.2% of adolescents aged 13 to 17.[6] By approximate comparison, 8.4% of typically developing early adolescents (13–14 year olds) had major depressive disorder or dysthymia in a large US representative study.[7]

A recent meta-analysis[8] found that individuals with ASD are approximately 4 times more likely to experience depression compared with the general population when age ranges are pooled. Significantly elevated lifetime depression rates in ASD are associated with the following:

- Increasing age (40.2% in adult samples vs 7.7% in samples <18 years old)
- Average to above average IQ (52.8% vs 12.2% when mean IQ is below average)
- Structured interviews to assess depression (28.5% vs 6.7% for other assessment instruments)
- Self-report (48.6% vs 14.4% via caregiver report)

Cooccurring depression has significant emotional, social, and behavioral consequences for individuals with ASD, including the following:

- Exacerbated impairments associated with ASD (eg, diminished social motivation and adaptive functioning)[1,9,10]
- Diminished quality of life, and increased caregiver burden, medication, and service use[11,12]

- Heightened physical (eg, gastrointestinal problems, seizures), emotional (eg, anxiety), and behavioral (eg, aggression, inattention) comorbidities[6,13]
- Increased suicidality in a population with elevated rates of suicidal ideation and attempts compared with the general population[14,15,16]

PHENOMENOLOGY OF DEPRESSION IN AUTISM SPECTRUM DISORDER

Individuals with ASD exhibit traditional *Diagnostic and Statistical Manual of Mental Disorders* (Fifth Edition)[17] depressive symptoms (eg, sadness, decreased pleasure in most activities, cognitive and somatic symptoms, and suicidality). As shown in **Table 1**, they may also exhibit more atypical presentations of depression[10,18,19] that focus on changes in engagement of special interests or other repetitive behaviors and decreases in adaptive behavior skills and self-care. Within the heterogeneous autism spectrum, depression presentation likely depends on a variety of factors, several covered below in the section on vulnerability factors. Although lacking prototypical benchmarks, the authors offer hypothetical "snapshots" of cases here:

- Cognitively able and socially motivated youth with ASD may experience sadness, increased irritability, anhedonia, sleep disturbance, diminished appetite, self-deprecatory thoughts, coupled with an exacerbation of their ASD symptoms (eg, more intense circumscribed interests and increased rigidity).
- Youth with ASD and intellectual disability may present with increased crying, self-injury, aggression, perseveration, weight gain or loss, and toileting accidents.

ASD and depression have overlapping features in several key areas (**Fig. 1**), most notably more constricted or flat affect and social withdrawal. Historically, this has led to diagnostic overshadowing, which has hindered awareness, characterization, and diagnostic precision of depression in ASD samples.

Little is known about the course of depression in children and adolescents with ASD, although preliminary data indicate that depression may persist longitudinally. Specifically, girls may show a steeper increase in depressive symptoms throughout adolescence, on par with typically developing girls, whereas boys with ASD may have elevated symptoms in school-aged years (compared with typically developing

---

Table 1
Symptom presentation of depression in autism spectrum disorder

Prototypical Depression Symptoms that Commonly Mark Depression in ASD	Depression Symptoms that May be More Specific to ASD
<ul><li>Depressed and/or irritable mood</li><li>Loss of pleasure in previously enjoyed activities</li><li>Hopelessness and tearfulness</li><li>Negative beliefs about oneself</li><li>Feelings of failure or worthlessness</li><li>Constricted affect</li><li>(Increased) Social withdrawal</li><li>Change in appetite (increased or decreased)</li><li>(Increased) Sleep problems</li><li>Poor concentration abilities</li><li>Lack of motivation</li><li>Thoughts about death or suicidal ideation</li></ul>	<ul><li>Increased irritability</li><li>Changes in circumscribed interests (CI):<ul><li>Decreased pleasure in CI</li><li>Increased intensity</li><li>Change to darker/morbid content</li></ul></li><li>Increased repetitive behaviors</li><li>Increased anxiety or insistence on sameness</li><li>Increase in aggression or self-injury</li><li>Regressive behavior</li><li>Decline in self-care</li></ul>

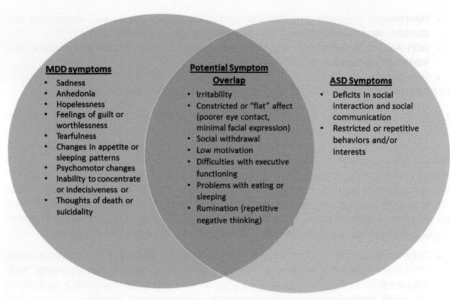

MDD symptoms
- Sadness
- Anhedonia
- Hopelessness
- Feelings of guilt or worthlessness
- Tearfulness
- Changes in appetite or sleeping patterns
- Psychomotor changes
- Inability to concentrate or indecisiveness or
- Thoughts of death or suicidality

Potential Symptom Overlap
- Irritability
- Constricted or "flat" affect (poorer eye contact, minimal facial expression)
- Social withdrawal
- Low motivation
- Difficulties with executive functioning
- Problems with eating or sleeping
- Rumination (repetitive negative thinking)

ASD Symptoms
- Deficits in social interaction and social communication
- Restricted or repetitive behaviors and/or interests

Fig. 1. Potential symptom overlap in major depressive disorder (MDD) and ASD.

children and with girls with ASD) that persist into adulthood.[20] Depressive symptoms may also be more likely to persist in children who are experiencing bullying or greater social communication difficulties.[21]

RISK FACTORS

Researchers have posited several potential vulnerability factors for depression in ASD. Most of these come from independent studies of ASD and of typically developing depressed samples, with no direct comparison of the 2 clinical populations. Very few studies have used longitudinal designs to capture the interplay between depressed mood and ASD symptoms over time. A summary of data is presented on potential candidate vulnerability factors associated with ASD and/or depression that may further the understanding of their cooccurrence.

Genetic/Neurobiological

- Higher familial rates of affective disorders have been reported in family members of individuals with autism, even before having a child with a developmental disability.[22]
- ASD, major depressive disorder, and other mental health conditions have been found to share common genetic variance.[23] Serotonin and dopamine gene variants have been linked to more severe depressive symptoms in children with ASD.[13]
- Atypical neural processes related to serotonin,[24] microglia (indicating inflammatory processes),[25] amygdala anatomy and function,[26] and other functional or connectivity disruptions[27] have been associated with both depression and ASD in independent samples.

Demographic and Individual Characteristics

- Age: Evidence suggests that the risk for depression in ASD increases in adolescence,[8,20,21] similar to patterns observed in the general population.[7] Adult ASD depression rates are significantly higher still than child rates in ASD[8] (several studies report lifetime depression rates ranging from 50% to 77% in adults with ASD[28,29]), which provides context for the importance of recognizing and treating this issue at younger ages.

- Sex/gender: It is still unclear whether girls with ASD are at a greater risk for depression than are boys, in line with general population findings.[30] Studies suggest that girls with ASD are at equal, greater, or less risk of developing depression than boys with ASD.[13,27] With emerging data on more frequent nonbinary interpretations of gender in youth with ASD, it will also be important to study how gender identity influences mood in this special population.[31]
- Intellectual and verbal ability: Individuals with lower ASD severity and average to above average IQ are at greater risk for depressive symptoms and suicidality.[8] This finding suggests that greater insight into their social difficulties might confer risk for depression, and/or depressive symptoms are more easily overlooked in individuals with lower verbal ability and intellectual disability.[27]
- Poor emotion regulation, and maladaptive coping strategies and/or thought patterns:
  ○ Children, adolescents, and transition-age youth with ASD have been reported to exhibit higher rates of negative self-perceptions (eg, guilt, shame, feelings of worthlessness), maladaptive coping strategies (eg, repetitive negative thinking), and perceived stress and inability to cope, all of which are associated with depression in the general population.[27]
  ○ Children with ASD who use adaptive coping strategies (ie, problem-solving, seeking social support) compared with those who engage in rumination and other maladaptive coping strategies appear to be at lower risk of depression.[32]
- Other psychiatric comorbidities: Depression is associated with the presence of additional psychiatric comorbidities, such as anxiety, in children and adolescents with ASD.[33]
- Social motivation: A desire to make meaningful connections paired with social communication impairments and negative social feedback in ASD could increase risk for depression.[34,35] In adults with ASD as a proxy, greater social interest was associated with loneliness,[36] and loneliness in turn has been associated with higher rates of depression and suicidality in individuals with ASD.[36–38]

External Variables that May Function as Vulnerability Factors for Depression in Autism Spectrum Disorder

- Socioeconomic status (SES): The limited research on SES and depression risk in ASD is inconclusive, with findings of no relationship or a significant positive relationship.[39–41]
- Social support: Adults with ASD who perceived greater social support and acceptance reported lower depressive symptoms,[42] whereas lower perceived social support and social satisfaction have been associated with elevated depressive symptoms.[38] The equivalent data in children are not known, but this suggested pathway may reasonably apply across the lifespan.
- Life stress/trauma: People with ASD tend to have higher rates of stressful life experiences, including stigma, bullying, and poor prospects for independence, employment, and romantic fulfillment.[43] Bullying and other stressful life experiences that were considered traumatic have been associated with depression in transition age youth and young adults with ASD in independent studies.[21,44]

DIAGNOSTIC EVALUATION OF DEPRESSION
Multimethod Multi-Informant Approach

Because diagnostic instruments for assessing depression in ASD have not yet been psychometrically validated, and given the diagnostic complexity due to symptom overlap, a multimethod, multi-informant approach is strongly recommended to assess symptoms across multiple contexts. This approach includes gathering information from the individual with ASD, parents, teachers, and other professionals. The psychiatric evaluation includes but it is not limited to assessing the following domains:

- Current and past psychiatric history, onset and phenotype of depressive symptoms, typical and atypical presentations, teasing apart overlapping symptoms between depression and ASD, presence of other cooccurring conditions
- Family history of affective disorders and other psychopathology
- Developmental history and current level of functioning
- Educational placement and supports
- Psychosocial history, which includes family functioning, trauma, and current stressful life events (eg, recent traumatic experiences, bullying, changes in the home environment, social support)
- Psychological and interpersonal functioning (eg, social interests, friendships, self-awareness of disability, isolation, recreational activities, ego strengths, self-attitude)
- Assessment of baseline behavior to determine recent behavioral changes and impact on functioning
- Medical history to rule out other conditions that may be contributing to depression (eg, anemia, hypothyroidism)
- Suicidal risk assessment
- Mental status examination

Special Diagnostic Considerations in Autism Spectrum Disorder

While conducting these assessments, clinicians are encouraged to keep in mind several factors that are unique to the diagnostic assessment in the ASD population. These factors include the following:

- Assessing symptom overlap between mood problems and autism (eg, irritability, sleep and eating problems, inconsistent eye contact, constricted affect, and social isolation) (see **Fig. 1**). Some symptoms may be part of the ASD, depression, or both. It is therefore important to carefully assess whether symptoms are new or are an exacerbation of baseline symptoms.
- Determining the validity of self-report: Social-communication deficits and inability to recognize and label emotions (ie, alexithymia)[45] may prevent individuals on the spectrum from identifying and expressing emotional states, causing depressive symptoms to be overlooked by family and clinicians.
- Using depression measures with caution: At this time, there is not enough evidence to determine if instruments designed for the general population may be valid to assess depressed mood in ASD.[46]
- Assessing for atypical presentations of depression in ASD (see **Table 1**).
- Evaluate for other comorbidities, particularly anxiety, gastrointestinal problems, seizures, and others known to cooccur with depression in ASD.[13]
- Screening for suicidality at every visit: Individuals with ASD are at high risk for suicidal thoughts and behaviors.[47] In addition to well-established suicidality

assessment practices, it is important to gauge impulsivity and the repetitive nature of thinking about death or self-harm in patients with ASD.

TREATMENT OF DEPRESSION IN AUTISM SPECTRUM DISORDER

Development of evidence-based practices for treating depression in ASD is an ongoing and emerging area of research. Preliminary evidence indicates the effectiveness of adapted psychotherapeutic interventions from the general population to the ASD population. Medications for depression in typically developing youth can be also considered, although data are lacking for their use in ASD.

Clinicians are encouraged to consider the following when making treatment decisions:

- Use a multimodal approach that tailors the intervention to the patient's needs and interests (the authors refer readers to these detailed case studies[27])
- Use a multidisciplinary care team with coordination of services across relevant systems (ie, home, social, educational, and vocational environments)
- Coordinate treatment modality with patient's level of cognitive functioning and social-emotional insight

Fig. 2 presents therapeutic options with consideration of the patient's cognitive and verbal abilities and social-emotional insight. As noted in the bottom band of **Fig. 2**, all patients may benefit from healthy living behaviors that have been shown to ameliorate and prevent depressive symptoms for the general population. Approaches that rely less on meta-cognitive skills (eg, behavioral activation [BA]) may be better initial choices for minimally verbal or intellectually disabled patients with depression. Finally, cognitive behavioral and interpersonal therapies may be more appropriate for individuals with requisite cognitive, social, and emotional insight. Importantly, these treatment options are not equivalently evidenced-based and must be considered of potential utility on a case-by-case basis.

Psychotherapeutic Treatments

Recent evidence suggests that *cognitive behavioral therapy* (CBT) can be effective in treating children and adolescents with comorbid ASD and depression.[48,49] CBT approaches focus on helping clients identify and change common unhelpful thoughts and behaviors to encourage improvement in mood and overall functioning.[50] Modifications to CBT protocols for ASD populations (see Kerns and colleagues[51]) include incorporating or considering the following:

- Psychoeducation to increase the individual's understanding of the depression diagnosis as a descriptor for maladaptive emotional symptoms (eg, prolonged sadness), physical symptoms (eg, fatigue, aberrant sleep patterns), and social consequences (eg, social withdrawal and isolation), which helps to identify core skills for symptom improvement
- Hands-on interactive activities (eg, role-playing, games)
- Visual analogue scales (eg, fear thermometer)
- Technology (eg, using telephone applications to monitor daily mood)
- Parent and family involvement
- Group therapy to foster a community of social support and accountability and to help the adolescent transition from family-centered support to peer support

The well-validated depression treatment protocol known as *behavioral activation or BA*[52] also may benefit youth on the spectrum. People with depression tend to isolate

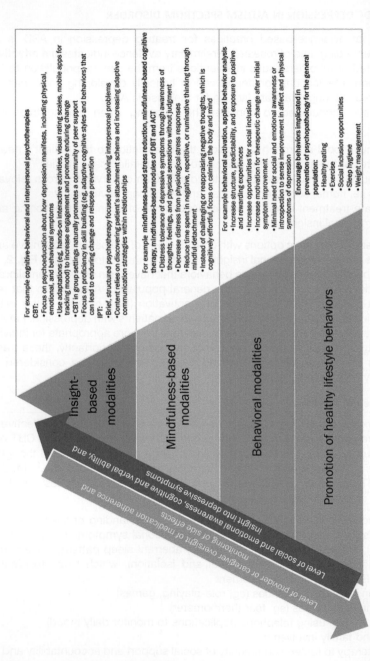

Fig. 2. Considerations in potential treatments for depression in ASD. These treatment modalities are neither equivalently nor thoroughly evidenced based at this point in time, particularly with regard to *youth* with ASD, and must be considered of potential utility on a case-by-case basis. ACT, acceptance and commitment therapy; DBT, dialectical behavioral therapy; IPT, interpersonal therapy.

themselves and withdraw from pleasant activities. Using BA, individuals work on modifying behavior to increase opportunities for rewarding and positive experiences, thus improving mood over time. With less emphasis on insight and cognitive work, BA might be considered a first-line treatment for patients with cooccurring intellectual disability and depression. In addition, BA may be particularly effective in the following circumstances:

- During transition periods (eg, moving, changing schools, transitioning into adulthood), because it provides structured activities to promote goal setting, to attain goals, and to mitigate tendencies for social withdrawal and isolation.[51]
- Patients with high levels of negative affect and minimal motivation for change. Increasing patient's access to rewarding experiences facilitates initial improvement in affect to provide hope and readiness to engage in other psychosocial interventions (eg, CBT).

Finally, some studies have provided support for *mindfulness-based interventions* in decreasing depressive symptoms in adults with ASD,[53,54] so results of child research on this modality are awaited. This approach is defined as being aware of thoughts, feelings, physical sensations, and experiences in the present moment, without judgment.[55] Through meditation exercises (eg, breathing, guided imagery, relaxation methods), patients learn to accept their feelings as a temporary state of mind, without overanalyzing the causes of their thoughts and emotions. Mindfulness interventions reduce maladaptive coping strategies, such as rumination, which is seen in ASD and in depressed individuals in the general population.[56,57] Although research is limited, mindfulness remains a promising treatment for reducing depression in ASD.

Psychopharmacological Treatments

Despite pharmacologic evidence supporting the use of selective serotonin reuptake inhibitors (SSRIs) for depression in typically developing youth,[58] evidence for their efficacy in children and adolescents with ASD is lacking. In fact, to date, there are no randomized controlled trials of antidepressant medications for the treatment of depression in children and adolescents with ASD. However, SSRIs are one of the most commonly prescribed classes of medications in individuals on the spectrum.[59] Existing studies examining the efficacy of SSRIs for other conditions (eg, repetitive behaviors) in youth ASD indicate high rates of BA (eg, impulsivity, aggression, disinhibition[60]; note that this is different from BA mentioned above as a therapeutic modality). Therefore, these medications should be prescribed cautiously for depression in youth with ASD with careful analysis of the risk/benefit ratio and close monitoring. Particular considerations when prescribing SSRIs include the following:

- Obtaining consent from the parent and from the individual with ASD if possible
- Eliciting a family history of bipolar disorder
- Starting with low doses and titrating slowly
- Routine monitoring of side effects, making every effort to elicit information from both the caregiver and individual with ASD
- Psychoeducation about medication side effects, with particular attention to providing parents with a clear plan about how to address BA and risk of mania should this occur
- Identifying objective treatment targets that can be tracked over time
- Establishing a timeline for assessing treatment efficacy, with a plan to taper and discontinue the medication if there is no benefit

SUMMARY AND FUTURE DIRECTIONS

Depression is common in youth with ASD, particularly for adolescents and those individuals with average or greater cognitive ability. Depression is associated with several negative outcomes, including functional impairments beyond those associated with autism itself and significant burden on the family system. Accurate screening and assessment of depression in people with ASD are complicated by uncertain validity of self-report, alexithymia and poor insight common to ASD, and overlapping symptoms between ASD and depression. Research is needed to elucidate the presentation of depression in people with ASD across age, gender, and ability ranges, in order to refine assessment practices for this commonly cooccurring disorder. In addition, identifying specific pathways to mood problems in this population will be important to understanding risk factors and contributing mechanisms, potentially informing targets for more precise and effective intervention.

REFERENCES

1. Ghaziuddin M, Ghaziuddin N, Greden J. Depression in persons with autism: implications for research and clinical care. J Autism Dev Disord 2002;32(4): 299–306.

2. Lainhart JE, Folstein SE. Affective disorders in people with autism: a review of published cases. J Autism Dev Disord 1994;24(5):587–601.

3. Mayes SD, Calhoun SL, Murray MJ, et al. Anxiety, depression, and irritability in children with autism relative to other neuropsychiatric disorders and typical development. Res Autism Spectr Disord 2011;5(1):474–85.

4. Simonoff E, Pickles A, Charman T, et al. Psychiatric disorders in children with autism spectrum disorders: prevalence, comorbidity, and associated factors in a population-derived sample. J Am Acad Child Adolesc Psychiatry 2008;47(8): 921–9.

5. Leyfer OT, Folstein SE, Bacalman S, et al. Comorbid psychiatric disorders in children with autism: interview development and rates of disorders. J Autism Dev Disord 2006;36(7):849–61.

6. Greenlee JL, Mosley AS, Shui AM, et al. Medical and behavioral correlates of depression history in children and adolescents with autism spectrum disorder. Pediatrics 2016;137(Suppl):S105–14.

7. Merikangas KR, He J, Burstein M, et al. Lifetime prevalence of mental disorders in U.S. adolescents: results from the National Comorbidity Survey Replication–Adolescent Supplement (NCS-A). J Am Acad Child Adolesc Psychiatry 2010; 49(10):980–9.

8. Hudson CC, Hall L, Harkness KL. Prevalence of depressive disorders in individuals with autism spectrum disorder: a meta-analysis. J Abnorm Child Psychol 2018. https://doi.org/10.1007/s10802-018-0402-1.

9. Magnuson KM, Constantino JN. Characterization of depression in children with autism spectrum disorders. J Dev Behav Pediatr 2011;32(4):332–40.

10. Stewart ME, Barnard L, Pearson J, et al. Presentation of depression in autism and Asperger syndrome: a review. Autism 2006;10(1):103–16.

11. Cadman T, Eklund H, Howley D, et al. Caregiver burden as people with autism spectrum disorder and attention-deficit/hyperactivity disorder transition into adolescence and adulthood in the United Kingdom. J Am Acad Child Adolesc Psychiatry 2012;51(9):879–88.

12. Joshi G, Wozniak J, Petty C, et al. Psychiatric comorbidity and functioning in a clinically referred population of adults with autism spectrum disorders: a comparative study. J Autism Dev Disord 2013;43(6):1314–25.

13. Menezes M, Robinson L, Sanchez MJ, et al. Depression in youth with autism spectrum disorders: a systematic review of studies published between 2012 and 2016. Rev J Autism Dev Disord 2018. https://doi.org/10.1007/s40489-018-0146-4.

14. Cassidy S, Bradley P, Robinson J, et al. Suicidal ideation and suicide plans or attempts in adults with Asperger's syndrome attending a specialist diagnostic clinic: a clinical cohort study. Lancet Psychiatry 2014;1(2):142–7.

15. Cassidy S, Rodgers J. Understanding and prevention of suicide in autism. Lancet Psychiatry 2017;4(6):e11.

16. Storch EA, Lewin AB, Collier AB, et al. A randomized controlled trial of cognitive-behavioral therapy versus treatment as usual for adolescents with autism spectrum disorders and comorbid anxiety: CBT for Adolescents with ASD and Anxiety. Depress Anxiety 2015;32(3):174–81.

17. American Psychiatric Association. Diagnostic and statistical manual of mental disorders: DSM-5. 5th edition. Arlington (VA): American Psychiatric Association; 2013. p. 2013.

18. Charlot L, Deutsch CK, Albert A, et al. Mood and anxiety symptoms in psychiatric inpatients with autism spectrum disorder and depression. J Ment Health Res Intellect Disabil 2008;1(4):238–53.

19. Chandrasekhar T, Sikich L. Challenges in the diagnosis and treatment of depression in autism spectrum disorders across the lifespan. Dialogues Clin Neurosci 2015;17(2):219–27.

20. Gotham K, Brunwasser SM, Lord C. Depressive and anxiety symptom trajectories from school age through young adulthood in samples with autism spectrum disorder and developmental delay. J Am Acad Child Adolesc Psychiatry 2015;54(5):369–76.e3.

21. Rai D, Culpin I, Heuvelman H, et al. Association of autistic traits with depression from childhood to age 18 years. JAMA Psychiatry 2018;75(8):835–43.

22. Bolton PF, Pickles A, Murphy M, et al. Autism, affective and other psychiatric disorders: patterns of familial aggregation. Psychol Med 1998;28(2):385–95.

23. Cross-Disorder Group of the Psychiatric Genomics Consortium. Identification of risk loci with shared effects on five major psychiatric disorders: a genome-wide analysis. Lancet 2013;381(9875):1371–9.

24. Muller CL, Anacker AMJ, Veenstra-VanderWeele J. The serotonin system in autism spectrum disorder: from biomarker to animal models. Neuroscience 2016;321:24–41.

25. Frick LR, Williams K, Pittenger C. Microglial dysregulation in psychiatric disease. Clin Dev Immunol 2013;2013:1–10.

26. Dichter GS, Damiano CA, Allen JA. Reward circuitry dysfunction in psychiatric and neurodevelopmental disorders and genetic syndromes: animal models and clinical findings. J Neurodev Disord 2012;4(1). https://doi.org/10.1186/1866-1955-4-19.

27. Gotham K, Pezzimenti F, Eydt-Beebe M, et al. Co-occurring mood problems in autism spectrum disorder. In: White S, Mazefsky C, Maddox B, editors. The Oxford Handbook of Psychiatric Comorbidity in Autism. Oxford, UK: Oxford University Press; In press.

28. Lugnegård T, Hallerbäck MU, Gillberg C. Psychiatric comorbidity in young adults with a clinical diagnosis of Asperger syndrome. Res Dev Disabil 2011;32(5): 1910–7.

29. Gotham K, Siegle G, Han G, et al. Pupil response to social-emotional materials is associated with rumination and depressive symptoms in adults with autism spectrum disorder. PLoS One 2018;13(8):e0200340.

30. Hankin BL, Abramson LY, Moffitt TE, et al. Development of depression from pre-adolescence to young adulthood: emerging gender differences in a 10-year longitudinal study. J Abnorm Psychol 1998;107(1):128–40.

31. van Schalkwyk GI, Klingensmith K, Volkmar FR. Gender identity and autism spectrum disorders. Yale J Biol Med 2015;88(1):81–3.

32. Rieffe C, De Bruine M, De Rooij M, et al. Approach and avoidant emotion regulation prevent depressive symptoms in children with an Autism Spectrum Disorder. Int J Dev Neurosci 2014;39:37–43.

33. Vasa RA, Kalb L, Mazurek M, et al. Age-related differences in the prevalence and correlates of anxiety in youth with autism spectrum disorders. Res Autism Spectr Disord 2013;7(11):1358–69.

34. Meyer JA, Mundy PC, Van Hecke AV, et al. Social attribution processes and comorbid psychiatric symptoms in children with Asperger syndrome. Autism 2006; 10(4):383–402.

35. Sterling L, Dawson G, Estes A, et al. Characteristics associated with presence of depressive symptoms in adults with autism spectrum disorder. J Autism Dev Disord 2008;38(6):1011–8.

36. Han GT, Tomarken AJ, Gotham KO. Social and non-social reward moderate the relation between autism symptoms and loneliness in adults with ASD, depression, and controls. Autism Res 2019. [Epub ahead of print].

37. Mazurek MO. Loneliness, friendship, and well-being in adults with autism spectrum disorders. Autism 2014;18(3):223–32.

38. Hedley D, Uljarević M, Foley K-R, et al. Risk and protective factors underlying depression and suicidal ideation in Autism Spectrum Disorder. Depress Anxiety 2018;35(7):648–57.

39. Gray K, Keating C, Taffe J, et al. Trajectory of behavior and emotional problems in autism. Am J Intellect Dev Disabil 2012;117(2):121–33.

40. Midouhas E, Yogaratnam A, Flouri E, et al. Psychopathology trajectories of children with autism spectrum disorder: the role of family poverty and parenting. J Am Acad Child Adolesc Psychiatry 2013;52(10):1057–65.e1.

41. Taylor JL, Seltzer MM. Changes in the autism behavioral phenotype during the transition to adulthood. J Autism Dev Disord 2010;40(12):1431–46.

42. Cage E, Di Monaco J, Newell V. Experiences of autism acceptance and mental health in autistic adults. J Autism Dev Disord 2018;48(2):473–84.

43. Henninger NA, Taylor JL. Outcomes in adults with autism spectrum disorders: a historical perspective. Autism 2013;17(1):103–16.

44. Taylor JL, Gotham KO. Cumulative life events, traumatic experiences, and psychiatric symptomatology in transition-aged youth with autism spectrum disorder. J Neurodev Disord 2016;8(1). https://doi.org/10.1186/s11689-016-9160-y.

45. Bird G, Cook R. Mixed emotions: the contribution of alexithymia to the emotional symptoms of autism. Transl Psychiatry 2013;3(7):e285.

46. Cassidy SA, Bradley L, Bowen E, et al. Measurement properties of tools used to assess depression in adults with and without autism spectrum conditions: a systematic review. Autism Res 2018;11(5):738–54.

47. Horowitz LM, Thurm A, Farmer C, et al. Talking about death or suicide: prevalence and clinical correlates in youth with autism spectrum disorder in the psychiatric inpatient setting. J Autism Dev Disord 2018;48(11):3702–10.
48. Keefer A, White SW, Vasa RA, et al. Psychosocial interventions for internalizing disorders in youth and adults with ASD. Int Rev Psychiatry 2018;30(1):62–77.
49. Santomauro D, Sheffield J, Sofronoff K. Depression in adolescents with ASD: a pilot RCT of a group intervention. J Autism Dev Disord 2016;46(2):572–88.
50. Beck AT, Rush AJ, editors. Cognitive therapy of depression. New York: Guilford Press; 1979. 13. Print.
51. Kerns CM, Roux AM, Connell JE, et al. Adapting cognitive behavioral techniques to address anxiety and depression in cognitively able emerging adults on the autism spectrum. Cogn Behav Pract 2016;23(3):329–40.
52. Jacobson NS, Martell CR, Dimidjian S. Behavioral activation treatment for depression: returning to contextual roots. Clin Psychol Sci Pract 2006;8(3):255–70.
53. Spek AA, van Ham NC, Nyklíček I. Mindfulness-based therapy in adults with an autism spectrum disorder: a randomized controlled trial. Res Dev Disabil 2013; 34(1):246–53.
54. Sizoo BB, Kuiper E. Cognitive behavioural therapy and mindfulness based stress reduction may be equally effective in reducing anxiety and depression in adults with autism spectrum disorders. Res Dev Disabil 2017;64:47–55.
55. Kabat-Zinn J. Mindfulness-based interventions in context: past, present, and future. Clin Psychol Sci Pract 2003;10:144–56.
56. Hayes SC. Acceptance and commitment therapy, relational frame theory, and the third wave of behavioral and cognitive therapies. Behav Ther 2004;35(4):639–65.
57. Jain S, Shapiro SL, Swanick S, et al. A randomized controlled trial of mindfulness meditation versus relaxation training: effects on distress, positive states of mind, rumination, and distraction. Ann Behav Med 2007;33(1):11–21.
58. March J, Silva S, Petrycki S, et al. Fluoxetine, cognitive-behavioral therapy, and their combination for adolescents with depression: treatment for adolescents with depression study (TADS) randomized controlled trial. JAMA 2004;292(7): 807–20.
59. Houghton R, Ong RC, Bolognani F. Psychiatric comorbidities and use of psychotropic medications in people with autism spectrum disorder in the United States. Autism Res 2017;10(12):2037–47.
60. King BH, Hollander E, Sikich L, et al. Lack of efficacy of citalopram in children with autism spectrum disorders and high levels of repetitive behavior: citalopram ineffective in children with autism. Arch Gen Psychiatry 2009;66(6):583–90.

When Night Falls Fast

Sleep and Suicidal Behavior Among Adolescents and Young Adults

Sara N. Fernandes, MA[a], Emily Zuckerman, BA[b],
Regina Miranda, PhD[c], Argelinda Baroni, MD[b],*

KEYWORDS

- Suicide • Sleep • Nightmares • Insomnia • Adolescent • Young adult

KEY POINTS

- Sleep disturbances, including insomnia and nightmares, are associated with suicidal behaviors in youth and predictive of future suicidal ideation.
- Data regarding hypersomnia, sleep apnea, and suicide risk in youth are mixed.
- Interconnected biological and psychological mechanisms may underlie the relationship between sleep and suicidal behaviors: executive functioning, hyperarousal, thwarted belongingness, and perceived burdensomeness, among others.

INTRODUCTION

Suicide is a leading cause of death worldwide; in the United States it is the tenth leading cause of death across the lifespan and the second leading cause of death among youth. Adolescents are at increased risk for both suicidal ideation and behaviors.[1,2] Notably, most youth who move from ideation to suicide planning do so within 1 year of the onset of their ideation.[3] Despite decades of research on risk factors for youth suicidal behavior, clinicians are not able to accurately predict or effectively prevent these catastrophic events.[4] Historically, many risk factor studies have focused on psychiatric diagnoses, distal and time-invariant risk factors such as history of child abuse, and demographic variables, which have not been useful in short-term detection and prediction of suicide risk.[4]

This article originally appeared in *Child and Adolescent Psychiatric Clinics*, Volume 30, Issue 1, January 2021.

Funding: This work was partially funded with grant MH120846.

[a] New York State Psychiatric Institute, Columbia University Irving Medical Center, 1051 Riverside Drive, Room 1600C, New York, NY 10032, USA; [b] Department of Child and Adolescent Psychiatry, NYU Langone Health, One Park Avenue, 7th Floor, New York, NY 10016, USA; [c] Department of Psychology, Hunter College and The Graduate Center, City University of New York, 695 Park Avenue, Room 611HN, New York, NY 10065, USA

* Corresponding author.

E-mail address: Argelinda.Baroni@nyulangone.org

Accordingly, it is critical to identify transdiagnostic and proximal suicide risk factors that can be objectively assessed and are amenable to interventions. Sleep problems, especially insomnia and nightmares, represent a promising area in suicide research and prevention.[4] This article discusses (1) what is known regarding the relationships between sleep symptoms and suicide, (2) potential mechanisms underlying these associations, and (3) assessments and treatments currently used in clinical practice.

SLEEP DISTURBANCES AND SUICIDAL IDEATION AND BEHAVIORS

Insomnia, short sleep duration, and nightmares have repeatedly been found to be associated with increased suicide risk (ie, ideation and/or behaviors, such as planning and attempts) in children, adolescents, and young adults, even if several limitations have been noted.[5–11] Main limitations include paucity of prospective studies and lack of use of reliable sleep measures; most studies have extracted a few sleep questions rather than using validated questionnaires focusing on sleep.[4,11]

Insomnia and Short Sleep Duration

Insomnia, common across all ages, includes difficulties going to sleep or staying asleep, accompanied by daytime dysfunction.[12] Large cross-sectional adolescent surveys show that experiencing insomnia or insufficient sleep duration is associated with increased rates of suicidal ideation after adjusting for covariates such as age, sex, socioeconomic status, depressive symptoms, and mood disorders.[4,6,13,14] A recent meta-analysis of cross-sectional data from 37,536 adolescents estimated that sleep disturbances substantially and significantly increase risk of suicidal ideation (odds ratio [OR], 2.35), plans (OR, 1.58) and attempts (OR, 1.92), with girls at higher risk of sleep-related suicide attempts than boys.[11]

Data from the Youth Risk Behavior Survey found that short sleep duration was associated with suicidal ideation and behaviors in a dose-dependent manner among 67,615 adolescents surveyed, independently of causes (eg, insomnia vs volitional sleep restriction). Adolescents who slept less than 6 hours (vs 8 hours) had more than 3 times higher odds of considering suicide, planning to attempt suicide, or attempting suicide, and more than 4 times higher odds of reporting an attempt that resulted in treatment.[15] Similarly, a recent review noted that an additional hour of sleep was associated with significantly decreased suicidal ideation among adolescents.[16] A study of adolescent monozygotic twins found short sleep durations to be related to both suicidal ideation and behaviors, adjusting for genetics and shared environments.[17] Similar results were found in studies linking insomnia with suicidal behaviors, including planning and attempts.[6,7,18,19] A study of adolescent suicide completers versus community controls found that the presence of insomnia, both within the week before death and within the current affective episode, significantly distinguished completers from controls, even after adjusting for affective disorders and depressive symptom severity.[18]

Moving beyond cross-sectional and self-report methods, prospective studies have also supported insomnia and short sleep duration as independent risk factors for future suicidal ideation and attempts.[11,20] A systematic review found that, in 7 of 10 studies, sleep problems significantly predicted suicidal ideation and behaviors among adolescents. However, a meta-analysis on the role of sleep in suicidal behaviors was inconclusive.[11] However, in one of the few studies that assessed sleep and suicide prospectively and proximally (after 1-week and 3-week periods) using both subjective and objective (ie, actigraphic) methods, insomnia significantly predicted future ideation among young adults.[20] Altogether, the literature supports insomnia as an independent risk factor for present and future suicidal ideation and behaviors. Accordingly, assessing insomnia subjectively and/or objectively may help clinicians determine an adolescent's current and future risk of suicidal ideation and behaviors. The literature supporting this conclusion spans a wide range of adolescent populations (eg, community based, nationally representative, and clinically severe), further supporting its potential use in a variety of clinical and community settings.[4]

Extended Sleep Time

Hypersomnia has also been associated with heightened suicide risk in adolescents.[16] However, the literature on hypersomnia is mixed, possibly because of inconsistent definitions across studies. One study found that extended sleep time (>10 hours) was associated with increased suicidal ideation and behaviors (ie, ideation, planning, and/or attempts; OR, 4.7) in adolescents,[21] whereas another noted that daytime sleepiness was associated with suicidal behaviors.[22] In a study comparing adolescent suicide completers and community controls, sleeping longer than usual yielded a significant group difference.[18] Incidentally, Diagnostic and Statistical Manual of Mental Disorders, Fifth Edition (DSM-5), defines hypersomnia as excessive daytime sleepiness and extended sleep periods as the main criteria.[12] At the same time, some studies have found no significant relation between longer sleep periods and suicidal behavior, and some have reported the opposite effect: that hypersomnia was protective.[6,23,24] Guo and colleagues[6] found that sleeping more than 9 hours (vs 7–9 hours) was associated with significantly higher odds of suicide attempts (OR, 2.5) in adolescents, but it was not associated with ideation. Of note, 9 hours is the normal sleep time for adolescents. In contrast, another study found that insomnia was related to suicidal ideation and attempts, but hypersomnia was not.[23] Moreover, Kim and colleagues[7] found that adolescents who self-reported typically spending 10 or more hours in bed had lower odds (OR, 0.61) of endorsing suicidal ideation and plans, compared with youth sleeping around 7 h/d. A few large, cross-sectional studies support a U-shaped relationship between suicidal behavior and sleep, with both short sleep periods and extended ones (>9 or 10 hours) being associated with more suicidal events (ideation and/or attempts).[16] Overall, more research is needed to understand the relationship between hypersomnia and suicidal behaviors and differentiate between total sleep time, total time in bed, and daytime sleepiness.

Sleep Regularity

Although less commonly studied than insomnia and sleep duration, sleep regularity and circadian rhythms have been found to be associated with increased suicide risk among adolescents and young adults.[20,25] Both self-report and actigraphy measures revealed that having highly variable sleep patterns was not only related to current suicidal ideation but also predictive of ideation 7 and 21 days later, adjusting for depressive symptoms and baseline ideation in young adults.[20] Intriguingly, sleep variability outperformed depressive symptoms in predicting future ideation. Similarly, sleep rhythm reversals (ie, sleeping during the day and being active at night) have been found to be associated with suicide attempts among adolescent outpatients.[23]

Obstructive Sleep Apnea

Pediatric obstructive sleep apnea is a common condition, with an estimated prevalence of 1% to 6% in the general population and 19% to 61% in obese children and adolescents.[26] It is included in the DSM-5 and should be suspected in youth with frequent loud snoring, witnessed apneas (pauses in nocturnal breathing), restless sleep, and mouth breathing.[12,27] Sleep apnea severely disrupts sleep continuity, and individuals with sleep apneas are functionally sleep deprived. Despite the high prevalence of obstructive sleep apnea, research regarding its relationship with suicide risk is scarce. Although a few large-scale and small-scale investigations among adults found significant associations between sleep apnea and suicide risk,[28–30] studies of children and adolescents have been mixed.[28] A recent survey of 746 children and adolescents that used daytime sleepiness as a proxy for sleep apnea found that obstructive sleep apnea was significantly associated with suicidal ideation even when adjusting for depressive symptoms and perceived stress.[24] This study suggests that sleep apnea is a significant independent risk factor for ideation in youth, with the limitation that the diagnosis did not include history of snoring or objective measures for sleep apnea. Similarly, a large (N = 7072), rigorous prospective study of adolescents found that excessive daytime sleepiness at baseline increased risk of ideation (OR, 1.6) and suicidal plans (OR, 2.6) 1 year later, whereas self-reported loud snoring did not.[31] Thus, the impact of sleep apnea and snoring on youth suicide risk is currently inconclusive, with initial evidence suggesting that excessive daytime sleepiness confers additional risk beyond other risk factors, such as depressive symptoms, anxiety, and perceived stress.

Nightmares

Nightmares are "extended, extremely dysphoric, and well-remembered dreams."[12] Clinicians often consider nightmares a feature of posttraumatic stress disorder (PTSD), but nightmares are often idiopathic, and frequent distressing nightmares are main features of nightmare disorder in the DSM-5 Sleep-Wake Disorder section.[12] Nightmares are usually described by frequency, level of distress caused, and chronicity.[32,33] Research examining nightmares in children and adolescents is limited,[34] but existing work suggests that nightmares are common, especially in younger youth. Approximately 22% to 28% of children aged 5 through 11 years experience nightmares, with a prevalence up to 41% for children in psychiatric care,[35,36] whereas 8% of older adolescents (15–18 years old) experience frequent nightmares.[35]

Nightmares have emerged as an important risk factor for suicidal behavior in adults.[10] Recent studies also support associations between nightmares and suicidal ideation and behaviors in adolescents and young adults, even when adjusting for mental disorder,[10,20,37,38] with a few exceptions.[10,11] A study of 503 college students found an association between nightmares and suicide attempts, even after adjusting for PTSD severity, highlighting that the morbidity of nightmares goes beyond PTSD.[39] A study of 50 inpatient adolescents showed an association between nightmares and suicidal ideation, independent of other sleep measures.[37] Two longitudinal studies suggested that nightmares precede both suicidal ideation and behaviors.[20,38] One study found that higher scores on a nightmare rating scale at baseline predicted increased ideation at 7-day and 21-day follow-ups in young adults,[20] and another study found that frequent nightmares increased the odds of suicidal behavior almost 2-fold (OR, 1.96) after 1 year among adolescents, even after adjusting for demographic factors and mental disorder.[38] Thus, available evidence suggests that nightmares are associated with increased risk of both suicidal ideation and attempts among adolescents and young adults.

POTENTIAL MECHANISMS IN THE RELATION BETWEEN SLEEP DISTURBANCES AND SUICIDE RISK

Several studies have examined biological and psychological factors that may account for the impact of sleep disturbances on suicide risk. Biological factors include executive functioning, frontal lobe processes, and hyperarousal, whereas psychological factors range from thwarted belonging, perceived burdensomeness, and acquired capability to specific cognitions and appraisals such as defeat, entrapment, rumination, hopelessness, and negative self-appraisals (**Fig. 1**).[40]

Executive Functioning

Sleep loss negatively affects executive functioning,[4] and executive function deficits have been associated with suicidal behavior. Accordingly, researchers suggest that insomnia and sleep disruptions may increase susceptibility to suicidal behavior via executive dysfunction.[4,11,41,42] Deficits in problem solving, decision making, attention, and impulse control have been found among suicide attempters and individuals with insomnia.[4,43–45] Likewise, insufficient sleep has been linked to impaired emotion regulation and heightened emotional reactivity, aspects of executive functioning linked to suicide risk.[4] Sleep restriction worsens mood and decreases adolescents' abilities to modulate negative emotions; these features have been found to be more severely impaired among adolescent suicide attempters compared with ideators,[46] as well as among adolescents with multiple attempts compared with 1-time attempters.[47] In adults, emotion regulation has been suggested to mediate the relationship between nightmares and suicidal behavior.[48]

Hyperarousal

Hyperarousal has also been linked to suicide risk. Studies have connected increased agitation, hyperarousal, and night awakenings with susceptibility to suicidal behaviors.[40,49–52] In addition, hyperarousal states can amplify suicidal ideation and risk in adults with high levels of capability for suicide, operationalized as lowered fear of death and increased tolerance for physical pain, per Joiner's (https://www.ncbi.nlm.nih.gov/pmc/articles/PMC5730496/) interpersonal theory of suicide.[40] Similarly, nightmares might interact with acquired capability to predict suicidal behavior via hyperarousal.[53] Altogether, pairing increased arousal with other deficits in executive functioning (ie, increased

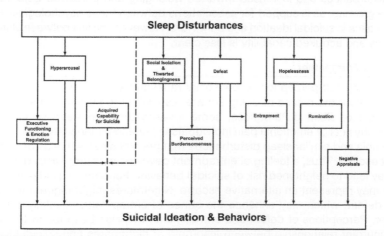

Sleep Disturbances

Hyperarousal · Social Isolation & Thwarted Belongingness · Defeat · Hopelessness

Acquired Capability for Suicide · Entrapment · Rumination

Executive Functioning & Emotion Regulation · Perceived Burdensomeness · Negative Appraisals

Suicidal Ideation & Behaviors

Fig. 1. Solid lines show pathways between sleep disturbances and suicidal ideation and behaviors via underlying biological and psychological mechanisms, as described in the text. Dotted lines show related pathways with mixed support from the literature, as described in the text. (*Adapted from* Littlewood D, Kyle SD, Pratt D, et al. Examining the role of psychological factors in relationship between sleep problems and suicide. Clin Psychol Rev 2017;54:10; with permission.)

impulsivity, decreased problem solving, and so forth) that accompany sleep disturbances may increase susceptibility to suicidal ideation and behaviors in adolescents.[4]

Thwarted Belonging, Perceived Burdensomeness, and Acquired Capability

The literature on psychological mechanisms underlying the impact of sleep disturbances on youth suicide risk is growing.[40] The interpersonal theory of suicide introduced 3 constructs that may determine suicide risk: thwarted belonging, perceived burdensomeness, and the aforementioned acquired capability for suicide.[40] Thwarted belonging represents feelings of loneliness, isolation, and lack of belonging, as well as limited social relationships. Perceived burdensomeness reflects individuals seeing themselves and their existence as a burden to family, friends, or society. The theory suggests that thwarted belonging and perceived burdensomeness lead to suicidal ideation, and people attempt suicide when they have also acquired the capability for suicide. The literature supports the idea that those with sleep disturbances and insomnia experience increased feelings of loneliness, isolation, and thwarted belonging.[9,54,55] Others are often asleep and unavailable at night, leaving those who are awake to feel more alone and without support. Insomnia has also been linked with increased perceived burdensomeness.[9,55] Thwarted belonging was found to mediate the association between insomnia and suicidal ideation in cross-sectional and longitudinal research with young adults.[56,57] Similarly, perceived burdensomeness mediated the relationship between insomnia and suicide risk in a cross-sectional study of adolescent inpatients.[55] However, studies investigating the links between sleep disturbances and acquired capability are scarce, particularly in adolescents, and the literature is mixed. For example, 2 studies found that insomnia was not associated with acquired capability in samples of young adults and adolescents, whereas it was positively associated with thwarted belongingness and perceived burdensomeness.[9,55] In contrast, a study involving mainly young adults found that insomnia and nightmares interacted with levels of acquired capability to predict concurrent suicidal ideation or attempts.[53] Altogether, data supporting a link between sleep disturbances and increased thwarted belonging and perceived burdensomeness are growing, as is support for associations between these psychological factors and increases in suicidal ideation and behaviors. However, the link between sleep disturbances and acquired capability is less clear.

Defeat and Entrapment

Defeat (ie, the self-perception of low social rank) and entrapment (ie, the desire to escape without the means of doing so) are also linked to suicidal behavior.[40,58] In the context of sleep disturbances, some investigators see sleep as an escape from the physical or emotional pain individuals experience during the day.[59] However, insomnia and similar sleep disturbances that prevent sleep serve as barriers that prevent escape. Thus, a feeling of entrapment develops or is emphasized, which, in turn, may lead to heightened risk of suicidal behavior. For some, suicide-related behaviors may represent an alternative escape. Nightmares might trigger the perception of defeat, which may enhance the sense of entrapment, resulting in suicidal behavior. Perceptions of defeat and entrapment have also been found to mediate the concurrent relationship between insomnia or nightmares and suicidal ideation among adolescents.[8]

Rumination, Hopelessness, and Negative Self-Appraisals

Other cognitions commonly explored in relation to suicide risk include rumination (ie, repetitive thinking about negative emotional states, their related causes, and their

Table 1
Screeners and assessments

	Format	Description
Suicide Risk		
Ask Suicide Screening Questions Tool	4-question screener for youth 10–24 y of age	Suicide risk screener designed for emergency departments, inpatient units, and outpatient care settings. Available in multiple languages at http://www.nimh.nih.gov/asq
Columbia Suicide Severity Rating Scale	17-item scale for children, adolescents, and adults	Suicide risk scale assessing past and present suicidal ideation and behaviors. Training and PDF versions for all ages and settings available at https://cssrs.columbia.edu/the-columbia-scale-c-ssrs/cssrs-for-communities-and-healthcare
Self-Injurious Thoughts and Behaviors Interview	5 screening items and up to (long form) 169 or (short form) 72 variable-format items for youth and young adults	Suicide risk structured interview assessing suicidal ideation, planning, gestures, attempts, and nonsuicidal self-injury. Available at https://nocklab.fas.harvard.edu/tasks
Sleep Disturbances		
BEARS	5-item screener for youth 2–12 y of age; based on parent and/or child reports	Clinical interview and/or self-report form assessing bedtime issues, excessive daytime sleepiness, awakenings and abnormal sleep behaviors, regularity and duration of sleep, and snoring. Available in original article[65]
Child Sleep Habits Questionnaire	45-item measure for youth 4–10 y of age; based on parent report	Parent-report measure designed to assess sleep disturbances, including bedtime issues, sleep-disordered breathing, daytime sleepiness, and parasomnias. Available in original article[80]
The Sleep Disturbance Scale for Children	26-item rating scale for youth 6–15 y of age; based on parent report	Likert-style rating scale designed to capture sleep disturbances in youth. Available in original article[81]
Children's Chronotype Questionnaire	27-item measure for youth 4–11 y of age; based on parent report	Parent-report measure assessing chronotype in youth. Available in original article[82]
Sleep diaries	Self-report tracking tool for all ages	Self-report tool for tracking sleep regularity and duration. Recommended for long-term care. Template available at http://yoursleep.aasmnet.org/pdf/sleepdiary.pdf
Nightmares		
Nightmare Distress Questionnaire	13-item measure for young adults and adults; has been used with adolescents	Self-report measure using Likert scales to assess distress and impact of nightmares. Available in original article[83]
Disturbing Dream and Nightmare Severity Index	5-item measure designed for adults; has been used with adolescents	Self-report measure assessing frequency, severity, and impact of nightmares. Available through the author[84]

potential consequences), feelings of hopelessness, and negative appraisals.[40] As previously highlighted, many sleep disturbances often involve lack of sleep and increased time awake at night. During these late hours, individuals are often without support or social interaction, while others are asleep and unavailable. These times can leave individuals susceptible to feelings of hopelessness and rumination. A study of 27,929 adolescents found that every hour of less sleep was associated with significantly heightened odds of experiencing sadness and hopelessness.[60] Hopelessness may also partially mediate the relationship between insomnia or nightmares and suicidal ideation.[40] Similarly, diminished sleep durations and sleep quality have been linked with increased rumination and related repetitive negative cognitions,[61–63] and rumination has been found to mediate the link between sleep disturbances and suicidal behavior.[63] Relatedly, both negative cognitive self-appraisals and dysfunctional attitudes toward sleep have been found to relate to suicidal ideation.[37,64] Negative sleep appraisals were even found to mediate associations between sleep disturbances and ideation in individuals with depressive disorders.[64] Altogether, lack of sleep seems to have a cascade effect on perceptions and cognitions that may increase susceptibility to suicidal ideation or behaviors.

APPLICATION TO CLINICAL CARE

Considering the literature's support that sleep disturbances are a modifiable risk factor for suicide in youth, it is imperative that effective and appropriate assessments for these phenomena be made available to clinicians and others. Screeners and assessments come in a variety of forms to adapt to various clinical and community settings: clinical interviews, self-report forms, and parent reports, among others. Resources for clinicians are summarized in **Table 1**. For sleep, the authors recommend a stepwise approach, starting with the BEARS (bedtime issues, excessive daytime sleepiness, awakenings and abnormal sleep behaviors, regularity and duration of sleep, and snoring) and proceeding with a more granular assessment if positive findings emerge from questionnaires or clinical interviews. Notably, using the BEARS in a primary pediatric setting increased detection of sleep disturbances 4-fold, compared with usual care.[65]

Although still untested, addressing sleep disturbances might ameliorate suicidal ideation and behaviors among children and adolescents. A few targeted studies of adults have found improvements in suicidal ideation by cognitive behavior therapy for insomnia (CBT-I) or hypnotics (1 trial used zolpidem and 1 mirtazapine).[4,66–69] No trials have been designed to measure change in suicidal behavior with specific interventions for insomnia or nightmares in youth, but a few trials have found improvements in mental health in youth receiving CBT-I.[70,71] Preliminary research on nightmares also suggests that imagery rehearsal therapy and exposure, relaxation, and rescripting therapy may be effective in reducing suicidal ideation in adults with nightmares.[72–74] Although there is some evidence that prazosin might reduce nightmares, 2 recent rigorous studies found that prazosin improved neither nightmares nor suicidal ideation in adult patients with PTSD.[75,76] However, there are no studies addressing suicidal ideation and nightmare treatment in youth, but imagery rehearsal therapy has been effectively adapted for adolescents.[77,78]

SUMMARY

Sleep problems, especially insomnia, short sleep duration, and chronic nightmares, are potential risk factors for suicidal ideation and behaviors in adolescents and young adults, and they often precede the onset of suicidal ideation or behaviors. Disturbed sleep is present across diagnoses and is modifiable.[4] As such, it represents a promising area in suicide prevention. Appropriate screening for sleep problems should be done systematically for all youth endorsing suicidal ideation or behaviors or with risk factors such as mood or trauma-related symptoms.[4] More work is needed to clarify the role of extended sleep periods, excessive daytime sleepiness, and the possible contribution of other sleep disorders to suicide risk. Nightmares are rarely explored or addressed beyond PTSD, but they seem to be an independent risk factor for suicide. Importantly, the association between sleep symptoms and suicidal ideation and behavior endures in most studies, even when demographic factors or mood symptoms are taken into account. Of note, the links between sleep disturbances and suicidal ideation and behaviors in younger children and preadolescents are rarely studied, and more research is needed in this area. Previous work suggests that sleep problems precede depression in children, and it is possible that disturbed sleep precedes suicidal ideation in younger children as well.[79] Further research is needed to understand the relationship between sleep disturbances and suicidal ideation and behaviors in children and adolescents, because improving sleep may represent one of the most tractable opportunities to address the problem of adolescent suicide.

CLINICS CARE POINTS

- Sleep disturbances are transdiagnostic, modifiable, and treatable.
- Screening for sleep disturbances in suicidal adolescents and vice versa is strongly encouraged, because sleep disturbances are associated with suicidal ideation and behaviors.
- Nightmares are often neglected symptoms associated with suicidal behaviors.
- Clinicians should consider a stepwise approach for assessing sleep, screening all youth with BEARS and then using questionnaires and clinical interviews if needed.
- Cognitive behavior therapies are effective in treating insomnia and nightmares.

DISCLOSURE

The authors have nothing to disclose.

REFERENCES

1. Balazs J, Miklosi M, Kereszteny A, et al. Adolescent subthreshold-depression and anxiety: psychopathology, functional impairment and increased suicide risk. J Child Psychol Psychiatry 2013;54(6):670–7.

2. Nock MK, Borges G, Bromet EJ, et al. Cross-national prevalence and risk factors for suicidal ideation, plans and attempts. Br J Psychiatry 2008;192(2):98–105.

3. Nock MK, Green JG, Hwang I, et al. Prevalence, correlates, and treatment of lifetime suicidal behavior among adolescents: results from the National Comorbidity Survey Replication Adolescent Supplement. JAMA Psychiatry 2013;70(3): 300–10.

4. Kearns JC, Coppersmith DDL, Santee AC, et al. Sleep problems and suicide risk in youth: a systematic review, developmental framework, and implications for hospital treatment. Gen Hosp Psychiatry 2020;63:141–51.

5. Baiden P, Tadeo SK, Tonui BC, et al. Association between insufficient sleep and suicidal ideation among adolescents. Psychiatry Res 2019;287:112579.

6. Guo L, Xu Y, Deng J, et al. Association between sleep duration, suicidal ideation, and suicidal attempts among Chinese adolescents: the moderating role of depressive symptoms. J Affect Disord 2017;208:355–62.

7. Kim JH, Park EC, Lee SG, et al. Associations between time in bed and suicidal thoughts, plans and attempts in Korean adolescents. BMJ Open 2015;5(9): e008766.

8. Russell K, Rasmussen S, Hunter SC. Insomnia and nightmares as markers of risk for suicidal ideation in young people: investigating the role of defeat and entrapment. J Clin Sleep Med 2018;14(5):775–84.

9. Nadorff MR, Anestis MD, Nazem S, et al. Sleep disorders and the interpersonal-psychological theory of suicide: independent pathways to suicidality? J Affect Disord 2014;152:505–12.

10. Bernert RA, Nadorff MR. Sleep disturbances and suicide risk. Sleep Med Clin 2015;10(1):35–9.

11. Liu JW, Tu YK, Lai YF, et al. Associations between sleep disturbances and suicidal ideation, plans, and attempts in adolescents: a systematic review and meta-analysis. Sleep 2019;42(6):zsz054.

12. American Psychiatric Association. Diagnostic and statistical manual of mental disorders (DSM-5®). Washington, DC: American Psychiatric Pub; 2013.

13. Kim Y, Kim K, Kwon HJ, et al. Associations between adolescents' sleep duration, sleep satisfaction, and suicidal ideation. Salud Mental 2016;39(4):213–9.

14. Park JH, Yoo JH, Kim SH. Associations between non-restorative sleep, short sleep duration and suicidality: findings from a representative sample of Korean adolescents. Psychiatry Clin Neurosci 2013;67(1):28–34.

15. Weaver MD, Barger LK, Malone SK, et al. Dose-dependent associations between sleep duration and unsafe behaviors among us high school students. JAMA Pediatr 2018;172(12):1187–9.

16. Chiu HY, Lee HC, Chen PY, et al. Associations between sleep duration and suicidality in adolescents: a systematic review and dose-response meta-analysis. Sleep Med Rev 2018;42:119–26.

17. Matamura M, Tochigi M, Usami S, et al. Associations between sleep habits and mental health status and suicidality in a longitudinal survey of monozygotic twin adolescents. J Sleep Res 2014;23(3):290–4.

18. Goldstein TR, Bridge JA, Brent DA. Sleep disturbance preceding completed suicide in adolescents. J Consult Clin Psychol 2008;76(1):84.

19. Kim SY, Sim S, Choi HG. High stress, lack of sleep, low school performance, and suicide attempts are associated with high energy drink intake in adolescents. PLoS One 2017;12(11):e0187759.

20. Bernert RA, Hom MA, Iwata NG, et al. Objectively assessed sleep variability as an acute warning sign of suicidal ideation in a longitudinal evaluation of young adults at high suicide risk. J Clin Psychiatry 2017;78(6):e678–87.

21. Fitzgerald CT, Messias E, Buysse DJ. Teen sleep and suicidality: results from the youth risk behavior surveys of 2007 and 2009. J Clin Sleep Med 2011;7(4):351–6.

22. Lopes MC, Boronat AC, Wang YP, et al. Sleep complaints as risk factor for suicidal behavior in severely depressed children and adolescents. CNS Neurosci Ther 2016;22(11):915–20.

23. McGlinchey EL, Courtney-Seidler EA, German M, et al. The role of sleep disturbance in suicidal and nonsuicidal self-injurious behavior among adolescents. Suicide Life Threat Behav 2017;47(1):103–11.

24. Tseng WC, Liang YC, Su MH, et al. Sleep apnea may be associated with suicidal ideation in adolescents. Eur Child Adolesc Psychiatry 2019;28(5):635–43.

25. Lee YJ, Cho SJ, Cho IH, et al. Insufficient sleep and suicidality in adolescents. Sleep 2012;35(4):455–60.
26. Andersen IG, Holm JC, Homøe P. Obstructive sleep apnea in obese children and adolescents, treatment methods and outcome of treatment - a systematic review. Int J Pediatr Otorhinolaryngol 2016;87:190–7.
27. Kaditis AG, Alonso Alvarez ML, Boudewyns A, et al. Obstructive sleep disordered breathing in 2- to 18-year-old children: diagnosis and management. Eur Respir J 2016;47(1):69–94.
28. Bishop TM, Ashrafioun L, Pigeon WR. The association between sleep apnea and suicidal thought and behavior: an analysis of national survey data. J Clin Psychiatry 2018;79(1):17m11480.
29. Choi SJ, Joo EY, Lee YJ, et al. Suicidal ideation and insomnia symptoms in subjects with obstructive sleep apnea syndrome. Sleep Med 2015;16(9):1146–50.
30. Kaufmann CN, Susukida R, Depp CA. Sleep apnea, psychopathology, and mental health care. Sleep Health 2017;3(4):244–9.
31. Liu X, Liu Z-Z, Wang Z-Y, et al. Daytime sleepiness predicts future suicidal behavior: a longitudinal study of adolescents. Sleep 2019;42(2):1–10.
32. Nielsen T, Zadra A. Idiopathic nightmares and dream disturbances associated with sleep–wake transitions. In: Kryger MH, Roth T, Dement WC, editors. Principles and practice of sleep medicine. 5th edition. Saunders; 2011. p. 1106–15.
33. Sandman N, Valli K, Kronholm E, et al. Nightmares: prevalence among the Finnish general adult population and war veterans during 1972-2007. Sleep 2013;36(7): 1041–50.
34. Munezawa T, Kaneita Y, Osaki Y, et al. Nightmare and sleep paralysis among Japanese adolescents: a nationwide representative survey. Sleep Med 2011;12(1): 56–64.
35. Simonds JF, Parraga H. Prevalence of sleep disorders and sleep behaviors in children and adolescents. J Am Acad Child Adolesc Psychiatry 1982;21(4): 383–8.
36. Salzarulo P, Chevalier A. Sleep problems in children and their relationship with early disturbances of the waking-sleeping rhythms. Sleep 1983;6(1):47–51.
37. Kaplan SG, Ali SK, Simpson B, et al. Associations between sleep disturbance and suicidal ideation in adolescents admitted to an inpatient psychiatric unit. Int J Adolesc Med Health 2014;26(3):411–6.
38. Liu X, Liu ZZ, Chen RH, et al. Nightmares are associated with future suicide attempt and non-suicidal self-injury in adolescents. J Clin Psychiatry 2019; 80(4):18m12181.
39. Nadorff MR, Nazem S, Fiske A. Insomnia symptoms, nightmares, and suicidal ideation in a college student sample. Sleep 2011;34(1):93–8.
40. Littlewood D, Kyle SD, Pratt D, et al. Examining the role of psychological factors in the relationship between sleep problems and suicide. Clin Psychol Rev 2017; 54:1–16.
41. Fortier-Brochu É, Beaulieu-Bonneau S, Ivers H, et al. Insomnia and daytime cognitive performance: a meta-analysis. Sleep Med Rev 2012;16(1):83–94.
42. Lo JC, Ong JL, Leong RL, et al. Cognitive performance, sleepiness, and mood in partially sleep deprived adolescents: the need for sleep study. Sleep 2016;39(3): 687–98.
43. Miranda R, Gallagher M, Bauchner B, et al. Cognitive inflexibility as a prospective predictor of suicidal ideation among young adults with a suicide attempt history. Depress Anxiety 2012;29(3):180–6.

44. Bridge JA, McBee-Strayer SM, Cannon EA, et al. Impaired decision making in adolescent suicide attempters. J Am Acad Child Adolesc Psychiatry 2012; 51(4):394–403.
45. Keilp JG, Gorlyn M, Russell M, et al. Neuropsychological function and suicidal behavior: attention control, memory and executive dysfunction in suicide attempt. Psychol Med 2013;43(3):539–51.
46. Zlotnick C, Donaldson D, Spirito A, et al. Affect regulation and suicide attempts in adolescent inpatients. J Am Acad Child Adolesc Psychiatry 1997;36(6):793–8.
47. Esposito C, Spirito A, Boergers J, et al. Affective, behavioral, and cognitive functioning in adolescents with multiple suicide attempts. Suicide Life Threat Behav 2003;33(4):389–99.
48. Ward-Ciesielski EF, Winer ES, Drapeau CW, et al. Examining components of emotion regulation in relation to sleep problems and suicide risk. J Affect Disord 2018;241:41–8.
49. Han KS, Kim L, Shim I. Stress and sleep disorder. Exp Neurobiol 2012;21(4): 141–50.
50. Dolsen MR, Cheng P, Arnedt JT, et al. Neurophysiological correlates of suicidal ideation in major depressive disorder: hyperarousal during sleep. J Affect Disord 2017;212:160–6.
51. Perlis ML, Grandner MA, Brown GK, et al. Nocturnal wakefulness as a previously unrecognized risk factor for suicide. J Clin Psychiatry 2016;77(6):e726–33.
52. Mars B, Heron J, Klonsky ED, et al. Predictors of future suicide attempt among adolescents with suicidal thoughts or non-suicidal self-harm: a population-based birth cohort study. Lancet Psychiatry 2019;6(4):327–37.
53. Hochard KD, Heym N, Townsend E. Investigating the interaction between sleep symptoms of arousal and acquired capability in predicting suicidality. Suicide Life Threat Behav 2017;47(3):370–81.
54. Kurina LM, Knutson KL, Hawkley LC, et al. Loneliness is associated with sleep fragmentation in a communal society. Sleep 2011;34(11):1519–26.
55. Zullo L, Horton S, Eaddy M, et al. Adolescent insomnia, suicide risk, and the interpersonal theory of suicide. Psychiatry Res 2017;257:242–8.
56. Chu C, Hom MA, Rogers ML, et al. Is insomnia lonely? exploring thwarted belongingness as an explanatory link between insomnia and suicidal ideation in a sample of South Korean university students. J Clin Sleep Med 2016;12(5):647–52.
57. Chu C, Hom MA, Rogers ML, et al. Insomnia and suicide-related behaviors: a multi-study investigation of thwarted belongingness as a distinct explanatory factor. J Affect Disord 2017;208:153–62.
58. O'Connor RC, Smyth R, Ferguson E, et al. Psychological processes and repeat suicidal behavior: a four-year prospective study. J Consult Clin Psychol 2013; 81(6):1137–43.
59. Littlewood DL, Gooding P, Kyle SD, et al. Understanding the role of sleep in suicide risk: qualitative interview study. BMJ Open 2016;6(8):e012113.
60. Winsler A, Deutsch A, Vorona RD, et al. Sleepless in Fairfax: the difference one more hour of sleep can make for teen hopelessness, suicidal ideation, and substance use. J Youth Adolesc 2015;44(2):362–78.
61. Pillai V, Steenburg LA, Ciesla JA, et al. A seven day actigraphy-based study of rumination and sleep disturbance among young adults with depressive symptoms. J Psychosom Res 2014;77(1):70–5.
62. Takano K, Iijima Y, Tanno Y. Repetitive thought and self-reported sleep disturbance. Behav Ther 2012;43(4):779–89.

63. Weis D, Rothenberg L, Moshe L, et al. The effect of sleep problems on suicidal risk among young adults in the presence of depressive symptoms and cognitive processes. Arch Suicide Res 2015;19(3):321–34.
64. McCall WV, Batson N, Webster M, et al. Nightmares and dysfunctional beliefs about sleep mediate the effect of insomnia symptoms on suicidal ideation. J Clin Sleep Med 2013;9(02):135–40.
65. Owens JA, Dalzell V. Use of the 'BEARS' sleep screening tool in a pediatric residents' continuity clinic: a pilot study. Sleep Med 2005;6(1):63–9.
66. Trockel M, Karlin BE, Taylor CB, et al. Effects of cognitive behavioral therapy for insomnia on suicidal ideation in veterans. Sleep 2015;38(2):259–65.
67. McCall WV, Benca RM, Rosenquist PB, et al. Reducing suicidal ideation through insomnia treatment (REST-IT): a randomized clinical trial. Am J Psychiatry 2019; 176(11):957–65.
68. Gandotra K, Chen P, Jaskiw GE, et al. Effective treatment of insomnia with mirtazapine attenuates concomitant suicidal ideation. J Clin Sleep Med 2018;14(5): 901–2.
69. Manber R, Bernert RA, Suh S, et al. CBT for insomnia in patients with high and low depressive symptom severity: adherence and clinical outcomes. J Clin Sleep Med 2011;7(6):645–52.
70. Trockel M, Manber R, Chang V, et al. An e-mail delivered CBT for sleep-health program for college students: effects on sleep quality and depression symptoms. J Clin Sleep Med 2011;7(3):276–81.
71. Blake MJ, Sheeber LB, Youssef GJ, et al. Systematic review and meta-analysis of adolescent cognitive–behavioral sleep interventions. Clin Child Fam Psychol Rev 2017;20(3):227–49.
72. Germain A, Nielsen T. Impact of imagery rehearsal treatment on distressing dreams, psychological distress, and sleep parameters in nightmare patients. Behav Sleep Med 2003;1(3):140–54.
73. Ellis TE, Rufino KA, Nadorff MR. Treatment of nightmares in psychiatric inpatients with imagery rehearsal therapy: an open trial and case series. Behav Sleep Med 2017;17(2):112–23.
74. Cogan CM, Lee JY, Cranston CC, et al. The impact of exposure, relaxation, and rescripting therapy for post-trauma nightmares on suicidal ideation. J Clin Psychol 2019;75(12):2095–105.
75. McCall WV, Pillai A, Case D, et al. A pilot, randomized clinical trial of bedtime doses of prazosin versus placebo in suicidal posttraumatic stress disorder patients with nightmares. J Clin Psychopharmacol 2018;38(6):618–21.
76. Raskind MA, Peskind ER, Chow B, et al. Trial of prazosin for post-traumatic stress disorder in military veterans. N Engl J Med 2018;378(6):507–17.
77. Krakow B, Sandoval D, Schrader R, et al. Treatment of chronic nightmares in adjudicated adolescent girls in a residential facility. J Adolesc Health 2001; 29(2):94–100.
78. St-Onge M, Mercier P, De Koninck J. Imagery rehearsal therapy for frequent nightmares in children. Behav Sleep Med 2009;7(2):81–98.
79. Gregory AM, Rijsdijk FV, Lau JY, et al. The direction of longitudinal associations between sleep problems and depression symptoms: a study of twins aged 8 and 10 years. Sleep 2009;32(2):189–99.
80. Owens JA, Spirito A, McGuinn M. The Children's Sleep Habits Questionnaire (CSHQ): psychometric properties of a survey instrument for school-aged children. Sleep 2000;23(8):1043–51.

81. Bruni O, Ottaviano S, Guidetti V, et al. The Sleep Disturbance Scale for Children (SDSC) construction and validation of an instrument to evaluate sleep disturbances in childhood and adolescence. J Sleep Res 1996;5(4):251–61.
82. Werner H, Lebourgeois MK, Geiger A, et al. Assessment of chronotype in four- to eleven-year-old children: reliability and validity of the Children's Chronotype Questionnaire (CCTQ). Chronobiol Int 2009;26(5):992–1014.
83. Belicki K. The relationship of nightmare frequency to nightmare suffering with implications for treatment and research. Dreaming 1992;2(3):143–8.
84. Krakow B, Melendrez D, Santana E, et al. Prevalence and timing of sleep disturbance in Cerro Grande Firestorm victims. Sleep 2001;24:A394–5.

Youth Depression in School Settings
Assessment, Interventions, and Prevention

Shashank V. Joshi, MD[a,b,*], Nadia Jassim, BS, MFA[a],
Nithya Mani, MD[b]

KEYWORDS

- Depression in schools • School-based mental health • Suicide prevention
- Well-being promotion • Depression prevention in schools

KEY POINTS

- School settings are where youth spend a significant amount of their waking hours and are ideal places for intervening when a depressive disorder is present.
- Depressive disorders have a high incidence in the school population. This can affect learning, social interactions, and classroom engagement.
- Educators can be the eyes and ears and serve as expert consultants for the clinician, who can in turn be the expert consultant to help educators engage effectively with all students, especially those affected by depression.
- Depressive symptoms usually manifest across home, social, and educational settings, and the range of interventions is often much broader in schools, where staff and school clinicians can help to implement instructional and behavioral strategies.
- Depression prevention programs and interventions that cultivate student and teacher well-being are part of emerging best practices in the school-based literature.

INTRODUCTION

For child and adolescent psychiatrists caring for youth with depressive disorders, educational settings are crucial environments to understand, and where possible, to actively engage.[1–4] Depressive disorders have a high incidence in the school population (about 27% of heterosexual youth and 63% of LGBT youth report feeling sad or

This article originally appeared in *Child and Adolescent Psychiatric Clinics*, Volume 28, Issue 3, July 2019.

Disclosure Statement: The authors report no financial conflicts regarding the content in this article.

[a] School Mental Health Team, Division of Child and Adolescent Psychiatry, Lucile Packard Children's Hospital @ Stanford, Stanford University School of Medicine, 401 Quarry Road, Stanford, CA 94305-5719, USA; [b] Lucile Packard Children's Hospital @ Stanford, Stanford University School of Medicine, 401 Quarry Road, Stanford, CA 94305-5719, USA

* Corresponding author. 401 Quarry Road, Stanford, CA 94305-5719.

E-mail address: svjoshi@stanford.edu

hopeless for at least 2 weeks in a row in 2016).[5] This can affect learning, social interactions, and classroom engagement. Teachers and other school staff can be key partners to help both clinicians and parents comprehend the social, educational, and cultural context where depressive symptoms may be present. Several interventions have been developed to help affected youth gain better access to the school curriculum, despite their depressive symptoms. Furthermore, prevention programs that focus on mental health promotion have shown promise in improving subjective well-being among youth.[3,6] As clinicians strive to understand the ecological and contextual factors in a student's life, careful attention should be paid to the *supporting alliance* among parents, teachers, and clinicians,[3] such that members of each of these groups can be resources for one another to best support youth affected by all mood conditions.[4] The supporting alliance is a concept that is based on the therapeutic alliance in mental health and applies to relationships among trusted adults in a young person's life. As mainstreaming in public schools has become more common, teachers are engaging with an ever-diversifying set of students. Mainstreaming requires that partnerships with parents, therapists, and other important adult figures be enhanced. If these relationships are strong and communication is easy and regular, teacher attrition and burnout can be prevented.[2,3]

Affected students are entitled to several educational interventions through both formal (legal) and informal mechanisms. Unfortunately, youth with depressive disorders are at high risk for school problems, including poor attendance, underachievement, and dropping out. When in the midst of a depressive episode, these students can find it especially hard to pay attention, think clearly, solve problems, recall information, or engage in group learning activities, let alone follow classroom rules.[4,7]

Previous work[8] has highlighted how depressive disorders can cause at least 3 types of problems for youth in school settings: those caused by the core symptoms themselves (eg, difficulty concentrating), those caused by secondary factors (eg, peer issues), and those associated with the treatment itself (eg, medication side effects or missed school with attending appointments). Youth with any mood condition may struggle with learning issues, and educators should strive to be aware of the additional layers of impaired concentration, reduced motivation, and emotional upheavals that mood conditions can create.[4,8]

Table 1 lists common issues seen in the classroom due to core symptoms of mood disorders; **Table 2** lists secondary factors that can contribute to problems in the classroom, and **Table 3** lists problems associated with treatment.[4,8]

Several online, social media, and book resources are available for both adults and peers who care for these youth as well as for the affected youth themselves, and these are listed at the end of this article for further reference (**Box 1**).

ASSESSMENT IN SCHOOL SETTINGS
Assessment

Identifying children at risk and diagnosing depression in the school setting can present unique challenges. For school-aged children, irritability or loss of interest can be the first signs of a depressive disorder. For teens, sad mood, sleep issues, weight changes, and thinking problems may be the predominant presenting symptoms.[9,10] For those who might appear quieter or withdrawn, these symptoms do not typically lead to disruptive behavior, and so these students may be overlooked.[9] Furthermore, students may feel isolated or stigmatized, making it harder for them to ask for help.

Given the difficulty in identifying students who are struggling, routine screening can be an effective and helpful tool.[11] Although there may be concerns about the feasibility

Table 1
Common problems caused by the core symptoms of a depressive disorder

Mood changes	• Extremes in mood (sad, angry, anxious) can be especially difficult to manage in school and can severely disrupt the learning process and experience of affected youth
Loss of interest	• May result in a lack of engagement in school activities • Negative cycle may ensue: not completing work leads to lower grades, which can lead to lower self-worth, loss of motivation, and withdrawal/absenteeism—leading the student to fall behind and feel so overwhelmed they cannot take the first step toward reengagement
Fatigue	• Sadness or sleep difficulties during depressive episodes can lead to fatigue and decreased school engagement
Concentration difficulties	• Especially frustrating for youth who would otherwise excel academically • Inability to focus and think clearly may be due to their depression or to a medication side effect
Agitation or tuning out	• Can be associated with a constant feeling of having to move (pacing, tapping fingers or feet, restless legs) and be disruptive to peers; tuning out can make a student feel as if they are going "in slow motion"

Reprinted with permission from A Clinical Handbook for the Diagnosis and Treatment of Pediatric Onset Mood Disorders, (Copyright ©2019). American Psychiatric Association. All Rights Reserved.

of screening every student, studies using school nurses show general acceptability of this practice.[12,13] A key consideration before screening is ensuring an adequate referral system exists for those found to need further assessment. Many screening tests are available and have been shown effective; ease of use and availability will likely determine widespread utilization (**Table 4**).

Table 2
Problems caused by secondary factors

Peer problems	• Among the most devastating and long lasting to youth in school settings • Associated with social isolation and withdrawal • As peer networks are ever-changing and sometimes fragile, turning down invitations for play dates or hanging out can result in no further invitations from a specific peer • Lost opportunities to play are also lost opportunities to learn and build social skills; affected students may fall further behind socially and be included less often by peer groups • Helping students to make social contacts with healthy and resilient peers with similar interests can help enhance mental health and build community
Other secondary problems	• Social isolation due to depressive disorders has downstream effects, for example, if a student spends the morning worrying about who to play with at recess, they will not be focused on the teacher's lessons • A student might act up just to avoid stressful times of day, for example, being sent to the office or detention may seem easier than facing one's social fears • School staff, parents, and clinicians need to be creative in efforts to understand problems like these in order to address them properly

Reprinted with permission from A Clinical Handbook for the Diagnosis and Treatment of Pediatric Onset Mood Disorders, (Copyright ©2019). American Psychiatric Association. All Rights Reserved.

Table 3
Problems caused by treatment

Medication side effects	• Range from nuisances to significant challenges • Side effects may be embarrassing (eg, falling asleep due to sedative effects) or uncomfortable (feeling thirsty, having dry mouth, or being dizzy and nauseous) • Medication titrations can be associated with headaches or drowsiness, further interfering with schoolwork
Other problems associated with treatment	• Once-daily dosing is ideal, but not always possible • School-administered medications may present challenges (school nurse availability, stigma regarding the need to leave class for medicine, logistical challenges [must obtain an "extra medication bottle" for school]) • Missing school activities for therapy/other appointments can cause a student who is already struggling to have even more problems

Reprinted with permission from A Clinical Handbook for the Diagnosis and Treatment of Pediatric Onset Mood Disorders, (Copyright ©2019). American Psychiatric Association. All Rights Reserved.

Once a student has been identified as having symptoms of depression, assessment by a mental health professional is essential to more fully evaluate and appropriately refer or treat the student. Despite its wide use, unstructured diagnostic interviews do not always correlate to standardized interviews.[21] Therefore, the gold standard for postscreening assessment would be a semistructured interview in conjunction with a broadband scale and caregiver interviews.[19] Although time

Box 1
Resources: useful school mental health web sites

1. Promising Practices Network on Children, Families, and Communities (http://www.promisingpractices.net/programs.asp); features summaries of programs and practices that have shown positive outcomes for children

2. Suicide Prevention Resource Center: Best Practices Registry for Suicide Prevention (http://www.sprc.org/featured_resources/bpr/index.asp)

3. National Center for School Mental Health (http://csmh.umaryland.edu): Up-to-date information about national school mental health training, practice, research, and policy

4. Center for Mental Health in Schools and Student/Learning Supports at University of California, Los Angeles (http://smhp.psych.ucla.edu): Clearinghouse of important mental health, school, and educational materials

5. Individuals With Disabilities Education Act (IDEA) Partnership (http://www.ideapartnership.org): Up-to-date information on changes in the IDEA parameters.

6. HEARD Alliance (Health Care Alliance for Response to Adolescent Depression; https://www.heardalliance.org): A collaborative Web site that features resources for suicide prevention and mental health promotion; features a best practice K-12 Toolkit for Mental Health Promotion and Suicide Prevention

7. National Child Traumatic Stress Network (http://www.nctsn.org): Contains very useful resources for educators to teach students with trauma, loss, and anxiety; also has useful tips for speaking with parents, children, and the media about the consequences of human-caused and natural disasters and resources for preventing burnout in educators

Data from Ref.[53]

Table 4
Screening instruments useful for assessing youth depression symptoms

Instrument	Description	Advantages
Quick Inventory of Depressive Symptoms self-report (QIDS-SR)	16-item scale; self-report	Suitable for use in adolescents; reliable in identifying symptoms of depression[14]
Patient Health Questionnaire (PHQ-9M)	9-item scale; self-report modified for adolescents	Good validity as a screener over the QIDS but may not have the same level or validity in tracking depressive symptoms[15]
Patient Health Questionnaire (PHQ-2)	2-item scale adapted from PHQ-9	Brief. Has sensitivity of 96% and specificity of 82% for detecting those who meet criteria for probable depression on PHQ-9[16]
Center for Epidemiologic Studies–Depression	20-item scale self-report	Widely used, suitable for adolescents; high internal consistency.[17] However, not as effective in studying well-being[18]
(Beck Depression Inventory for Youth)	20-item scale rating scale	High internal consistency; validity and reliability have been established for depression[19]
Kessler-10 and Kessler-6	10-item scale of psychological distress with a 6-item scale embedded	Good precision for assessing psychological distress; can differentiate anxiety from depression[20]

intensive, this is the ideal way to elicit information about the student's symptoms, psychosocial environment, and subjective history. Trauma-informed assessments will ensure that posttraumatic stress disorder symptoms masking as depression will not be missed.[22]

Classroom Interventions

Classroom interventions by mental health professionals are not done individually, but rather should incorporate the school staff and use an already fostered relationship. As consultants, mental health professionals should follow the 3R's of school consultation as outlined by Bostic and Rauch.[23] First, one must pay close attention to the relationships that need to be built. For consultation to be effective, a trusting partnership must be fostered between the larger social system in a student's life, including parents, therapists, and school staff.[3] Second, recognition of the human motivation, specifically the motives and concerns that may hinder promotion of depression awareness in schools, is imperative. In order to make an intervention, it is important for a mental health provider to use their understanding of staff motivation to collaborate and align with multiple professionals who have different but potentially overlapping goals.[24] Last, a consultant should support the staff in generating responses to difficult events or situations. Providing staff with new skills to support and teach affected students, finding common goals to unite students, parents, and staff, and helping to identify a path to achieve these goals are necessary to empower those within the school to feel comfortable with these interventions.[4] In addition, mental health professionals can be an important resource in helping parents advocate for their child to get the school accommodations they need through an appropriate individualized education plan (IEP), 504 Plan, or other classroom interventions. In order to develop this relationship, it is essential to spend individual time with the parents as part of the consultation to address any concerns they may have.[4]

Table 5 highlights the educational implications and classroom strategies for students who struggle with Depressive Disorders.

TREATMENT IN SCHOOL SETTINGS

A systematic review of depression prevention and treatment programs[27] found support for prevention and early intervention programs in schools, most of which are based on cognitive behavioral therapy (CBT). Indicated approaches appear to produce the strongest results, with universal and selective trials also having positive effects. An example of a time-limited individual treatment with strong evidence for use in school populations is interpersonal therapy, adapted for adolescents (IPT-A).[28] In a study that spanned 5 school health clinics in New York City, adolescents treated with IPT-A showed greater symptom reduction and improvement in overall functioning compared with treatment as usual. The core components of IPT-A include 3 phases of treatment delivered over 12 weeks. The adapted-for-teens version differs from adult IPT in that it is shorter (12 weeks vs 16–20 weeks), adds a parent component, and focuses less on the sick role. The treatment manual is clear and concise, and focuses on current interpersonal issues that are most important to adolescents, including grief, interpersonal disputes, role transitions, and interpersonal deficits.

PREVENTION STRATEGIES

Several programs have shown promise as preventative in the development of depression.

Examples of school-based depression prevention programs have been summarized nicely in a review by Calear.[9] The investigator suggests important factors to be considered before implementing a depression prevention program in schools, such as consideration of target audience (universal prevention directed to all students; indicated prevention directed to students with elevated symptoms of depression, or selected prevention directed only at students identified as being at high-risk of developing depression); program scheduling, support and protocols for referrals, and the assurance of full buy-in from school administrative leaders. Specific programs that are aimed at preventing depression and increasing mental health awareness are listed in **Table 6** and include the RAP-Kiwi, MoodGYM, Penn Resiliency Program, IPT-AST, Stress Inoculation Training, Brain Driver Education, and Positive Action programs. Other approaches with growing empirical support focus on mindfulness and resilience. Several scholarly reviews highlight how these programs can be implemented for children, adolescents, and young adults.[37–40]

An example of a best practices universal prevention classroom curriculum is Break Free From Depression (BFFD).[41] The goal of BFFD is to raise student awareness and knowledge about depression and to highlight risk factors working against help-seeking behaviors for the students themselves or others. The material consists of a PowerPoint lecture with interactive student components, a documentary film, and a group-guided facilitation activity regarding depression in youth. The BFFD curriculum includes a detailed facilitator's guide and supplementary materials. There is also a group discussion about stigma and other barriers against getting help, how the teens

Table 5
Educational manifestations of depressive disorders and classroom strategies

Educational Manifestations	Instructional Strategies and Classroom Accommodations
Fluctuations in mood, energy, and motivation that may be seasonal or cyclical	During times of low mood, energy, and motivation, reduce academic workload and demands; adjust accordingly when mood, energy, and motivation increase
Difficulty concentrating or completing assignments	Provide students with books on tape or recorded instructions when concentration is low
Difficulty understanding complex instructions; challenges reading long written passages of text	Break assignments into smaller sections and monitor student progress, checking comprehension periodically
Difficulty with prompt arrival and "readiness to learn" in the early morning due to difficulty sleeping	Accommodate late arrivals by arranging for separate workspace if needed; ensure that IEP or 504 Plan accounts for this, especially relevant during medication changes
Easily frustrated and prone to sadness, embarrassment, or anger	Identify a place where student can go for privacy until they can regain control
Difficulty with social skills, boundaries, and peer relationships	Seat student next to peers whom the student feels would be helpful to their classroom functioning, with changes made as needed
Fluctuations in cognitive and physical abilities and presence of side effects, especially with medication changes	Adjust the homework and in-class work to prevent overload; adjust for need for frequent hydration and bathroom breaks
Impaired planning, organizing, and abstract reasoning	Provide skills training with occupational therapist, school psychologist, or learning specialist to improve these
Prone to heightened sensitivity to perceived criticism and may react emotionally over seemingly small things	Create a plan for self-calming strategies (journaling, listening to music, drawing, walking out of class/running classroom errands at designated intervals)
May experience high levels of anxiety that interfere with their ability to logically assess a situation; difficulty or shame/self-doubt in communicating educational needs	Have a "lead school staff" whom the student knows and trusts the most: a guidance counselor, administrator, teacher, or other staff member who could be honest with the student to assist during times of high distress and be the single point of communication
Marked decreases in interest in school work and activities; especially problematic for group assignments	Group student with peers whom the student feels is helpful to their classroom functioning, with changes made as needed
Fluctuations in cognitive and physical abilities and presence of side effects, especially with medication changes	Adjust the homework and in-class load to prevent the student from becoming overwhelmed; adjust for need for frequent hydration and bathroom breaks

(continued on next page)

Table 5 (continued)	
Grades may drop significantly due to lack of interest, loss of motivation, or excessive absences	Adjust expectations accordingly and meet with student, parent, and guidance counselor regularly to review progress; be flexible and realistic about educational goals (school failures and unmet expectations can exacerbate depressive symptoms)
Prone to "all-or-none" thinking (all bad or all good)	Keep a record of accomplishments to show to student at low points

Data from Refs.[5,25,26]

in the film negotiated and overcame these barriers, and what finally worked for them. Students are encouraged to seek help for themselves or their peers through a discreet and simple form that is given in each session.[42]

Other examples of depression awareness and suicide prevention curricula for high schools include More Than Sad: Teen Depression, More Than Sad: Preventing Teen Suicide (American Foundation for Suicide Prevention, 2010), and Linking Education and Awareness of Depression and Suicide (Suicide Awareness Voices of Education, 2008).

These interventions collectively highlight how clinicians can be helpful not only for diagnosing and treating depressive disorders in the school setting but also for serving as partners or implementers of best practice curricula to promote mental health, well-being, and education about the signs and symptoms of mood conditions to mitigate risk from developing serious depressive disorders. Prior research[42] has led to recommendations against 1-and-done presentations or assemblies that focus on depression or suicide prevention, because they may not be effective in changing knowledge over the long term or help-seeking behavior. Moreover, students (and school staff or parents) ought to have opportunities for questions, reflection, follow-up and support as needed. Thus, all of the curricula described in this section should be delivered over multiple sessions and monitored for effect.

An example of an evidence-supported program to enhance teacher self-efficacy in engaging with high-risk students is the Kognito: At Risk for Educators Program. It features interactive role-play simulations that build awareness, knowledge, and skills about mental health and suicide prevention, preparing educators in K12 settings to recognize and intervene with students in psychological distress, and, if needed, connect them with support services.[43] Because teachers are the most present adults directing the learning environment, it is important to engage with them early and often in order to build a healthy and long-lasting supporting alliance. When children are younger, it may be quite easy for parents/guardians to engage with school staff through volunteering or chaperoning a school field trip, for example. It gets harder to stay engaged as a parent, as youth progress through middle and high school. Parent strategies for engaging with school staff can be found at https://community.understood.org/school-services/f/working-with-teachers.

THE SOCIOCULTURAL MILIEU OF TREATMENTS IN THE SCHOOL SETTING

In schools, culture influences important areas that are central to mental health, such as behavioral expectations and tolerance, language, emotion, attention, attachment,

Table 6 Examples of evidence-supported depression prevention and mental health awareness programs developed for schools	
RAP-Kiwi[29]	Eleven-session manual-based program derived from cognitive-behavioral therapy, delivered by teachers; ages 13–15; depression scores were reduced significantly more by RAP-Kiwi than by placebo and were effective across cultural subgroups, at follow-up, postgroup, and 18 mo
MoodGYM[30]	Interactive, Web-based intervention designed to prevent and decrease depression symptoms; presented by classroom teacher for 1 h weekly over 5 wk, based on CBT; contains information, animated demonstrations, quizzes, and homework exercises; ages 13–17
Penn Resiliency Program[31]	Twelve-session group intervention for students aged 10–14; teaches CBT and problem-solving skills; widely researched and supported by 8 RCTs showing significantly positive results; among the most broadly researched depression prevention programs. Ten school-based trials for ages 10–14 y have been conducted since 2001. Significant effects found in 8 of the trials after follow-up. Delivery by teachers, mental health professionals, and graduate students[24]
Interpersonal Therapy, Adolescent Skills Training (IPT-AST)[32]	Based on IPT; goal is to prevent depression by teaching social and communication skills necessary to develop and maintain positive relationships; 2 individual and 8 group sessions for students 11–16 y old; significant positive results reported at 3- and 6-mo follow-ups in the areas of handling interpersonal role disputes, navigating role transitions, and addressing interpersonal deficits
Stress Inoculation Training[33]	Based on CBT; provides individual and group therapy for 15–18 y olds; 9–13 sessions delivered weekly with a 3-phase stress inoculation model: Conceptualization phase, skill acquisition phase, skill application phase; techniques taught include cognitive restructuring, problem solving, and relaxation. At least 2 universal school-based trials have found significant results
Brain Drivers Education[34,35] (https://www.massgeneral.org/psychiatry/assets/pdfs/school-psych/Brain-Drivers-Education-Operators-Guide.pdf)	Based on CBT; developed by a child and adolescent psychiatrist at the Massachusetts General Hospital School Psychiatry Program at Harvard Program and an educator in the Boston schools; evidence-informed curriculum on emotional self-regulation; uses elements of CBT, DBT, and other widely accepted approaches for achieving well-being and healthy interpersonal relationships. Pilot study showed significant positive results regarding emotion regulation and conflict resolution; most students found the curriculum useful for their everyday lives
Positive Action[36]	An evidence-based educational program that promotes intrinsic learning and cooperation among peers; links positive actions to positive self-perception; adapted for various grade levels; shown to increase academic achievement and reduce problem behaviors. Intervention topics address mental health, physical health, behavior, family, academics, and substance use; designed for teachers to run in as little as 15 min per school day

Abbreviations: CBT, cognitive behavioral therapy; DBT, dialectical behavioral therapy; RCT, randomized controlled trials.

Modified from Calear AL. Depression in the classroom: considerations and strategies. Child Adolesc Psychiatr Clin N Am 2012;21(1):138; with permission.

traumatic experiences, conduct, personality, motivation, limit setting, and other aspects of teaching in general. Cultural context plays an important role not only in structuring the school environment in which youth with emotional and behavioral disorders function but also in the way such children and teens are understood and treated.[44,45]

Teachers play a crucial role in promoting the overall health and academic engagement of their students, in addition to their social and emotional learning and development.

As McCullough and Quinlan[46] have highlighted:

Without a more direct focus on teacher well-being, the proposed strategies for promoting youth happiness may be futile, especially if the adults with whom they interact with most during the school day feel emotionally exhausted and overworked. Accordingly, Hills and Robinson[47] emphasized that "teachers need to be the first to put on their oxygen masks prior to supporting their students' social and emotional wellness" (p. 104).[6]

As parents engage with schools to advocate for accommodations for their children with mood conditions, it is important to know what their rights and resources are. In the United States, the main laws of relevance are the Individuals with Disabilities Education and Improvement IDEA, and section 504 of the Rehabilitation Act of 1973. A useful site that summarizes relevant information is https://www.understood.org/en/school-learning/special-services/504-plan/the-difference-between-ieps-and-504-plans.

FROM PREVENTION TO STATE POLICY AND A NEW LAW

In 2016, California became one of the first states to require that all public school districts serving students in grades 7 to 12 develop a suicide prevention board policy and administrative regulations. A model suicide prevention policy has been developed by the California Department of Education,[48] and a K12 Toolkit for Mental Health Promotion and Suicide Prevention[49] lists evidence-supported suicide prevention programs and social-emotional learning strategies that can begin even earlier than middle school, such as the Good Behavior Game (GBG), Promoting Alternative Thinking Strategies (PATHS),[50] and others that are especially suited for middle and older teens (Sources of Strength).[51] GBG is a classroom game where elementary school children are rewarded for displaying appropriate on-task behaviors during instructional times. It has shown long-term benefits in multiple social and emotional domains by strengthening inhibition, extending self-regulation, and improving social emotional scaffolding, in addition to being associated with significantly decreased suicide risk in later school years by those who participated in this game while in elementary school.[52] PATHS has shown effectiveness in enhancing the educational process and promoting social and emotional competencies in elementary school youth, while also reducing aggression and behavior problems.[4]

Sources of Strength is a universal suicide prevention program that builds protective influences and reduces the likelihood that vulnerable youth will become suicidal. It trains students as peer leaders and connects them with adult advisors at school and in the community. These trusted adults support the peer leaders in conducting well-defined messaging activities that aim to change peer group norms that influence coping practices and problem behaviors (eg, self-harm, drug use, unhealthy sexual practices). The program has benefits for both suicide prevention and well-being promotion. In an 18-school randomized controlled trial (RCT), Wyman and colleagues[51] demonstrated that the program led to changes in norms across the full population of high school students after 4 months of school-wide messaging.

SUMMARY

In this article, evidence-supported programs and approaches that to address depression in schools are highlighted. The process of school stakeholder buy-in and the cultivation of a supporting alliance among school staff, clinician, and parent are essential. A review of assessment tools, intervention strategies, and prevention programs is complemented by approaches that focus on well-being promotion. Virtual role-play software can assist teachers in implementing practical tools for responding to students in need, developing classroom management strategies for those in crisis, and referring them to resources. Programs such as the GBG in elementary schools and Sources of Strength in secondary schools can be used as school-wide positive behavior and suicide prevention programs and may also have important downstream prevention benefits in reducing adolescent risk-taking behaviors more broadly.[4] Finally, the importance of positive student-teacher relationships is emphasized in order to promote healthy school functioning and both student and teacher well-being.[46,47,49]

REFERENCES

1. Results from the 2016 national survey on drug use and health (NSDUH). Available at: https://www.nimh.nih.gov/health/statistics/major-depression.shtml. Accessed February 11, 2019.

2. Suldo SM. Promoting student happiness: positive psychology interventions in schools. New York: Guilford Press; 2016.

3. Feinstein NF, Fielding K, Udvari-Solner A, et al. The supporting alliance in child and adolescent treatment: enhancing collaboration between therapists, parents and teachers. Am J Psychother 2009;63(4):319–44.

4. Joshi SV, Jassim N. School-based interventions for mood disorders. In: Singh MK, editor. A clinical handbook for the diagnosis and treatment of pediatric onset mood disorders. Washington, DC: Amer Psychiatric Press, Inc; 2019.

5. Centers for Disease Control and Prevention. Youth risk behavior survey 2017. Available at: https://www.cdc.gov/healthyyouth/data/yrbs/index.htm. Accessed February 11, 2019.

6. Rettew D, Satz I, Joshi SV. Teaching well-being: from kindergarten to child psychiatry training programs. Child Adolesc Psychiatr Clin N Am 2019;28(2):267–80.

7. Evans DW, Andrews LW. If your adolescent has depression or bipolar disorder-an essential resource for parents. New York: Oxford Univ Press; 2005. p. 198.

8. Fristad M, Goldberg Arnold JS. Raising a moody child: how to cope with depression and bipolar disorder. New York: Guilford Press; 2004. p. 260.

9. Calear AL. Depression in the classroom: considerations and strategies. Child Adolesc Psychiatr Clin N Am 2012;21:135–44.

10. Lewinsohn PM, Rohde P, Seeley JR. Treatment of adolescent depression: frequency of services and impact on functioning in young adulthood. Depress Anxiety 1998;7:47–52.

11. Williams SB, O'Connor EA, Eder M, et al. Screening for child and adolescent depression in primary care settings: a systematic evidence review for the US preventive services task force. Pediatrics 2009;123:e716–35.

12. Carnevale T. An integrative review of adolescent depression screening instruments: applicability for use by school nurses. J Child Adolesc Psychiatr Nurs 2011;24:51–7.

13. Allison VL, Nativio DG, Mitchell AM, et al. Identifying symptoms of depression and anxiety in students in the school setting. J Sch Nurs 2014; 30(3):165–72.

14. Bernstein IH, Rush AJ, Trivedi MH, et al. Psychometric properties of the quick inventory of depressive symptomatology in adolescents. Int J Methods Psychiatr Res 2010;19(4):185–94.

15. Nandakumar AL, Vande Voort JL, Nakonezny PA, et al. Psychometric properties of the patient health questionnaire-9 modified for major depressive disorder in adolescents. J Child Adolesc Psychopharmacol 2019;29(1):34–40.

16. Richardson LP, Rockhill C, Russo JE, et al. Evaluation of the PHQ-2 as a brief screen for detecting major depression among adolescents. Pediatrics 2010; 125:e1097–103.

17. Radloff LS. The use of the center for epidemiologic studies depression scale in adolescents and young adults. J Youth Adolesc 1991;20:149–66.

18. Siddawaya AP, Wood AM, Taylorb PJ. The Center for Epidemiologic Studies-Depression (CES-D) scale measures a continuum from well-being to depression: testing two key predictions of positive clinical psychology. J Affect Disord 2017; 213:180–6.

19. D'Angelo EJ, Augenstein T. Developmentally informed evaluation of depression: evidence-based instruments. Child Adolesc Psychiatr Clin N Am 2012;21: 279–98.

20. Kessler RC, Andrews G, Colpe LJ, et al. Short screening scales to monitor population prevalences and trends in non-specific psychological distress. Psychol Med 2002;32:959–76.

21. Jensen-Doss A. Practice involves more than treatment: how can evidence-based assessment catch up to evidence-based treatment? Clin Psychol Sci Pract 2011; 18:173–7.

22. Craig SE. Reaching and teaching children who hurt. Baltimore (MD): Brookes; 2008.

23. Bostic JQ, Rauch PK. The 3 R's of school consultation. J Am Acad Child Adolesc Psychiatry 1999;38(3):339–41.

24. Waxman RP, Weist MD, Benson DM. Toward collaboration in the growing education–mental health interface. Clin Psychol Rev 1999;19(2):239–53.

25. Chokroverty L. 100 questions and answers about your child's depression or bipolar disorder. Sudbury (MA): Jones and Bartlett; 2010. p. 203.

26. California Department of Education. Placer Co. Office of education and Minnesota association for children's health: a guide to student mental health and wellness in California. St. Paul (MN): Minnesota Association for Children's Health; 2014.

27. Calear AL, Christensen H. Systematic review of school-based prevention and early intervention programs for depression. J Adolesc 2010;33:429–38.

28. Mufson LH, Dorta KP, Olfson M, et al. Effectiveness research: transporting interpersonal psychotherapy for depressed adolescents (IPT-A) from the lab to school-based health clinics. Clin Child Fam Psychol Rev 2004;7(4):251–61.

29. Merry S, McDowell H, Wild CJ, et al. A randomized placebo-controlled trial of a school-based depression prevention program. J Am Acad Child Adolesc Psychiatry 2004;43(5):538–47.

30. Twomey C, O'Reilly G. Effectiveness of a freely available computerized cognitive behavioural therapy programme (MoodGYM) for depression: meta-analysis. Aust N Z J Psychiatry 2016. Available at: https://moodgym.com.au/info/about. Accessed February 11, 2018.

31. Gillham JE, Reivich KJ, Freres DR, et al. School-based prevention of depressive symptoms: a randomized controlled study of the effectiveness and specificity of the Penn Resiliency Program. J Consult Clin Psychol 2007;75:9–19.
32. Young JF, Mufson L, Davies M. Efficacy of interpersonal psychotherapy-adolescent skills training: an indicated preventive intervention for depression. J Child Psychol Psychiatry 2006;47(12):1254–62.
33. Hains AA, Ellmann SW. Stress inoculation training as a preventative intervention for high school youths. J Cogn Psychother 1994;8(3):219–28, 230–232.
34. Khan CK, Patterson AD, Joshi SV. Brain driver education: teaching kids emotion regulation skills through an innovative and integrative curriculum; presented at annual meeting of the Amer Acad of Child Adolesc Psychiatry. San Diego, October 20–25, 2014.
35. Blumenfeld K, Bostic JQ, Potter MP, et al. Massachusetts General Hospital. Brain Drivers Education. 2005. Available at: https://www.massgeneral.org/psychiatry/assets/pdfs/school-psych/Brain-Drivers-Education-Operators-Guide.pdf. Accessed February 11, 2019.
36. Lewis KM, DuBois DL, Bavarian N, et al. Effects of positive action on the emotional health of urban youth: a cluster-randomized trial. J Adolesc Health 2013;53:706–11. Available at: https://www.positiveaction.net/research-outcomes. Accessed February 11, 2019.
37. Chi X, Bo A, Liu T, et al. Effects of mindfulness-based stress reduction on depression in adolescents and young adults: a systematic review and meta-analysis. Front Psychol 2018;9:1034.
38. Dray J, Bowman J, Wolfenden L, et al. Systematic review of universal resilience interventions targeting child and adolescent mental health in the school setting. Syst Rev 2015;4:186.
39. Zoogman S, Goldberg SB, Hoyt WT, et al. Mindfulness interventions with youth: a meta-analysis. Mindfulness (N Y) 2015;6:290–302.
40. Dunning DL, Griffiths K, Kuyken W, et al. The effects of mindfulness-based interventions on cognition and mental health in children and adolescents: a meta-analysis of randomised controlled trials. J Child Psychol Psychiatry 2019;60(3):244–58.
41. Boston Children's Hospital neighborhood partnerships program: break free from depression curriculum, revised. 2017. Available at: https://www.openpediatrics.org/course/break-free-depression. Accessed February 11, 2019.
42. Joshi SV, Hartley SN, Kessler M, et al. School-based suicide prevention: content, process, and the role of trusted adults and peers. Child Adolesc Psychiatr Clin N Am 2015;24(2):353–70.
43. Long MW, Albright G, McMillan J, et al. Enhancing educator engagement in school mental healthcare through digital simulation professional development. J Sch Health 2018;88:651–9.
44. Malik M, Lake J, Lawson W, et al. Culturally adapted pharmacotherapy and the integrative formulation. Child Adolesc Psychiatr Clin N Am 2010;19(4):791–814.
45. Lin K-M, Smith MW, Ortiz V. Culture and psychopharmacology. Psychiatr Clin North Am 2001;24(3):523–38.
46. McCullough M, Quinlan D. Universal strategies for promoting student happiness. In: Suldo SM, editor. Promoting student happiness: positive psychology interventions in schools. New York: Guilford Press; 2016. p. 103–21.
47. Hills KJ, Robinson A. Enhancing teacher well-being: put on your oxygen masks! Communique 2010;39:1–17.

48. California Department of Education. Model youth suicide prevention policy. 2017. Available at: https://www.cde.ca.gov/ls/cg/mh/suicideprevres.asp. Accessed September 22, 2018.
49. Joshi SV, Lenoir L, Ojakian M, et al. K-12 mental health promotion and suicide prevention Toolkit 2017. p. 300. Available at: http://www.heardalliance.org/help-toolkit/. Accessed February 11, 2019.
50. Promoting alternative thinking strategies (PATHS):information on classroom applications. Available at: http://www.pathstraining.com/main/curriculum/. Accessed July 2, 2018.
51. Wyman PA, Brown CH, LoMurray M, et al. An outcome evaluation of the Sources of Strength suicide prevention program delivered by adolescent peer leaders in high schools. Am J Public Health 2010;100(9):1653.
52. PAX Good Behavior Game: information on scientific basis. Available at: https://www.goodbehaviorgame.org/pax-science. Accessed July 2, 2018.
53. Bostic JQ, Hoover SA. School consultation. In: Martin A, Bloch MH, Volkmar F, editors. Lewis's child & adolescent psychiatry: a comprehensive textbook. 5th edition. Philadelphia: LWW; 2018. p. 956–74.

Depression in Justice-involved Youth

Sarah Mallard Wakefield, MD[a],*, Regina Baronia, MD[b],
Stephanie Brennan, MD[c]

KEYWORDS

- Juvenile justice • Justice-involved youth • Depression • Treatment

KEY POINTS

- Justice-involved youth experience high rates of child maltreatment and involvement in the child welfare system.
- Justice-involved youth experience high rates of mental disorder, including major depression.
- Successful treatment of justice-involved youth requires early screening and referral for evidence-based services.
- Multisystemic therapy and cognitive behavior therapies, among others, offer effective strategies for decreasing mental disorder along with recidivism for justice-involved youth.
- Juvenile mental health courts provide oversight for screening, referral, and consistency in care.

INTRODUCTION

In 2017, law enforcement nationwide made 809,700 arrests of persons younger than 18 years.[1] According to the National Center for Juvenile Justice Juvenile Court Statistics, in 2016, 79% of justice-involved youth were 10 to 15 years of age.[2] Exceedingly high rates of mental health diagnoses are consistently found when justice-involved youth are surveyed worldwide,[3–9] with up to 100% of youth reporting criteria consistent with at least 1 mental health diagnosis.[8] Multiple mental health diagnoses are common for justice-involved youth. Drerup and colleagues[10] identified criteria for 1 mental health diagnosis in 92% of boys and 97% of girls. Thirty-four percent of boys and 60% of girls met criteria for 3 or more mental health diagnoses.

This article originally appeared in *Child and Adolescent Psychiatric Clinics*, Volume 28, Issue 3, July 2019.
Disclosures: None.
a Department of Psychiatry, School of Medicine, Texas Tech University Health Sciences Center, 3601 4th Street, STOP 8103, Lubbock, TX 79430, USA; b Department of Psychiatry, Texas Tech University Health Sciences Center, 3601 4th Street, STOP 8103, Lubbock, TX 79430, USA; c Department of Pediatrics, Texas Tech University Health Sciences Center, 3601 4th Street, STOP 9406, Lubbock, TX 79430, USA
* Corresponding author.
E-mail address: sarah.wakefield@ttuhsc.edu

In the National Comorbidity Survey Adolescent Supplement, 10,123 youth aged 13 to 17 years were studied from 2001 to 2004.[11] Youth with any psychiatric disorder were more likely to commit a crime, including violent crime, than youth without a psychiatric diagnosis.[11] Additional studies have also shown that a mental health diagnosis increased the likelihood of juvenile justice involvement, especially in the absence of an effective caregiver,[12] and that a lifetime diagnosis of depression is predictive of future juvenile justice involvement.[13]

The rate of diagnoses seems to increase with increasing involvement in the juvenile justice system.[14] Youth processed in adult courts have higher prevalence of psychiatric disorders than incarcerated adults.[15] Mental health diagnosis has been correlated with an 80% increased rate of recidivism compared with individuals without a mental health diagnosis,[12] and, for justice-involved youth, symptoms of mental illness have been found to persist into adulthood.[16]

It may make sense that justice-involved youth have higher rates of mental health diagnoses when considering diagnoses of conduct disorder and oppositional defiant disorder. However, justice-involved youth also have a higher prevalence of depression than what is expected in the general population. A study of 350 youth involved in family court, juvenile detention, residential facilities, and juvenile court found that 49.4% of youth met criteria for depressive disorder.[17] These symptoms are common in justice-involved youth and are typically present on first arrest. Burke and colleagues[3] found that 74% of first-time juvenile offenders met criteria for a mental health disorder, and female youth in the justice system have higher rates of depression than justice-involved youth boys.[6,18,19] Thoughts of suicide and suicidal behaviors are common in justice-involved youth and increase with greater contact with the justice system. Stokes and colleagues[20] identified a history of depression, sexual abuse, and other trauma as the most common predictors of suicidal thoughts and behaviors in justice-involved youth.

CAUSES OF DEPRESSION IN JUSTICE-INVOLVED YOUTH

It is more the rule than the exception that justice-involved youth are also youth involved in the child welfare system. For all youth who came before the juvenile court in Washington's King County, 67% had prior contact with the child welfare system. The percentage increased to 89% for youth with 3 or more contacts with the juvenile court.[21] In Los Angeles County, the number who had at least 1 referral to the child welfare system for maltreatment increased to 83%. Seventy percent of these youth were referred to the child welfare system before age 10 years, and 43% before age 5 years.[22] Youth who come in contact with the justice system have had 5 child welfare referrals on average.[22,23]

Justice-involved youth have astoundingly high rates of abuse history compared with the general population.[3,24–26] More than 67% of boys and more than 75% of girls report physical abuse, and more than 10% of boys and 40% of girls report sexual abuse.[24] Justice-involved youth with histories of trauma experience an average of 5 distinct traumas, most of which are experienced in the first 5 years of life.[25]

A history of abuse in justice-involved youth has been associated with nearly every type of psychiatric disorder.[24] Justice-involved youth who have experienced trauma present with both internalizing and externalizing symptoms,[25] and maltreatment has proved a strong direct correlate with depression for this population.[27] In a study of 350 youth involved in family court, juvenile detention, residential facilities, and juvenile court, 94% reported a history of 1 or more traumas, and 45.7% of the overall population met criteria for posttraumatic stress disorder (PTSD).[17] The average number of traumas reported by these youth was 5.4, which correlated with an 8-fold increase in PTSD diagnosis, a 7-fold increase in a depressive disorder diagnosis, and a 6-fold increase in history of substance abuse compared with those youth with history of only 1 traumatic event.

Justice-involved female youth seem to have a higher rate of major depressive disorder over time compared with boys,[28] although similar rates of trauma exposure exist between girls and boys. Girls report significantly higher rates of sexual abuse,[25] up to 6 times the sexual abuse and severe physical abuse rates reported by boys.[24] Female youth also report higher rates of posttraumatic symptoms compared with boys.[6,18,19] For girls, sexual abuse is associated with every psychiatric diagnosis[24] but is particularly associated with PTSD, depressive disorders, increased likelihood of suicidal behaviors, running away, and substance abuse.[29] Surveys of 186 juvenile justice–involved girls indicated that a history of physical and emotional abuse also predicted depressive symptoms.[30]

For boys, maltreatment has been associated with every psychiatric diagnosis except anxiety disorders.[24] Jencks and Leibowitz[31] studied predictors of depression in male youth charged with a sexual offense and found that depressed affect was most strongly predicted by history of emotional abuse and exposure to multiple traumas. Traumatic brain injury (TBI) is more common in youth involved in the juvenile justice system than in youth in the general population, but justice-involved male youth are more likely to report a history of TBI than girls involved in the juvenile justice system.[16] A history of trauma predicts future symptoms of mental illness for black, white, and Hispanic justice-involved youth.[32] There are no significant differences in rates of depression based on ethnicity.[19]

Despite their traumatized past, only about 20% of justice-involved youth accessed mental health services over a 3-year period. A diagnosis of oppositional defiant disorder was most likely to precipitate contact with mental health services. Justice-involved youth meeting criteria for depression, anxiety disorders, and attention-deficit/hyperactivity disorder were less likely to have accessed mental health services.[3] Eighty-five percent of justice-involved youth reported at least 1 barrier to accessing mental health services. Most frequent barriers included the belief that the problem would resolve on its own, uncertainty of where to find help, difficulty in accessing help, fear of others' perceptions, and cost.[33] Brady and colleagues[34] (2014) outlined "structurally embedded stressors" in school, community, and home environments, in addition to inadequate resources, as a cause for systems to focus on child behavior rather than on depressive symptoms. This approach may lead to the impulse to punish rather than treat children who present with externalizing symptoms.

Family and social modeling may also mitigate or exacerbate depressive symptoms for justice-involved youth. Family support has been shown to reduce reports of depressive symptoms.[30] Even nonparent family members, especially siblings and extended family, are important emotional supports for teens.[35] Children receiving mental health services in the community are more likely to become justice-involved if their living situations are disrupted.[36] As the number of living transitions increase, they have more significant justice involvement. Delinquency in adolescents with depression has also been associated with affiliation with other justice-involved youth and lack of prosocial involvement.[37]

ASSESSMENT AND INTERVENTION

Justice-involved youth have high rates of mental illness symptoms. Most symptoms are present on first arrest, and symptoms likely contribute to the behaviors that led to arrest. Effective care for these youth lies in an overall system of early identification, accurate assessment, and evidence-based intervention. This system has been corre-lated with reduced symptom burden as well as reduced recidivism.[38]

On the continuum of prevention and treatment strategies, the first step is to prevent youth from becoming involved in the justice system. Schools and primary care clini-cians are on the front lines for these children where they can screen for trauma early and often. When a youth is referred for assessment within the special education sys-tem, to their primary care clinician, or for a mental health evaluation, better interven-tions are needed than just recognizing externalizing symptoms. Clinicians must work to peel back the layers with effective screening and evaluation to expose the true cause of the youth's behaviors.

Children living in communities with high rates of "structurally embedded stressors"[34] should be targets of prevention programs. Although many exist, there are 2 specific community-based programs, 1 targeting female youth and 1 targeting boys, and these have been correlated with improvement in symptoms of children with high-risk behaviors. The Girls Advocacy Project (GAP) is a 6-month strengths-based program set in the female youth's natural community environment.[39] GAP was found to be significantly associated with greater resilience, and decreased engagement in violence, crime, and substance abuse. In addition, GAP was associ-ated with decreased depression, anxiety, and anger symptoms. The Stop Now and Plan (SNAP) program is an education and skill-building intervention for boys 6 to 11 years of age with antisocial behaviors.[40] SNAP showed reduction in aggression, externalizing behaviors, depression, and number of other future criminal charges.

Dembo and colleagues[41] studied health risk behavior among 777 newly justice-involved youth, both male and female, and suggested that grouping newly incarcer-ated youth based on lower, higher, and highest health risk would allow for best use of limited resources. Dembo and colleagues[41] found high rates of depression among newly arrested youth, consistent with current literature, and cited a "critical need" for "front end, juvenile justice intake facilities to provide behavioral and public health screening, with treatment follow up on newly arrested youth." History of trauma expo-sure, abuse, and polyvictimization are all linked to higher rates of behavioral and mental health symptoms[42] and should be included in early screening efforts at first contact with the justice system. Youth should also be screened for a history of TBI,[16] gang involvement,[43] substance abuse, and mental health symptoms. The Mas-sachusetts Youth Screening Instrument-Second Version (MAYSI-2) seems to be a useful screening tool for justice-involved youth.[6] The MAYSI-2 is a brief screening tool that can be administered by law enforcement officials without professional training to assess immediate mental health needs of children 12 to 17 years of age.[44] The MAYSI-2 screens for current suicidal ideation, substance abuse, as well as symptoms that may correlate with a mental health diagnosis and warrant referral for more comprehensive mental health assessment and treatment.

Once identified, linking justice-involved youth with mental health services has shown improvement in overall mental health symptoms, including decreased depres-sive, anxiety, and psychotic symptoms, and improved family function, school function, and frequency of dangerous behaviors toward others.[45] Recidivism decreased from 72% to 29% when services were received for longer than just 1 month.

Several interventions have shown efficacy in studies targeting justice-involved youth. Multisystemic therapy (MST) has decades of research supporting use in youth and families at high risk of justice involvement and as an alternative to incarceration for those who have already made contact.[46] MST is a family and community-based inter-vention through which the youth and family unit receive therapeutic interventions and social supports in their immediate communities.[47] When held to the standard of the original model, MST has shown efficacy in reducing recidivism at a cost saving to the system at large.[48] Sheidow and colleagues[49] adapted MST for "emerging adults" (MST-EA) with serious mental illness and justice system involvement and published a pilot study of 57 subjects who met this description. MST-EA was correlated with improvement in mental health symptoms and decrease in recidivism at discharge.

Other interventions with diagnosis-specific indications, such as cognitive behavior therapy (CBT), would be expected to decrease symptoms in justice-involved youth with that diagnosis. CBT is also correlated with lower recidivism rates for justice-involved youth when delivered in either the community or residential setting.[50–57] A meta-analysis suggested that CBT, even when delivered in a group setting, is correlated with a reduction in depressive symptoms in justice-involved youth.[58] Aggression replacement therapy (ART) is a 10-week CBT program that is listed as an effective program by the Office of Juvenile Justice and Delinquency Prevention.[59] ART has shown both reduced recidivism and cost savings when delivered competently to justice-involved youth.[60] Dialectical behavioral therapy (DBT) uses a CBT framework and focuses on improving self-regulating skills to deal with difficult situations.[61] When delivered in a comprehensive system-wide fashion, DBT is associated with large cost savings compared with youth detention.[62] Olafson and colleagues[63] found significant reduction in posttraumatic stress, depression, and anger symptoms following trauma-focused group treatment in juvenile justice residential facilities using the Trauma and Grief Component Therapy for Adolescents and Think Trauma intervention training for all staff at the residential facility.

Multidimensional treatment foster care (MTFC) is an intensive therapeutic intervention used instead of and to reduce placement in residential treatment centers.[64] Youth are placed in foster care with highly trained foster parents who deliver a consistent therapeutic environment of positive reinforcement; appropriate supervision; and clear, consistent, nonviolent limit setting. MTFC is correlated with reduction in delinquent behaviors in addition to reduction in depressive symptoms and suicidal thoughts compared with youth in congregate care.[65,66] MTFC seems to have the most dramatic effect for youth with the highest severity of depressive symptoms,[66] with benefits lasting into adulthood.[65]

Juvenile mental health courts (JMHCs) are an increasingly popular method for linking justice-involved youth with mental health services. JMHC is a regularly scheduled special docket, typically with a less formal interaction style, and age-appropriate screening and assessment for mental health needs.[67] Youth are involved in JMHCs for 1 year on average. The first JMHC was established in 1998 in Pennsylvania and courts continue to increase in number around the country. At the time of this publication, at least 41 such courts are in existence in 15 states. JMHCs vary in design. About half of the current courts allow all youth with a diagnosed mental health disorder to participate, and most include youth with both misdemeanor and felony charges. JMHCs assess youth for mental health needs and facilitate access to mental health services through a closely supervised probation program including individual outpatient treatment, family therapy, and case management.[68] Despite varying design, most current JMHCs share some characteristics, including team-based approach to case review, specialized probation officers trained in mental health, system-wide accountability, graduated incentives, and sanctions.[67]

SUMMARY

The relationship of juvenile justice involvement and mental health diagnosis is complex. It is clear that justice-involved youth are at exceedingly high risk of trauma exposure; multisystem involvement; and mental health distress, including depression.[17] Justice-involved youth carry with them both a high symptom burden and a high cost to society.[10] Both could be reduced through evidence-based prevention, screening, and treatment strategies. Prevention strategies should be targeted toward communities and families with high risk of justice involvement. Screening for trauma and mental health symptoms should be part of typical school practice and primary care visits with subsequent access to community health and mental health services.[11] Routine mental health screening and assessment of adolescents entering juvenile justice should be universal.[10] Great care should be taken to support families of justice-involved youth through family-focused programs within the youth's community when safe. Youth in residential facilities should have access to family support,[35] and families should engage in training modules focused on promoting successful youth reentry. Disruptions in treatment programs, clinical care providers, and effective medication should be limited as much as possible as youth move through the juvenile justice system. JMHCs can be an effective mechanism for advocacy, increasing access to care and improving family involvement in care.

Effective treatment of mental disorders may reduce future justice involvement, whereas lack of treatment increases the likelihood of justice involvement into adulthood.[69] Multiple effective programs exist to improve the lives of justice-involved youth and subsequently decrease the cost to society of detaining and adjudicating these youth within the juvenile justice system. These youth, who carry such a high burden of adverse childhood experiences, benefit from and deserve clinical thoughtfulness, attention, and effective care.

REFERENCES

1. Office of juvenile justice and delinquency prevention statistical briefing book. Available at: https://www.ojjdp.gov/ojstatbb/crime/qa05101.asp?qaDate=2017. Accessed January 20, 2019.

2. Hockenberry S, Puzzanchera C. Juvenile court statistics 2016. Pittsburgh (PA): National Center for Juvenile Justice; 2018.

3. Burke JD, Mulvey EP, Schubert CA. Prevalence of mental health problems and service use among first-time juvenile offenders. J Child Fam Stud 2015;24(12): 3774–81.

4. Ghazali SR, Chen YY, Aziz HA. Childhood maltreatment and symptoms of PTSD and depression among delinquent adolescents in Malaysia. J Child Adolesc Trauma 2018;11(2):151–8.

5. Poyraz Fındık OT, Rodopman Arman A, Erturk Altınel N, et al. Psychiatric evaluation of juvenile delinquents under probation in the context of recidivism. Psychiatr Clin Psychopharmacology 2018. https://doi.org/10.1080/24750573.2018. 1505282.

6. Van Damme L, Grisso T, Vermeiren R, et al. Massachusetts Youth Screening Instrument for mental health needs of youths in residential welfare/justice institutions: identifying gender differences across countries and settings. J Forensic Psychiatr Psychol 2016;27(5):645–64.

7. Lemos I, Faísca L. Psychosocial adversity, delinquent pathway and internalizing psychopathology in juvenile male offenders. Int J Law Psychiatry 2015;42-43: 49–57.

8. Gretton HM, Clift RJW. The mental health needs of incarcerated youth in British Columbia, Canada. Int J Law Psychiatry 2011;34(2):109–15.

9. Maniadaki K, Kakouros E. Social and mental health profiles of young male offenders in detention in Greece. Crim Behav Ment Health 2008;18(4):207–15. Cited 17 times.

10. Drerup LC, Croysdale A, Hoffmann NG. Patterns of behavioral health conditions among adolescents in a juvenile justice system. Prof Psychol Res Pract 2008; 39(2):122–8. Cited 19 times.

11. Coker KL, Smith PH, Westphal A, et al. Crime and psychiatric disorders among youth in the US population: an analysis of the national comorbidity survey-adolescent supplement. J Am Acad Child Adolesc Psychiatry 2014; 53(8):888–98.

12. Yampolskaya S, Chuang E. Effects of mental health disorders on the risk of juvenile justice system involvement and recidivism among children placed in out-of-home care. Am J Orthopsychiatry 2012;82(4):585–93.

13. Mallet CA, Dare PS, Seck MM. Predicting juvenile delinquency: the nexus of childhood maltreatment, depression and bipolar disorder. Crim Behav Ment Health 2009;19(4):235–46.

14. Kinner SA, Degenhardt L, Coffey C, et al. Complex health needs in the youth justice system: a survey of community-based and custodial offenders. J Adolesc Health 2014;54(5):521–6.

15. Washburn JJ, Teplin LA, Voss LS, et al. Psychiatric disorders among detained youths: a comparison of youths processed in juvenile court and adult criminal court. Psychiatr Serv 2008;59(9):965–73.

16. Vaughn MG, Salas-Wright CP, Delisi M, et al. Prevalence and correlates of psychiatric disorders among former juvenile detainees in the United States. Compr Psychiatry 2015;59:107–16.

17. Rosenberg HJ, Vance JE, Rosenberg SD, et al. Trauma exposure, psychiatric disorders, and resiliency in juvenile-justice-involved youth. Psychol Trauma 2014; 6(4):430–7.

18. Conrad SM, Queenan R, Brown LK, et al. Psychiatric symptoms, substance use, trauma, and sexual risk: a brief report of gender differences in marijuana-using juvenile offenders. J Child Adolesc Subst Abuse 2017;26(6):433–6.

19. Vincent GM, Grisso T, Terry A, et al. Sex and race differences in mental health symptoms in juvenile justice: the MAYSI-2 national meta-analysis. J Am Acad Child Adolesc Psychiatry 2008;47(3):282–90.

20. Stokes ML, McCoy KP, Abram KM, et al. Suicidal ideation and behavior in youth in the juvenile justice system: a review of the literature. J Correct Health Care 2015; 21(3):222–42.

21. Halemba G, Siegel G. Doorways to delinquency: multi-system involvement of delinquent youth in King County (Seattle, WA). Pittsburgh (PA): National Center for Juvenile Justice; 2011.

22. McCroskey J, Herz D, Putnam-Hornstein E. Crossover youth: Los Angeles county probation youth with previous referrals to child protective services. Children's data network. Available at: http://foster-ed.org/crossover-youth-los-angeles-county-probation-youth-with-previous-referrals-to-child-protective-services/. Accessed January 30, 2019.

23. Hobbs AM, Peterson J. Youth re-entering Lancaster County after commitment to a state youth rehabilitation center. Omaha (NE): Juvenile Justice Institute University of Nebraska at Omaha; 2012. Available at: https://www.unomaha.edu/college-of-public-affairs-and-community-service/juvenile-justice-institute/reports-and-publications/index.php. Accessed January 30, 2019.

24. King DC, Abram KM, Romero EG, et al. Childhood maltreatment and psychiatric disorders among detained youths. Psychiatr Serv 2011;62(12):1430–8.
25. Dierkhising CB, Ko SJ, Woods-Jaeger B, et al. Trauma histories among justice-involved youth: findings from the national child traumatic stress network. Eur J Psychotraumatol 2013;4(1):20274.
26. Abram KM, Washburn JJ, Teplin LA, et al. Posttraumatic stress disorder and psychiatric comorbidity among detained youths. Psychiatr Serv 2007;58(10):1311–6.
27. Wanklyn SG, Day DM, Hart TA, et al. Cumulative childhood maltreatment and depression among incarcerated youth: impulsivity and hopelessness as potential intervening variables. Child Maltreat 2012;17(4):306–17.
28. Teplin LA, Welty LJ, Abram KM, et al. Prevalence and persistence of psychiatric disorders in youth after detention: a prospective longitudinal study. Arch Gen Psychiatry 2012;69(10):1031–43.
29. Tossone K, Wheeler M, Butcher F, et al. The role of sexual abuse in trauma symptoms, delinquent and suicidal behaviors, and criminal justice outcomes among females in a juvenile justice diversion program. Violence Against Women 2018; 24(8):973–93.
30. Goodkind S, Ruffolo MC, Bybee D, et al. Coping as a mediator of the effects of stressors and supports on depression among girls in juvenile justice. Youth Violence Juv Justice 2009;7(2):100–18.
31. Jencks JW, Leibowitz GS. The impact of types and extent of trauma on depressive affect among male juvenile sexual offenders. Int J Offender Ther Comp Criminol 2018;62(5):1143–63.
32. Caldwell-Gunes RM, Romero VI, Silver NC. The relationship between trauma and mental health issues among African American, white, and Hispanic male juvenile offenders. Am J Forensic Psychol 2015;33(2):21–38.
33. Abram KM, Paskar LD, Washburn JJ, et al. Perceived barriers to mental health services among youths in detention. J Am Acad Child Adolesc Psychiatry 2008;47(3):301–8.
34. Brady SS, Winston W, Gockley SE. Stress-related externalizing behavior among African American youth: How could policy and practice transform risk into resilience? J Soc Issues 2014;70(2):315–41.
35. Johnson JE, Esposito-Smythers C, Miranda R, et al. Gender, social support, and depression in criminal justice-involved adolescents. Int J Offender Ther Comp Criminol 2011;55(7):1096–109. Cited 15 times.
36. Graves KN, Frabutt JM, Shelton TL. Factors associated with mental health and juvenile justice involvement among children with severe emotional disturbance. Youth Violence and Juvenile Justice 2007;5(2):147–67. Cited 20 times.
37. Mellin EA, Fang H-N. Exploration of the pathways to delinquency for female adolescents with depression: implications for cross-systems collaboration and counseling. J Addict Offender Couns 2010;30(2):58–72. Cited 1 time.
38. Underwood LA, Washington A. Mental illness and juvenile offenders. Int J Environ Res Public Health 2016;13(2):1–14.
39. Javdani S, Allen NE. An ecological model for intervention for juvenile justice-involved girls: development and preliminary prospective evaluation. Fem Criminol 2016;11(2):135–62.
40. Burke JD, Loeber R. The effectiveness of the stop now and plan (snap) program for boys at risk for violence and delinquency. Prev Sci 2014;16(2):242–53.
41. Dembo R, Faber J, Cristiano J, et al. Health risk behavior among justice involved male and female youth: exploratory, multi-group latent class analysis. Subst Use Misuse 2017;52(13):1751–64.

42. Ford JD, Grasso DJ, Hawke J, et al. Poly-victimization among juvenile justice-involved youths. Child Abuse Negl 2013;37(10):788–800.

43. King KM, Voisin DR, Diclemente RJ. The relationship between male gang involvement and psychosocial risks for their female juvenile justice partners with non-gang involvement histories. J Child Fam Stud 2015;24(9):2555–9.

44. MAYSI 2. In National youth screening and assessment partners. Available at: http://www.nysap.us/MAYSI2.html. Accessed January 30, 2019.

45. Lyons JS, Griffin G, Quintenz S, et al. Clinical and forensic outcomes from the Illinois mental health juvenile justice initiative. Psychiatr Serv 2003;54(12):1629–34.

46. Henggeler SW, Melton GB, Smith LA. Family preservation using multisystemic therapy: an effective alternative to incarcerating serious juvenile offenders. J Consult Clin Psychol 1992;60(6):953–61.

47. Henggeler SW. Multisystemic therapy: an overview of clinical procedures, outcomes, and policy implications. Child Psychol Psychiatr Rev 1999;4(1):2–10.

48. Henggeler SW, Melton GB, Brondino MJ, et al. Multisystemic therapy with violent and chronic juvenile offenders and their families: the role of treatment fidelity in successful dissemination. J Consult Clin Psychol 1997;65(5):821–33.

49. Sheidow AJ, McCart MR, Davis M. Multisystemic therapy for emerging adults with serious mental illness and justice involvement. Cogn Behav Pract 2016;23(3): 356–67.

50. Andrews DA, Zinger I, Hoge RD, et al. Does correctional treatment work?: a clinically relevant and psychologically informed meta-analysis. Criminology 1990; 28(3):369–404.

51. Izzo RL, Ross RR. Meta-analysis of rehabilitation programs for juvenile delinquents: a brief report. Crim Justice Behav 1990;17(1):134–42.

52. Lipsey MW. Juvenile delinquency treatment: a meta-analysis inquiry into the variability of effects. In: Cook TD, Cooper H, Cordray DS, et al, editors. Meta-analysis for explanation: a casebook. New York: Russell Sage; 1992. p. 83–127.

53. Lipsey MW, Chapman G, Landenberger NA. Cognitive-behavioral programs for offenders. Ann Am Acad Polit Soc Sci 2001;578:144–57.

54. Lipsey MW, Landenberger NA. Cognitive-behavioral interventions. In: Welsh BC, Farrington DP, editors. Preventing crime: what works for children, offenders, victims and places. New York: Springer; 2006. p. 57–71.

55. Lipsey MW, Landenberger NA, Wilson SJ. Effects of cognitive-behavioral programs for criminal offenders. Nashville (TN): Center for Evaluation Research and Methodology, Vanderbilt Institute for Public Policy Studies; 2007.

56. Pearson FS, Lipton DS, Cleland CM, et al. The effects of behavioral/cognitive-behavioral programs on recidivism. Crime Delinquen 2002;48(3):476–96.

57. Wilson DB, Bouffard LA, Mackenzie DL. A quantitative review of structured, group-oriented, cognitive-behavioral programs for offenders. J Crim Justice Behav 2005;32(2):172–204.

58. Townsend E, Walker D-M, Sargeant S, et al. Systematic review and meta-analysis of interventions relevant for young offenders with mood disorders, anxiety disorders, or self-harm. J Adolesc 2010;33(1):9–20.

59. Office of Juvenile Justice and Delinquency Prevention Model Programs Guide. Available at: https://www.ojjdp.gov/mpg/Topic/Details/79. Accessed January 30, 2019.

60. Barnoski R. Outcome evaluation of Washington State's research-based programs for juvenile offenders. Olympia (WA): Washington State Institute for Public Policy; 2004.

61. Whitbeck B. A review of research and literature addressing evidence-based and promising practices for gang-affiliated and violent youth in juvenile institutions and detention centers. JRA literature review. 2010. Report 2.23. Available at: https://www.altsa.dshs.wa.gov/sites/default/files/SESA/rda/documents/research-2-23.pdf. Accessed January 30, 2019.
62. Aos S, Lieb R, Mayfield J, et al. Benefits and costs of prevention and early intervention programs for youth. Olympia (WA): Washington State Institute for Public Policy; 2004.
63. Olafson E, Boat BW, Putnam KT, et al. Implementing trauma and grief component therapy for adolescents and think trauma for traumatized youth in secure juvenile justice settings. J Interpers Violence 2018;33(16):2537–57.
64. Fisher PA, Gilliam KS. Multidimensional treatment foster care: an alternative to residential treatment for high risk children and adolescents. Interv Psicosoc 2012;21(2):195–203.
65. Kerr DCR, Degarmo DS, Leve LD, et al. Juvenile justice girls' depressive symptoms and suicidal ideation 9 years after multidimensional treatment foster care. J Consult Clin Psychol 2014;82(4):684–93.
66. Harold GT, Kerr DCR, van Ryzin M, et al. Depressive symptom trajectories among girls in the juvenile justice system: 24-month outcomes of an RCT of multidimensional treatment foster care. Prev Sci 2013;14(5):437–46.
67. Callahan L, Steadman HJ, Gerus L. Seven common characteristics of juvenile mental health courts. Delmar (NY): Policy Research Associates; 2013.
68. Callahan L, Cocozza J, Steadman HJ, et al. A national survey of US juvenile mental health courts. Psychiatr Serv 2012;63(2):130–4.
69. Jurma AM, Tocea C, Iancu O, et al. Psychopathological symptoms in adolescents with delinquent behavior. Rom J Leg Med 2014;22(3):193–8.

Depression in Children and Adolescents Involved in the Child Welfare System

Michael W. Naylor, MD[a],*, Sarah M. Wakefield, MD[b],
Wynne Morgan, MD[c], Alka Aneja, MD[d]

KEYWORDS

• Child welfare system • Foster care • Child maltreatment • Depression • Treatment

KEY POINTS

• Child maltreatment is associated with psychopathology in children and adolescents, including major depression, suicidal behavior, and nonsuicidal self-injurious behavior.

• Child maltreatment is associated with a more severe and chronic course of depression with poor treatment response compared with patients with depression with no history of maltreatment.

• Involvement with the child welfare system presents an additional risk for the development of psychopathology, independent of maltreatment.

• Trauma-focused cognitive behavioral therapy has been shown to be effective in the treatment of trauma-related symptoms and to relieve symptoms of depression.

• Successful treatment of youth in the child welfare system requires the clinician to collaborate with other care providers and stakeholders to help plan and implement youth care.

INTRODUCTION

Child maltreatment presents a significant public health challenge. Exposure to childhood adversity has been linked to an array of adverse health outcomes in adulthood,[1] and is strongly associated with the onset of psychiatric illness during adolescence.[2,3]

This article originally appeared in *Child and Adolescent Psychiatric Clinics*, Volume 28, Issue 3, July 2019.
Disclosure Statement: None.
[a] Department of Psychiatry, University of Illinois at Chicago, Institute for Juvenile Research, 1747 West Roosevelt Road, M/C 747, Room 155, Chicago, IL 60608, USA; [b] School of Medicine, Texas Tech University Health Sciences Center, Texas Tech University, 3601 4th Street, STOP 8103, Lubbock, TX 79430, USA; [c] Division of Child and Adolescent Psychiatry, Department of Psychiatry, University of Massachusetts Medical School, 55 Lake Avenue North, Worcester, MA 01655, USA; [d] Department of Psychiatry, Fremont Hospital, 39001 Sundale Drive, Fremont, CA 94538, USA
* Corresponding author.
E-mail address: mnaylor@uic.edu

Child maltreatment is common. In 2016, there was an estimated 4,100,000 reports of child maltreatment involving 7,400,000 children nationally. Approximately 55.1 per 1000 children experienced maltreatment. Nearly 75% of victims were neglected, 18.2% were physically abused, and 8.5% were sexually abused.[4] A prospective cohort study of a nationally representative probability sample of adolescents documented a high prevalence of self-reported child maltreatment. Supervision neglect was the most common (41.5%), followed by physical assaults by parents or caregivers (28.4%), physical neglect (11.8%), and contact sexual abuse by 4.5%.[5]

An extensive body of literature documents the association between child maltreatment and depression. Adolescents and adults with a history of physical and sexual abuse are at an increased risk for lifetime major depression compared with those not maltreated.[6,7] Child maltreatment is a risk factor even for patients whose first episode of depression presents later in life.[8]

Age of exposure to child maltreatment affects the development of depression, with early childhood being a time of unique vulnerability.[9] There is a "dosage effect" in that youth who experienced more types of maltreatment or a series of abusive episodes, as opposed to a single incident, endorsed greater severity of depression, anxiety, hopelessness, and suicidal ideation.[7,10–12]

Childhood maltreatment is associated with poor outcomes in patients with depression who have more severe depression, psychotic subtype, recurrent and chronic depression, decreased rates of remission of depression and high rates of suicidal behavior.[13–15]

Child maltreatment also confers an increased risk of suicidal thoughts and behaviors in adolescents, even after controlling for depression severity. These findings are consistent across gender, racial, and ethnic lines.[16] A history of child maltreatment is associated with an earlier age of onset of suicidal ideation and behavior.[17]

A history of child maltreatment has a deleterious effect on response to treatment. Adolescents with a history of sexual or physical abuse are less responsive to cognitive behavioral therapy (CBT) for depression than patients without.[18,19] Childhood maltreatment is associated with a lower probability of response to antidepressant pharmacotherapy in depressed adults.[20]

Involvement with the child welfare system presents an additional risk for the development of psychopathology, independent of maltreatment. By definition, most children involved in the child welfare system have experienced child maltreatment. Various risk factors have been implicated in children's involvement in the child welfare system, including caregiver substance abuse and depression, caregiver history of child abuse, lack of social supports for the caregiver, and impaired child development.[21] In addition, children in the child welfare system are considerably more likely than other children to experience parental incarceration, and are more likely than children living in poverty to be exposed to adverse childhood experiences.[22]

Poverty is a powerful risk factor for both child maltreatment and involvement in the child welfare system. Poverty can predispose to child abuse and neglect through parental stress. The incidence of child maltreatment is nearly 6 times higher for children in low socioeconomic status families compared with other children. The incidence of physical and sexual abuse is 3 times higher, and the incidence of physical neglect nearly 9 times higher, in poor families. Furthermore, children placed in foster care are largely from economically disadvantaged families. In 2011, 12.9 per 1000 children in the overall population were in child welfare agency-initiated out-of-home placement. The rate of out-of-home placement was considerably higher (nearly 6 of every 100 children) for children from poor families.[23]

The increased risk of mental health issues is present at a child's first contact with the child welfare system. Youth investigated for possible child maltreatment demonstrate high levels of psychopathology. In one study, 48% of children demonstrated emotional and behavioral problems severe enough to warrant referral to mental health services.[24] A second study found high rates of depression (9%), suicidality (13.9%), anxiety (13.5%), and attention-deficit/hyperactivity disorder. Girls were more likely to report depression than boys.[25]

Rates of mental illness and depression are even higher for children whose maltreatment has been substantiated and are in the custody of the child welfare system. A meta-analysis of 8 studies of children in the child welfare system found that 49% of foster children were identified as having a current mental illness and 11% with depressive disorders.[26] Rates of psychiatric disorders are higher in older adolescents. McMillen and colleagues[11] found that 61% of older youth in foster care had at least one psychiatric disorder during their lifetime. The prevalence of major depression was 3 times higher than rates from a community sample.

The adverse impact of involvement with the child welfare system persists even after foster children leave foster care. Compared with peers in the general population, adolescent and young adult alumni of the child welfare system were more likely to be depressed, to have been hospitalized for suicide attempts, and to be hospitalized for serious psychiatric illnesses including depression. Adolescents and young adults who had been in long-term foster care had the worst outcomes.[27,28]

Factors specific to the child welfare experience, associated with the development of emotional and behavioral disorders in children in the foster care system, include multiple and sudden placement moves and childcare provider alienation.[29] Placement instability has been associated with both short- and long-term mental and behavioral symptoms, independent of maltreatment characteristics.[30] An authoritarian parenting style is associated with internalizing problems in foster children.[31]

Type of placement determines the rate of emotional and behavioral disturbances in children involved with the child welfare system. Children placed in kinship care have greater placement stability, fewer behavior and emotional problems, and enhanced well-being than those placed in nonkinship foster care.[32,33] Children in foster care do better than those in institutional settings.[34]

Although diagnostic criteria for depressive disorder are unchanged for children and adolescents who have experienced child maltreatment, care must be taken not to over diagnose depression in this population. As described by Griffin and colleagues,[35] several symptoms of child traumatic stress overlap with those of depression, including self-injurious behaviors in response to trauma-related stimuli, social withdrawal, affective numbing, and impaired sleep.

Causes of Depression in Children in the Foster Care System

As McLaughlin[36] has pointed out, it can be challenging to assimilate the data regarding the specific causes of these difficulties because of the variation in definitions used in recent research. Perinatal exposure to substance use, maternal stress and mental illness symptoms; exposure to maltreatment and placement instability are risk factors for the future development of depression for children involved in the child welfare system and will be the subject of greater exploration.

Perinatal exposure to stress

Children typically come into contact with the child welfare system owing to concerns of abuse or neglect by their primary caretakers. Caretakers who abuse or neglect a child may be suffering from mental health symptoms, and youth in foster care may have higher rates of exposure to mental illness and substance use, often beginning in utero. Brain development is most rapid during the fetal period.[37] Maternal prenatal stress, including that due to depression during pregnancy, adversely affects fetal development and is an established risk factor for preterm birth and low birth weight.[38] Preterm birth and low birth weight have been associated with neurocognitive, socioemotional, and behavioral difficulties.[39] Mothers with a history of prenatal depression and anxiety are 1.5 to 2 times more likely to have a child with behavioral difficulties.[40] Bornstein and colleagues[41] reported that preschool-aged children with lower levels of socioemotional development had more internalizing and externalizing behaviors at ages 10 and 14 years.

There are several postulated mechanisms for the disruption of neonatal development by maternal stress. Welberg and colleagues[42] and Wyrwoll and colleagues[43] have demonstrated that maternal stress is correlated with reduced enzymatic activity of the placenta increasing fetal exposure to maternal stress hormones, in turn resulting in a lifelong risk for anxiety. Increased exposure to cortisol in utero may alter the development of the hypothalamic pituitary adrenal axis in the developing fetus.[44] Maternal prenatal stress has also been associated with restriction in uterine blood supply,[43] resulting in changes in the normal patterns and volume of circulation in the fetal brain.[45] In addition, maternal stress is associated with a higher risk of pre-eclampsia[46,47] and accompanying increases of placental corticotropin-releasing hormone. Increased levels of corticotropin-releasing hormone are associated with both preterm delivery and a negative effect on hypothalamic pituitary adrenal axis development, risk factors for future difficulty with socioemotional, and behavioral functioning.[48]

The prenatal environment and early attachment patterns are independent predictors of future socioemotional development in children. Although prenatal exposure to maternal stress can expose a child to early developmental risk, the quality of the attachment relationship after birth can predict future psychosocial function.[49] Parenting stress is associated with emotional and behavioral disorders in children as young as 3 years of age, especially in children with insecure attachment relationships with the primary caregiver.[50] This risk seems to be mitigated by a secure attachment relationship between the primary caregiver and child.

Maltreatment

Poly-victimization, or exposure to multiple types and frequent events of maltreatment, is the norm, not the exception, for youth involved in the child welfare system.[51] Greater severity of maltreatment predicts greater number of mental and behavioral symptoms in foster care youth.[52] It may be that the frequency, duration, severity, and exposure to different types of maltreatment differentiates maltreated children and adolescents involved in the child welfare system from maltreated youth not engaged in the child welfare system.[53]

As noted, maltreatment has long been associated with maladaptive effects on development in children. Green and colleagues[54] demonstrated that 45% of child psychiatric disorders are the likely result of adverse experiences in childhood. Prevention of these sequelae is precisely the goal of the child welfare system. Maltreatment has been linked with deficits in many areas of neurobiological and socioemotional development, including high rates of cognitive, motor, and language delays.[55,56] More specifically, it is important to screen children engaged in the welfare system for depression because maltreatment is associated with future development of depressive disorders.[57]

The neurobiological underpinnings of the link between maltreatment and depression are unclear and deserve additional study. Depression may be linked to difficulties in the processing of rewards and threats with reduced reward sensitivity.[58] Maltreatment may affect the development of these neurobiological pathways. McEwen[59] introduced the concept of allostatic loading as an explanation for a link between stress and future maladaptive response. Allostasis is the body's way of adapting to current stress and maintaining homeostasis. In the short term, homeostasis is achieved through alteration of stress hormones, including adrenaline and cortisol, but comes at a future cost of "overload" to the body's stress response system.

Genetic polymorphism and epigenetic modifications have been found to interact with trauma, affecting the risk of depression especially at critical neurodevelopmental periods.[60] Several studies have found that abuse during these critical neurodevelopmental periods can affect brain circuitry, endocrinologic function, immune system, and the physiologic reaction to stress.[61,62]

Placement issues

The most unique stressors for children involved in the child welfare system are those related to placement. Stressors may include separation from nonabusive supports, including siblings, teachers, and school counselors, and also the familiar neighborhood.

Instability of placement, the quality of placement, and uncertainty related to future placement or reunification may affect a child's future socioemotional function. McGuire and colleagues[63] reported that "placement stability is critical for mental health of youth in foster care, regardless of type, severity, or frequency of their maltreatment experience." Placement instability, defined as moves that do not result in a child's permanent placement,[64] is typical of a child's experience in the child welfare system.[65] Changes in placement are made for a variety of reasons, but are typically related to behavioral or medical problems outside the skill range of the placement.[66,67] The number of placement changes varies across different settings. Rubin and colleagues[68] reported that about one-third of youth in foster care have 3 or more placement changes. Pecora and colleagues[69] found that one-third of foster children reported 8 or more changes, whereas McGuire and colleagues[63] reported the average number of placement changes was 9. Placement instability contributes to depressive, anxiety, and aggressive symptoms in youth involved in the child welfare system.[70] These symptoms increase over time for youth in out-of-home placement compared with youth who remain in their home of origin.[71]

Treatment

Trauma-focused CBT (TF-CBT), consisting of 9 components: psychoeducation, relaxation skills, affective modulation skills, cognitive coping skills, trauma narration and processing, in vivo mastery of trauma reminders, conjoint youth-parent sessions, and enhancing safety and future development delivered through weekly sessions (typically 12–16 sessions) to children and their caregivers (when available), has been studied extensively and is the primary psychotherapeutic intervention for children and adolescents with symptoms referable to traumatic stress because of child maltreatment. It has been shown to be more effective than treatment-as-usual and wait-list controls in reducing symptoms of posttraumatic stress disorder (PTSD), anxiety, hyperarousal and depression.[72] With modifications, the interventions are effective for preschool-aged children with a history of maltreatment.[73,74] TF-CBT has been shown to be effective in community-based clinics for intimate partner violence[75] and in residential treatment facilities for adjudicated youth.[76] Therapeutic benefits were found to persist after 1 year, with some symptoms continuing to improve. A higher baseline severity of internalizing and depressive symptoms was predictive of children who continued to meet diagnostic criteria for PTSD at the 12-month follow-up.[77] Preliminary data suggest that TF-CBT can be delivered remotely via telemedicine without deleterious impact on effectiveness.[78]

In a Cochran review, Gillies found that children and adolescents who received psychological therapies (CBT, eye movement desensitization and reprocessing therapy, narrative therapy, supportive therapy) after a trauma were less likely to be diagnosed with PTSD, and had fewer symptoms of PTSD up to a month after treatment, compared with those who received no treatment, highlighting the importance for youth in the child welfare system to have access to therapeutic interventions. Of the therapeutic modalities compared, CBT showed moderate evidence that it may be more effective in reducing PTSD symptoms at 1 month, although no therapies showed evidence of reduced symptoms past a month.[79] Significantly, CBT for depression seemed to be less effective for patients with depression with a history of physical and sexual abuse.[18,19,80]

Multiple treatments are available for child welfare involved children and families. Providers can search for specific interventions and their respective evidence bases through the California Evidence-Based Clearinghouse for Child Welfare (CEBC). The CEBC was established to help identify, select, and implement evidence-based child welfare practices to improve child and family well-being and increase permanency. The CEBC Program Registry provides information on evidence-based and non-evidence-based child welfare-related practices. The CEBC rates these practices on a 5-point scale ranging from "Well-Supported by Research Evidence" to "Concerning Practice" that potentially present a risk of harm to clients served, based on the available research evidence.[81]

Pharmacotherapy

Very little research has been done to examine the effectiveness of pharmacotherapy in the treatment of depression of children with a history of maltreatment. Seedat and colleagues[82] conducted a 12-week open label study of a fixed dose of citalopram in 8 adolescents with PTSD. They reported a statistically significant decrease in severity of PTSD, with improvement in re-experiencing, hyperarousal, and avoidance, but no improvement in self-reported symptoms of depression. In a second study, Seedat and colleagues[83] compared the response of 24 children and adolescents with 14 adults with PTSD with an 8-week open trial of citalopram. Both groups demonstrated significant reduction in severity of PTSD and Clinical Global Impressions (CGI) ratings. Adolescents had a significantly greater improvement in hyperarousal symptoms. Although there was significant comorbidity with major depression in both groups, the investigators did not study the impact of citalopram on depression severity. A double-blind placebo-controlled study of children and adolescents with PTSD randomized to sertraline (n = 67) or placebo (n = 62) failed to show an advantage for sertraline over placebo in mean change in total PTSD symptoms severity, CGI improvement score, or change in depression severity, as measured by the CDRS-R. Older adolescents showed greater improvement than younger adolescents.[84] In a small placebo-controlled study examining the benefit of adding sertraline to TF-CBT, Cohen and colleagues[85] found that all patients showed significant improvement in PTSD and anxiety symptoms, and total psychopathology measures over time, but there were no significant differences between patients receiving TF-CBT and sertraline and those receiving TF-CBT and placebo on any of these measures. Patients on sertraline showed greater improvement in Children's Global Assessment Scale scores than those receiving placebo.

SUMMARY

Youth involved with the child welfare system are often involved in other child-serving systems, such as the criminal justice system, and special educational programs through their schools. Clinicians working with foster children must understand their role vis-à-vis these other child-serving systems and collaborate with care providers and other stakeholders to help plan and implement a youth's care, and to obtain information from various sources on their functioning and response to services. Clinicians should monitor the youth's functioning in the various areas of their lives, including school, peer relationships, and functioning at home and in the community, with the goal of enhancing placement permanence.[86,87]

REFERENCES

1. Felitti VJ, Anda RF, Nordenberg D, et al. Relationship of childhood abuse and household dysfunction to many of the leading causes of death in adults. The adverse childhood experiences (ACE) study. Am J Prev Med 1998;14:245–58.

2. McLaughlin KA, Green JG, Gruber MJ, et al. Childhood adversities and first onset of psychiatric disorders in a national sample of US adolescents. Arch Gen Psychiatry 2012;69:1151–60.

3. Edwards VJ, Holden GW, Felitti VJ, et al. Relationship between multiple forms of childhood maltreatment and adult mental health in community respondents: results from the adverse childhood experiences study. Am J Psychiatry 2003; 160:1453–60.

4. U.S. Department of Health and Human Services, Administration for Children and Families, Administration on Children, Youth and Families. Children's Bureau. Child Maltreatment; 2016. Available at: https://www.acf.hhs.gov/sites/default/files/cb/cm2016.pdf. Accessed October 18, 2018.

5. Hussey JM, Chang JJ, Kotch JB. Child maltreatment in the United States: prevalence, risk factors, and adolescent health consequences. Pediatrics 2006;118: 933–42.

6. Widom CS, DuMont K, Czaja SJ. A prospective investigation of major depressive disorder and comorbidity in abused and neglected children grown up. Arch Gen Psychiatry 2007;64:49–56.

7. Pillay AL, Schoubben-Hesk S. Depression, anxiety, and hopelessness in sexually abused adolescent girls. Psychol Rep 2001;88:727–33.

8. Comijs HC, van Exel E, van der Mast RC, et al. Childhood abuse in late-life depression. J Affect Disord 2013;147:241–6.

9. Dunn EC, Nishimi K, Gomez SH, et al. Developmental timing of trauma exposure and emotion dysregulation in adulthood: are there sensitive periods when trauma is most harmful? J Affect Disord 2018;227:869–77.

10. Miller AB, Jenness JL, Oppenheimer CW, et al. Childhood emotional maltreatment as a robust predictor of suicidal ideation: a 3-year multi-wave, prospective investigation. J Abnorm Child Psychol 2017;45:105–16.

11. McMillen JC, Zima BT, Scott LD Jr, et al. Prevalence of psychiatric disorders among older youths in the foster care system. J Am Acad Child Adolesc Psychiatry 2005;44:88–95.

12. Danielson CK, de Arellano MA, Kilpatrick DG, et al. Child maltreatment in depressed adolescents: differences in symptomatology based on history of abuse. Child Maltreat 2005;10:37–48.

13. Holshausen K, Bowie CR, Harkness KL. The relation of childhood maltreatment to psychotic symptoms in adolescents and young adults with depression. J Clin Child Adolesc Psychol 2016;45:241–7.

14. Gaudiano BA, Zimmerman M. The relationship between childhood trauma history and the psychotic subtype of major depression. Acta Psychiatr Scand 2010;121: 462–70.

15. Nanni V, Uher R, Danese A. Childhood maltreatment predicts unfavorable course of illness and treatment outcome in depression: a meta-analysis. Am J Psychiatry 2012;169:141–51.

16. King CA, Merchant CR. Social and interpersonal factors relating to adolescent suicidality: a review of the literature. Arch Suicide Res 2008;12:181–96.

17. Dunn EC, McLaughlin KA, Slopen N, et al. Developmental timing of child maltreatment and symptoms of depression and suicidal ideation in young adulthood: results from the national longitudinal study of adolescent health. Depress Anxiety 2013;30:955–64.

18. Shamseddeen W, Asarnow JR, Clarke G, et al. Impact of physical and sexual abuse on treatment response in the treatment of resistant depression in adolescent study (TORDIA). J Am Acad Child Adolesc Psychiatry 2011;50:293–301.

19. Barbe RP, Bridge JA, Birmaher B, et al. Lifetime history of sexual abuse, clinical presentation, and outcome in a clinical trial for adolescent depression. J Clin Psychiatry 2004;65:77–83.

20. Klein DN, Arnow BA, Barkin JL, et al. Early adversity in chronic depression: clinical correlates and response to pharmacotherapy. Depress Anxiety 2009;26: 701–10.

21. English DJ, Thompson R, White CR. Predicting risk of entry into foster care from early childhood experiences: a survival analysis using LONGSCAN data. Child Abuse Negl 2015;45:57–67.

22. Turney K, Wildeman C. Adverse childhood experiences among children placed in and adopted from foster care: evidence from a nationally representative survey. Child Abuse Negl 2017;64:117–29.

23. Pelton LH. The continuing role of material factors in child maltreatment and placement. Child Abuse Negl 2015;41:30–9.

24. Burns BJ, Phillips SD, Wagner HR, et al. Mental health need and access to mental health services by youths involved in child welfare: a national survey. J Am Acad Child Adolesc Psychiatry 2004;43:960–70.

25. Heneghan A, Stein REK, Hurlburt MS, et al. Mental health problems in teens investigated by U.S. child welfare agencies. J Adolesc Health 2013;52:634–40.

26. Bronsard G, Alessandrini M, Fond G, et al. The prevalence of mental disorders among children and adolescents in the child welfare system: a systematic review and meta-analysis. Medicine 2016;95:e2622.

27. Vinnerljung B, Hjern A, Lindblad F. Suicide attempts and severe psychiatric morbidity among former child welfare clients-a national cohort study. J Child Psychol Psychiatry 2006;47:723–33.

28. Dregan A, Brown J, Armstrong D. Do adult emotional and behavioural outcomes vary as a function of diverse childhood experiences of the public care system? Psychol Med 2011;41:2213–20.

29. Hillen T, Gafson L. Why good placements matter: pre-placement and placement risk factors associated with mental health disorders in pre-school children in foster care. Clin Child Psychol Psychiatry 2015;20:486–99.

30. Proctor LJ, Skriner LC, Roesch S, et al. Trajectories of behavioral adjustment following early placement in foster care: predicting stability and change over 8 years. J Am Acad Child Adolesc Psychiatry 2010;49:464–73.

31. Fuentes MJ, Salas MD, Bernedo IM, et al. Impact of the parenting style of foster parents on the behaviour problems of foster children. Child Care Health Dev 2015;41:704–11.

32. Rubin DM, Downes KJ, O'Reilly AL, et al. Impact of kinship care on behavioral well-being for children in out-of-home care. Arch Pediatr Adolesc Med 2008; 162:550–6.

33. Winokur M, Holtan A, Batchelder KE. Kinship care for the safety, permanency, and well-being of children removed from the home for maltreatment. Cochrane Database Syst Rev 2014;(1):CD006546.

34. McLaughlin KA, Zeanah CH, Fox NA, et al. Attachment security as a mechanism linking foster care placement to improved mental health outcomes in previously institutionalized children. J Child Psychol Psychiatry 2012;53:46–55.

35. Griffin G, McClelland G, Holzberg M, et al. Addressing the impact of trauma before diagnosing mental illness in child welfare. Child Welfare 2011;90:69–89.

36. McLaughlin KA. Future direction in childhood adversity and youth psychopathology. J Clin Child Adolesc Psychol 2016;45:361–82.

37. Joseph R. Fetal brain behavior and cognitive development. Dev Rev 2000;20: 81–98.

38. Bussieres E-L, Tarabulsy GM, Pearson J, et al. Maternal prenatal stress and infant birth weight and gestational age: a meta-analysis of prospective studies. Dev Rev 2015;36:179–99.

39. Grote NI, Bridge JA, Gavin AR, et al. A meta-analysis of depression during pregnancy and the risk of preterm birth, low birth weight, and intrauterine growth restriction. Arch Gen Psychiatry 2010;67:1012–24.

40. Madigan S, Oatley H, Racine N, et al. A meta-analysis of maternal prenatal depression and anxiety on child socioemotional development. J Am Acad Child Adolesc Psychiatry 2018;57:645–57.

41. Bornstein MH, Hahn C-S, Haynes OM. Social competence, externalizing, and internalizing behavioral adjustment from early childhood through early adolescence. Dev Psychopathol 2010;22:717–35.

42. Welberg LAM, Thrivikraman KV, Plotsky PM. Chronic maternal stress inhibits the capacity to up-regulate placental 11B-hydroxysteroid dehydrogenase type 2 activity. J Endocrinol 2005;186:R7–12.

43. Wyrwoll CS, Homes MC, Seckl JR. 11beta-hydroxysteroid dehydrogenases and the brain: from zero to hero, a decade of progress. Front Neuroendocrinol 2011;32:265–86.

44. O'Donnell K, O'Connor T, Glover V. Prenatal stress and neurodevelopment of the child: focus on the HPA axis and role of the placenta. Dev Neurosci 2009;31: 346–51.

45. Sjostrom K, Valentin L, Thelin T, et al. Maternal anxiety in late pregnancy and fetal hemodynamics. Eur J Obstet Gynecol Reprod Biol 1997;74:149–55.

46. Landsbergis PA, Hatch MC. Psychosocial work stress and pregnancy induced hypertension. Epidemiology 1996;7:346–51.

47. Hobel CJ, Dunkel-Schetter C, Roesch SC, et al. Maternal plasma corticotropin-releasing hormone associated with stress at 20 weeks' gestation in pregnancies ending in pre-term delivery. Am J Obstet Gynecol 1999;180(Suppl 2):S257–63.

48. Hostinar CE, Gunnar MR. Future directions in the study of social relationships as regulators of the HPA axis across development. J Clin Child Adolesc Psychol 2013;42:564–75.
49. McGoron L, Gleason MM, Smyke AT, et al. Recovering from early deprivation: attachment mediates effects of caregiving on psychopathology. J Am Acad Child Adolesc Psychiatry 2012;51:683–93.
50. Tharner A, Luijk MPCM, van IJzendoorn MH, et al. Infant attachment, parenting stress, and child emotional and behavioral problems at age 3 years. Parenting 2012;12:261–81.
51. Turner HA, Finkelhor D, Ormrod R. Poly-victimization in a national sample of children and youth. Am J Prev Med 2010;38:323–30.
52. Jackson Y, Gabrielli J, Fleming K, et al. Untangling the relative contribution of maltreatment severity and frequency to type of behavioral outcome in foster youth. Child Abuse Negl 2014;38:1147–59.
53. Hambrick EP, Oppenheim-Weller S, N'zi AM, et al. Mental health interventions for children in foster care: a systematic review. Child Youth Serv Rev 2016;70:65–77.
54. Green JG, McLaughlin KA, Berglund P, et al. Childhood adversities and adult psychopathology in the national comorbidity survey replication (NCS-R) I: associations with first onset of DSM-IV disorders. Arch Gen Psychiatry 2010;62:113–23.
55. Pears KC, Kim HK, Fisher PA. Psychosocial and cognitive functioning of children with specific profiles of maltreatment. Child Abuse Negl 2008;32:958–71.
56. Cicchetti D. Socioemotional, personality, and biological development: illustrations from a multilevel developmental psychopathology perspective on child maltreatment. Annu Rev Psychol 2016;67:187–211.
57. Danese A, Moffitt TE, Harrington H, et al. Adverse childhood experiences and adult risk factors of age-related disease: depression, inflammation, and clustering of metabolic risk markers. Arch Pediatr Adolesc Med 2009;163:1135–43.
58. Insel T, Cuthbert B, Garvey M, et al. Research domain criteria (RDoC): toward a new classification framework for research on mental disorders. Am J Psychiatry 2010;167:748–51.
59. McEwen BS. Allostasis and allostatic load Implications for neuropsychopharmacology. Neuropsychopharmacology 2000;22:108–24.
60. Williams LM, Gatt JM, Schofield PR, et al. 'Negativity bias' in risk for depression and anxiety: brain-body fear circuitry correlates, 5-HTT-LPR and early life stress. Neuroimage 2009;47:804–14.
61. McGee RA, Wolfe DA, Yuen SA, et al. The measurement of maltreatment: a comparison of approaches. Child Abuse Negl 1995;19:233–49.
62. Kaffman A, Meaney MJ. Neurodevelopmental sequelae of postnatal maternal care in rodents: clinical and research implications of molecular insights. J Child Psychol Psychiatry 2007;48:224–44.
63. McGuire A, Cho B, Huffhines L, et al. The relation between dimensions of maltreatment, placement instability, and mental health among youth in foster care. Child Abuse Negl 2018;86:10–21.
64. Fisher PA, Mannering AM, Van Scoyoc A, et al. A translational neuroscience perspective on the importance of reducing placement instability among foster children. Child Welfare 2013;92:9–36.
65. Farmer EMZ, Wagner HR, Burns BJ, et al. Treatment foster care in a system of care: sequences and correlates of residential placements. J Child Fam Stud 2003;12:11–25.

66. James S. Why do foster care placements disrupt? An investigation of reasons for placement change in foster care. Soc Serv Rev 2004;78:601–27.
67. Seltzer RR, Johnson SB, Minkovitz CS. Medical complexity and placement outcomes for children in foster care. Child Youth Serv Rev 2017;83:285–93.
68. Rubin DM, Alessandrini EA, Feudtner C, et al. Placement stability and mental health costs for children in foster care. Pediatrics 2004;113:1336–41.
69. Pecora PJ, Kessler RC, Williams J. Findings from the Northwest foster care alumni study. Seattle (WA): Casey Family Programs; 2015.
70. Newton RR, Litrownik AJ, Landsverk JA. Children and youth in foster care: disentangling the relationship between problem behaviors and number of placements. Child Abuse Negl 2000;24(10):1363–74.
71. Lawrence CR, Carlson EA, Egeland B. The impact of foster care on development. Dev Psychopathol 2006;18:57–76.
72. Gillies D, Taylor F, Gray C, et al. Psychological therapies for the treatment of post traumatic stress disorder in children and adolescents. Evid Based Child Health 2013;8:1004–116.
73. Cohen JA, Mannarino AP. A treatment outcome study for sexually abused preschool children: initial findings. J Am Acad Child Adolesc Psychiatry 1996;35: 42–50.
74. Scheeringa MS, Weems CF, Cohen JA, et al. Trauma-focused cognitive-behavioral therapy for posttraumatic stress disorder in three-through six year-old children: a randomized clinical trial. J Child Psychol Psychiatry 2011;52: 853–60.
75. Cohen JA, Mannarino AP, Iyengar S. Community treatment of posttraumatic stress disorder for children exposed to intimate partner violence: a randomized controlled trial. Arch Pediatr Adolesc Med 2011;165:16–21.
76. Cohen JA, Mannarino AP, Jankowski K, et al. A randomized implementation study of trauma-focused cognitive behavioral therapy for adjudicated teens in residential treatment facilities. Child Maltreat 2016;21:156–67.
77. Mannarino AP, Cohen JA, Deblinger E, et al. Trauma-focused cognitive-behavioral therapy for children: sustained impact of treatment 6 and 12 months later. Child Maltreat 2012;17:231–41.
78. Stewart RW, Orengo-Aguayo RE, Cohen JA, et al. A pilot study of trauma-focused cognitive-behavioral therapy delivered via telehealth technology. Child Maltreat 2017;22:324–33.
79. Gillies D, Maiocchi L, Bhandari AP, et al. Psychological therapies for children and adolescents exposed to trauma. Cochrane Database Syst Rev 2016;(10):CD012371.
80. Lewis CC, Simons AD, Nguyen LJ, et al. Impact of childhood trauma on treatment outcome in the treatment for adolescents with depression study (TADS). J Am Acad Child Adolesc Psychiatry 2010;49:132–40.
81. California Evidence-Based Clearinghouse for Child Welfare (CEBC). Available at: http://www.cebc4cw.org/. Accessed November 12, 2018.
82. Seedat S, Lockhat R, Kaminer D, et al. An open trial of citalopram in adolescents with post-traumatic stress disorder. Int Clin Psychopharmacol 2001;16:21–5.
83. Seedat S, Stein DJ, Ziervogel C, et al. Comparison of response to a selective serotonin reuptake inhibitor in children, adolescents, and adults with posttraumatic stress disorder. J Child Adolesc Psychopharmacol 2002;12:37–46.
84. Robb AS, Cueva JE, Sporn J, et al. Sertraline treatment of children and adolescents with posttraumatic stress disorder: a double-blind, placebo-controlled trial. J Child Adolesc Psychopharmacol 2010;20:463–71.

85. Cohen JA, Mannarino AP, Perel JM, et al. A pilot randomized controlled trial of combined trauma-focused CBT and sertraline for childhood PTSD symptoms. J Am Acad Child Adolesc Psychiatry 2007;46:811–9.
86. American Academy of Child and Adolescent Psychiatry. A guide for community serving child agencies on psychoatropic medications for child & adolescents 2012. Available at: https://www.aacap.org/App_Themes/AACAP/docs/clinical_practice_center/systems_of_care/Psychopharm_in_SOC_Feb_2012.pdf. Accessed November 19, 2018.
87. Lee T, Fouras G, Brown R. Practice parameter for the assessment and management of youth involved with the child welfare system. J Am Acad Child Adolesc Psychiatry 2015;54:502–17.

Depression in Maltreated Children and Adolescents

Michael D. De Bellis, MD, MPH[a],*, Kate B. Nooner, PhD[b],
Jeanette M. Scheid, MD, PhD[c], Judith A. Cohen, MD[d]

KEYWORDS

- Depressive disorders • Maltreatment • Children • Adolescents • Suicide
- Self-injury • Selective serotonin reuptake inhibitors (SSRIs)
- Trauma-focused cognitive behavior therapy

KEY POINTS

- Child maltreatment affects 9.1 to 17.1 of every 1000 US children and adolescents. Maltreated youth are at high risk for depression but may present with more externalizing symptoms.
- Clinicians should screen their young patients for past or ongoing trauma and maltreatment.
- Maltreated youth are at high risk for treatment-resistant depression caused by comorbid posttraumatic stress disorder, which can be overlooked without a trauma-informed approach.
- Combination treatment with selective serotonin reuptake inhibitors and cognitive behavior therapy (CBT) with a trauma-informed approach should be considered for depressed maltreated youth.
- Behavioral management can be integrated with trauma-focused CBT to treat the externalizing disorders that commonly occur in maltreated depressed youth.

INTRODUCTION

Depressive disorders are common consequences of experiencing child maltreatment. Depressive disorders herein termed depression, are defined in the Diagnostic and Statistical Manual of Mental Disorders-5 (DSM-5), under the chapter "Depressive Disorders," as major depressive disorder, persistent depressive disorder (formerly

This article originally appeared in *Child and Adolescent Psychiatric Clinics*, Volume 28, Issue 3, July 2019.
[a] Healthy Childhood Brain Development and Developmental Traumatology Research Program, Department of Psychiatry and Behavioral Sciences, Duke University Medical Center, Box 104360, Durham, NC 27710, USA; [b] Department of Psychology, University of North Carolina Wilmington, 601 South College Road, TL 2074, Wilmington, NC 28409, USA; [c] Department of Psychiatry, Michigan State University, 909 Wilson Road, East Lansing, MI 48824, USA; [d] Drexel University College of Medicine, Allegheny Health Network, 4 Allegheny Center, 8th Floor, Pittsburgh, PA 15212, USA
* Corresponding author.
E-mail address: michael.debellis@duke.edu

Clinics Collections 11 (2021) 147–160
https://doi.org/10.1016/j.ccol.2020.12.036

dysthymia), disruptive mood dysregulation disorder, other specified depressive disorder, and unspecified depressive disorder.[1] The diagnostic criteria for a major depressive disorder did not change from the DSM fourth edition text revision (DSM-IV-TR).[2] This critical review of depression in maltreated youth includes literature from DSM-IV-TR and DSM-5. Maltreated youth may also have 3 types of depressive disorders listed under the chapters "Anxiety Disorders" in DSM-IV-TR and "Trauma- and Stressor-Related Disorders," in the DSM-5, namely adjustment disorder with depressed mood, adjustment disorder with mixed anxiety and depressed mood, and adjustment disorder with mixed disturbance of emotions and conduct.[3] Adjustments disorders do not have enough symptoms to meet other DSM diagnostic criteria and occur in response to an identified stressor. Adjustments disorders can be acute, with symptoms occurring less than 3 months, or chronic, with symptoms occurring more than 3 months.

A literature search of PubMed and PsychINFO articles published from 2000 to 2018 using keywords and MeSH terms "depression" (and DSM-5 terms for depressive disorders), "maltreatment" "emotional, physical or sexual abuse," "neglect," "childhood," "child," and "adolescence" were crossed individually with "incidence," "prevalence," "assessment," "practice parameters," "evidence-based treatment," "psychopharmacology," "psychotherapy," "medications," "suicide, and " self-injury," which were limited to the English language, were reviewed and selected for this article. Our criteria were that the articles be peer reviewed and methodologically sound. When reviews were needed to summarize important information, meta-analyses or peer-reviewed reviews published by depression or maltreatment researchers were cited.

CHILD MALTREATMENT

Child maltreatment is defined by law (The Child Abuse Prevention and Treatment Act) and investigated by Child Protective Services (CPS) as physical, sexual, or emotional abuse, and/or neglect by a caregiver that results in harm, potential for, or threat of harm to a child.[4] CPS usually codes emotional abuse or physical neglect in youth who witness interpersonal or domestic violence. According to the National Child Abuse and Neglect Data System, each year 3 million referrals are made to CPS, involving 6 million children. Of these, fewer than 700,000 youth, about 9.1 of every 1000 children, are identified as victims, with 75% classified as neglect, 16% as physical abuse, and 9% sexual abuse.[5] Perpetrators are mainly biological parents (88%), and about half of the perpetrators are female.[5] Parental factors such as substance use disorder (SUD), history of maltreatment, and depression are the strongest risk factors for abusing or neglecting a child.[5] At greatest risk are children, aged 0 to 4 years, because 80% of the 1545 maltreatment-related fatalities in 2011 resulted from neglect, physical abuse, or their combination.[6]

The actual US child abuse and neglect rates are likely higher than official reports. The National Incidence Study of Child Abuse and Neglect 4 estimated rates of child abuse and neglect by US caretakers in 2005 to 2006 to be 17.1 of every 1000 children (approximately 1.25 million children).[7] The National Incidence Study applied 2 definitional standards: a harm standard, restricted to children who were harmed by child abuse and neglect, and the endangerment standard, for children not yet harmed, but at high risk of being harmed. Most states apply only the harm standard in their official reports.

CHILD MALTREATMENT IS A MAJOR RISK FACTOR FOR YOUTH AND ADULT DEPRESSION

Maltreated children have greater rates of depression, posttraumatic stress disorder (PTSD), behavioral problems, suicidal thoughts, suicide attempts, self-injury, and

SUDs compared with nonmaltreated youth.[8] In a meta-analysis of adults with histories of child maltreatment, all forms of abuse and neglect increased the odds ratio of having depression from 2 to 3.00.[9] Emotional abuse, with an odds ratio of 3.53, most strongly increased depression risk.[9] Although the 12-month prevalence rate of depression in the United States is 7%,[1] the depression rate in maltreated individuals is estimated to be 24.7%. In the Longitudinal Studies of Child Abuse and Neglect, a study of 638 at-risk youth, emotional abuse also showed the strongest association to depression in girls, whereas emotional neglect was the strongest predictor of depression in boys.[10] Widom and colleagues[11] (2007) found that child abuse and neglect before age 11 years was associated with an increased risk for depression in young adulthood (odds ratio, 1.51) compared with those without maltreatment histories from similar sociodemographic backgrounds. Depression in abused and neglected youth had a much earlier age of onset (between ages 5 and 10 years) than depression in nonmaltreated youth.[11] A challenge for detecting depression in maltreated youth is that emotional abuse or emotional neglect may not be reported to CPS or the police. Thus, it is important for clinicians to screen their young patients for past or ongoing maltreatment. When maltreatment is identified, prompt referral to early evidence-based trauma-focused treatment (described later) may be a potent strategy for curtailing or preventing the onset of later depression in those youth for whom it is not already present.

DEPRESSED YOUTH SHOULD BE ASSESSED FOR MALTREATMENT HISTORY, TYPE OF DEPRESSION, AND THE PRESENCE OF OTHER DIAGNOSTIC AND STATISTICAL MANUAL OF MENTAL DISORDERS-5 AXIS I COMORBIDITY
Depression Definitions

Another challenge in identifying depression in maltreated youth is that core symptoms of depression are similar to the core symptoms of distress that are commonly seen in maltreated youth. Even though the symptoms overlap, it is important to account for maltreatment exposure when diagnosing and treating depressive disorders. A major depressive episode includes having depressed/irritable mood or loss of interest or pleasure, for the same 2-week period for most of the day/nearly every day, along with at least 4 of the following symptoms:

1. Significant decreased or increased appetite with weight loss, or failure to make expected weight for developmental stage or weight gain
2. Insomnia or hypersomnia early every day
3. Psychomotor agitation or retardation
4. Fatigue or loss of energy
5. Feelings of worthlessness or inappropriate guilt
6. Poor concentration or indecision
7. Recurrent thoughts of death, suicidal ideation, plan, or attempt

   Core symptoms of a persistent depressive disorder (dysthymia) include having clinically significant depressed/irritable mood for 1 year or more along with at least 2 symptoms of depressive disorder or 1 symptom of depressive disorder and chronic feelings of hopelessness. Core symptoms of a disruptive mood dysregulation disorder (DMDD), include a period of 12 months or more of severe temper outbursts that are inconsistent with developmental stage and occur on average 2 to 3 times a week, along with persistent irritable mood in at least 2 settings.[1] Although there are few published studies on the incidence or prevalence of DMDD in maltreated youth, there is significant overlap of DMDD with oppositional defiant disorder (ODD) and attention-deficit/hyperactivity disorder (ADHD).[12] Some maltreatment researchers posit that DMDD is similar in clinical presentation to developmental trauma disorder, not present in the DSM-5, and may represent PTSD symptoms of reenactment and irritability.[13] There are no evidence-based treatments for either disorder, so treatment should focus on evidence-based treatments for depression along with PTSD, ODD, and ADHD, as appropriate.

ASSESSING MALTREATMENT AND TRAUMA IN YOUTH

Depressed maltreated youth should be assessed for current and past maltreatment experiences and other traumas. One method for asking about adverse experiences is to normalize the question as can be found in structured clinical interviews, which includes informing youth and parents separately that good and bad things happen to everyone and asking what each believes is the worst thing that happened in the youth's life and why. For young children, asking them to draw a picture of the best and worst things in their lives may be helpful. In maltreated youth, depression is commonly comorbid with PTSD, ODD, ADHD, separation anxiety disorder (particularly in cases of intimate partner violence toward primary caregiver) in children, as well as conduct disorder and alcohol use disorder (AUD) and SUD in adolescents. There are many structured clinical interviews (some are free of charge) and self-reports listed in **Table 1** that outline methods of asking questions about maltreatment, other adverse child experiences, and DSM-5 axis I disorders. In maltreated youth, multiple trauma exposures may be present. It is important to document the age of onset, duration, and offset of these events and identify the impact of these events on the child's emotional, cognitive, and behavioral development.

RISK FACTORS FOR DEPRESSION IN MALTREATED CHILDREN

Children of depressed parents have a 2-fold increased risk for depression and those with at least 1 parent and grandparent with depression are at highest risk.[14] Parental depression, PTSD, and SUDs increase the risk of having a child who is reported for maltreatment.[15] Other direct risk factors for depression in youth with high familial depression risk include irritability, fear behaviors, externalizing symptoms or anxiety before first depressive episode, economic disadvantage, and recent psychosocial adversity (eg, being bullied, death in family, parental conflict).[16] These risk factors for depression are commonly seen in maltreated youth.

REPORTING CHILD MALTREATMENT

When assessing the impact of potential maltreatment during a comprehensive clinical examination, it is important to first outline the limits of confidentiality. If a child or adolescent responds in the affirmative to the maltreatment or other traumatic stress questions, the clinician must follow up appropriately according to the clinical guidelines of the setting that the child is in and in full accordance with mandatory child abuse reporting laws. It is recommended that clinicians identify resources in the community to address any urgent concerns associated with trauma disclosure as part of setting up clinical services (eg, child abuse reporting lines, domestic violence shelters, emergency room access). In cases in which a clinician is mandated to report maltreatment, the youth's safety is the first concern. In most cases, clinicians can make a report in a transparent way. Reporting maltreatment after explaining the laws, the clinician's legal obligations, and the need for youth and family safety does not have to result in ending the clinician's treatment relationship with the youth and the family.

Table 1
Interviews and self-reports for assessment of diagnoses, maltreatment, and other traumatic experiences in children and adolescents

Measure	What It Assesses	Given to?	Age (y)	Where to Obtain the Measure
National Child Traumatic Stress Network Measure Review of assessment instruments	This user-friendly Web site lists a database for trauma-informed mental health screenings, assessments for clinicians to use with parents, children, and adolescents, including interviews and self-reports	Interviews and self-reports	Infancy to −18	https://www.nctsn.org/treatments-and-practices/screening-and-assessments/measure-reviews/all-measure-reviews
Diagnostic Infant and Preschool Assessment	Standardized assessment of 11 traumatic life events, PTSD, major depressive disorder, ADHD, separation anxiety disorder, and generalized anxiety disorder	Child's caregiver	Birth to 6	http://www.midss.org/sites/default/files/dipa_version_11_17_10.pdf
The Preschool Age Psychiatric Assessment	Structured interview that assesses different types of traumas and adverse life events, including various types of child abuse and neglect and the age at which each event was experienced, as well as developmentally sensitive version of PTSD and for diagnosing psychiatric disorders in preschool children	Child's caregiver	2–5	http://devepi.duhs.duke.edu/papa.html
Kiddie Schedule for Affective Disorders and Schizophrenia – Present and Lifetime Version for DSM-5	Semistructured interview that assesses 12 different types of trauma, including various types of child abuse and neglect and the age at which each event was experienced, as well as PTSD, and all major axis I disorders	Caregiver and youth as interview or computerized self-report	3–18	https://www.kennedykrieger.org/patient-care/faculty-staff/joan-kaufman

(continued on next page)

Table 1
(continued)

Measure	What It Assesses	Given to?	Age (y)	Where to Obtain the Measure
Child PTSD Symptom Scale for DSM-5	Self-report instrument or clinical interview that assesses DSM-5 symptoms for PTSD	Youth self-report or interview	7–18	https://www.ncbi.nlm.nih.gov/pubmed/28820616
UCLA PTSD Reaction Index for DSM-5	A comprehensive trauma history profile for many discrete forms of trauma, including abuse, neglect, bullying, and community violence, and the age at which each event was experienced. Includes a PTSD scale for DSM-5	Caregiver and youth as interview or self-report	7–18	https://www.reactionindex.com/index.php/
Trauma Symptom Checklist for Children	Self-report instrument that assesses PTSD and related problems, such as depressive, anxiety, and dissociative symptoms	Youth self-report	8–16	https://www.parinc.com/Products/Pkey/461
The Child and Adolescent Psychiatric Assessment	Structured interview that assesses different types of trauma and adverse life events, including various types of child abuse and neglect and the age at which each event was experienced, as well as PTSD and all major axis I disorders	Caregiver and youth interview	9–18	http://devepi.duhs.duke.edu/capa.html
Childhood Trauma overall mental health Questionnaire	Assesses childhood physical abuse, sexual abuse, emotional abuse, emotional neglect, and physical neglect	Youth self-report	12 to adulthood	http://www.pearsonclinical.com/psychology/products/100000446/childhood-trauma-questionnaire-a-retrospective-self-report-ctq.html

Abbreviation: UCLA, University of California, Los Angeles.

Youth may not disclose ongoing maltreatment until a therapeutic alliance is built, which may take place many months after treatment initiation. Educating caregivers and their youth about these systems and the urgent need for child safety usually leads to cooperation with CPS investigations and maintaining the youth and family in treatment.

ESTABLISHING THE DIAGNOSIS OF DEPRESSION AND TREATMENT PLAN

Depressed maltreated youth should be screened for symptom severity and assessed for safety pertaining to child abuse and neglect, suicide, and homicide, which could indicate the need for CPS/police involvement or a higher level of care. Clinicians can use the mood disorder sections of the interviews or depression, irritability or anxiety, self-reports, or other rating scales listed in **Table 1** to serve as a baseline that can be used to examine the effectiveness of the treatment plan. Hospitalization is a short-term stabilization strategy for youth whose level of function is severely impaired, who may be suicidal or homicidal (eg, secondary to severe irritability), who have depressive symptoms with psychosis, or would benefit from an inpatient environment because of unstable family support and inability to adhere to outpatient treatment.

Given that maltreated youth are more likely to have medical issues than nonmaltreated youth,[17] it is important for depressed youth to have a medical evaluation to rule out medical causes of depression. The American Academy of Child and Adolescent Psychiatry has a practice parameter for the assessment and treatment of children and adolescents with depressive disorders.[18] Medical disorders (eg, hypothyroidism, sleep disorders, mononucleosis, anemia, cancer, autoimmune diseases, premenstrual dysphoric disorder, chronic fatigue syndrome, vitamin deficiencies involving folic acid, and side effects of medications) should be ruled out as part of the treatment plan. If there is a history of physical abuse or head injury involving loss of consciousness, head computed tomography or MRI of the brain may be indicated to rule out an organic cause for depression. The medical evaluation can be completed as inpatient or outpatient depending on the youth's severity of depression and individual needs.

The treatment of depression is usually divided into 3 phases: acute, continuation, and maintenance.[18] The acute phase involves stabilization of dangerous behaviors, and initial evaluation, which includes an assessment of child maltreatment and other ongoing stressors, family support, family conflict, parental mental disorder, school function, and peer relationships. These factors should be assessed because they can contribute to persistence or desistence of depression and may need to be addressed in the youth's treatment. The aim of the acute phase is full remission of depression (a period of ≥ 2 weeks and < 2 months with no or few depressive symptoms) or recovery (a period of > 2 months with no depressive symptoms). Continuation treatment is required for depressed youths to secure a successful treatment response during the acute phase and prevent depression relapses. New stressors can put maltreated youth with a history of depression at high risk for relapse or recurrence of depression, including suicidal, homicidal, and self-injurious thoughts and behaviors. Maintenance treatment is used to prevent recurrences in youth who have had a more severe, recurrent, and chronic depressive disorder. Because maltreated youth are more likely to have a severe and recurrent form of depression with poor prognosis,[19] treatment planning should include all 3 phases, including psychotherapy that includes learning cognitive and behavioral strategies to manage ongoing stressors to prevent the recurrence of depression symptoms, including suicidality. **Fig. 1** represents a working guideline for the treatment of maltreated youth with depression.

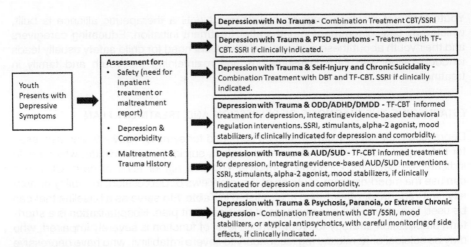

Fig. 1. Guideline for treating maltreated youth with depression. AUD, alcohol use disorder; CBT, cognitive behavioral therapy; DBT, dialectical behavior therapy; SUD, substance use disorder; TF-CBT, trauma-focused cognitive behavioral therapy.

COMBINED PSYCHOTHERAPY AND PSYCHOPHARMACOLOGY TREATMENT ARE THE EVIDENCE-BASED TREATMENTS FOR DEPRESSION IN YOUTH AND SHOULD BE THE FIRST APPROACH FOR MALTREATED DEPRESSED YOUTH

A landmark study, The Treatment for Adolescents with Depression Study (TADS), showed that, in adolescents (aged 12–17 years), combined treatment with fluoxetine (a selective serotonin reuptake inhibitor [SSRI]) and cognitive behavior therapy (CBT) with an 86% response rate, compared with 81% for fluoxetine alone and 81% for CBT alone, was judged to be superior to either treatment alone at 36 weeks after treatment initiation, and the combination treatment was also associated with decreased suicidal ideation compared with fluoxetine treatment alone.[20] Maltreated depressed youth in the TADS study showed better outcomes with combined treatment than with CBT alone.[21] According to a meta-analysis of 13 pediatric trials involving 3004 children and adolescents that examined the SSRIs fluoxetine, paroxetine, sertraline, citalopram, and escitalopram, SSRIs showed the greatest benefits within the first 4 weeks of treatment initiation and then had a smaller benefit compared with studies in adults thereafter.[22] Another meta-analysis compared 34 antidepressant trials, including 5260 children and adolescents and 14 antidepressant treatments (amitriptyline, citalopram, clomipramine, desipramine, duloxetine, escitalopram, fluoxetine, imipramine, mirtazapine, nefazodone, nortriptyline, paroxetine, sertraline, and venlafaxine) and found that only fluoxetine was statistically significantly more effective than placebo.[23] Fluoxetine was better tolerated and imipramine, venlafaxine, and duloxetine had more discontinuations because of adverse events compared with placebo.

The Treatment of SSRI-Resistant Depression in Adolescents (TORDIA) trial defined treatment-resistant depression as clinically significant depression that has not responded to acute treatment with a SSRI.[24] In this randomized controlled trial of a clinical sample of 334 patients aged 12 to 18 years with a primary diagnosis of major depressive disorder who had not responded to 2 months of SSRI treatment, patients were randomized to 12 weeks of (1) switch to a second, different SSRI (paroxetine, citalopram, or fluoxetine, 20–40 mg); (2) switch to a different SSRI plus CBT; (3) switch to venlafaxine (150–225 mg); or (4) switch to venlafaxine plus CBT. The combination of CBT and a switch to another antidepressant resulted in a higher rate of clinical response than did a medication switch alone, and venlafaxine was not tolerated as well as other SSRIs.[24] By 24 weeks, patients in the TORDIA study, who showed remission of depression, also showed reductions in symptoms of anxiety, ADHD, disruptive behavior disorders symptoms,[25] and parent-child conflict.[26] The patients with a history of physical abuse had a lower rate of response to combination treatment in the TORDIA study, and those without maltreatment histories showed the best outcomes.[27]

There are several evidence-based therapies for the treatment of depression: CBT, whose focus is on increasing behavioral activation and decreasing negative cognitive distortions; interpersonal psychotherapy, whose focus is on shifting the patient's outlook and interaction in key relationships and interpersonal life events; and supportive therapy. All show improvement in youth depression, with a moderate effect size.[28] Data from a recent meta-analysis of 13 randomized trials of 796 children and adolescents showed that computer-based and Internet-based cognitive behavioral treatments decreased anxiety and depressive symptoms and may be an attractive treatment alternative to regular face-to-face treatment.[29] Although all of these treatments have been used with maltreated youth with depression, maltreated youth are less likely to access psychotherapy resources and have more limited computer access than nonmaltreated youth.[30]

TREATMENT OF DEPRESSED MALTREATED YOUTH WITH POSTTRAUMATIC STRESS DISORDER SYMPTOMS

Child maltreatment becomes biologically embedded in the stress systems of its victims, leading to cognitive deficits, high rates of depression, PTSD, other mental disorders, immune dysregulation, and adverse brain development.[31–33] Clinicians may consider treating depressed maltreated youth with PTSD symptoms and an identified trauma with a trial of trauma-focused CBT (TF-CBT) as a first-line treatment. TF-CBT includes psychoeducation, learning parenting skills, relaxation training, affective modulation, cognitive restructuring, and behavioral coping skills. After these skills are mastered, trauma narration and processing to correct cognitive distortions and in vivo mastery of traumatic reminders are implemented. Then conjoint child and parent sessions and safety planning skills are addressed. A critical review suggests that TF-CBT is the best evidence-based treatment of maltreated youth.[34] Behavioral management strategies can easily be integrated with TF-CBT to treat the behavioral regulation problems that commonly occur in traumatized children (ADHD, ODD) (see Ref.[35]). Information about therapist training and certification in TF-CBT is available at https://tfcbt.org. The National Child Traumatic Stress Network Learning Collaboratives (NCTSN), whose mission is "to raise the standard of care and improve access to services for traumatized children, their families and communities throughout the United States" (www.nctsn.org) is an excellent trauma-informed resource for clinicians working with maltreated youth with depression. If depression is severe, SSRIs can be offered, with careful monitoring of suicidality.

TREATMENT OF DEPRESSED MALTREATED YOUTH WITH SELF-INJURY AND SUICIDALITY

Dialectical behavior therapy (DBT), a cognitive behavioral, evidence-based, multimodal, outpatient treatment that involves individual, group treatment, and life skills coaching, is effective for reducing self-injury and suicidality as well as depression and PTSD.[36] DBT was modified for adolescents with borderline personality disorder traits and was found to be more effective than enhanced usual care in reducing self-harm, suicidal ideation, and depression.[37] DBT is a promising treatment of maltreated adolescents with depression, self-injury, and suicidality.

TREATMENT OF DEPRESSED MALTREATED YOUTH WITH EXTERNALIZING DISORDERS

There are important evidence-based interventions for disruptive behavioral disorders and for antisocial behaviors in youth with early trauma (eg, multisystemic therapy[38]). The American Academy of Child and Adolescent Psychiatry established practice parameters for the assessment and treatment of children and adolescents with ADHD,[39] ODD, and conduct disorder.[40] Many of these interventions can be integrated into TF-CBT or evidence-based treatments for depression and undertaken concurrently as part of a community treatment approach. Psychostimulants have a moderate to large effect and the alpha-2 agonist, guanfacine, a small to moderate effect on oppositional behavior, conduct problems, and aggression in youth with ADHD, with and without ODD or conduct disorder.[41] Stimulants may improve mood and decrease irritability, outbursts, and DMDD symptoms.[42] The Center for Education and Research on Mental Health Therapeutics Treatment of Maladaptive Aggression in Youth consensus guidelines include the possibility of using second-generation antipsychotic medications for psychosis or severe aggression only after a comprehensive assessment, treatment as indicated for underlying disorders, in combination with evidence-based behavioral interventions and with regular monitoring and planned taper/discontinuation as soon as feasible.[43] Intensive case management may be necessary to address significant behavioral symptoms.

TREATMENT OF DEPRESSED MALTREATED YOUTH WITH ALCOHOL AND SUBSTANCE USE DISORDERS

Maltreatment is a strong risk factor for developing AUD and SUD in adolescents and adults.[44,45] Depression in maltreated youth is highly comorbid with AUD and SUD. It is important to ask about tobacco, alcohol, marijuana, and other drug use as described in the assessments outlined in **Table 1**. Adolescents may "self-medicate" symptoms (eg, sad/irritable mood, insomnia) of depression with substances. Toxicology tests are indicated in an assessment of depression if the clinician is concerned about AUD/SUD. The American Academy of Child and Adolescent Psychiatry has a practice parameter for the assessment and treatment of child and adolescents with substance use disorders.[46] This practice parameter has detailed descriptions on the types of formal screening tools that can be helpful in AUD/SUD assessment. These recommendations for the formal evaluation and the ongoing assessment of SUD include toxicologic tests of bodily fluids, such as urine, to detect the presence of specific substances. Toxicologic tests may assist in making a differential diagnosis because some substances (eg, cannabis, alcohol) may cause depressive symptoms and, once an individual is sober, the depression may remit. According to this practice parameter, treatment of AUD/SUD must be evidence based, should be done in the least restrictive setting that is safe and effective, should involve family/caregivers and family therapy, should be comprehensive (eg, including treatment of comorbid disorders, educational/vocational issues, or addressing legal issues), and may involve medications to treat cravings or the underlying depression that may have led to AUD/SUD.

Seeking Safety is an evidence-based treatment model that emphasizes safety, integration of trauma and AUD/SUD issues, coping skills, and hope, and consistently shows positive outcomes in adolescents and adults with interpersonal trauma histories.[47] If a depressed adolescent has these problems, then referral for this evidence-based treatment is appropriate. Further information can be sought at www.seekingsafety.org. A modified version of TF-CBT, Risk Reduction through Family Therapy, has been shown in a small randomized controlled trial to significantly reduce substance abuse and trauma symptoms in traumatized youth with significant substance use.[48]

FACTORS TO EXPLORE IF EVIDENCE-BASED TREATMENTS ARE NOT ALLEVIATING DEPRESSION IN MALTREATED YOUTH

Caregivers and youth may complain about ineffectiveness of medications that were previously effective. It is always important to reevaluate the target symptoms and differential diagnosis when this occurs. There are several possible reasons for treatment resistance:

1. Noncompliance with drug regimen as prescribed
2. Unrealistic expectations of what a medication will and will not do to change mood and behaviors
3. New onset of maltreatment or increase in chronic stressors that may lead to increased depression
4. Significant side effects, such as akathisia or sleepiness
5. A medical issue
6. Growth spurts/increased drug metabolism during adolescence may require dose increase
7. The need to change to another medication, drug class, or type of CBT may be indicated
8. PTSD/trauma symptoms that have not been addressed or that emerge during treatment

SUMMARY

This article outlines approaches for the treatment of depression in maltreated children and adolescents. At the time of this writing, combination treatment with SSRIs and CBT with a trauma-informed approach should be considered for depressed maltreated youth. Behavioral management can be integrated with TF-CBT to treat the externalizing disorders that commonly occur in maltreated depressed youth. However, randomized clinical trials of depressed maltreated youth are needed to make progress and help guide maltreated youth to recovery.

REFERENCES

1. American Psychiatric Association. Depressive disorders. In: Diagnostic and statistical manual of mental disorders: fifth edition. Arlington (VA): American Psychiatric Publishing; 2013. p. 155–88.
2. American Psychiatric Association. Mood disorders. In: Diagnostic and statistical manual of mental disorders: fourth edition text revision. Washington, DC: American Psychiatric Press; 2000. p. 345–428.
3. American Psychiatric Association. Trauma- and stressor-related disorders. In: Diagnostic and statistical manual of mental disorders: fifth edition. Arlington (VA): American Psychiatric Publishing; 2013. p. 265–90.
4. Leeb RT, Paulozzzi L, Melanson C, et al. Child maltreatment surveillance: uniform definitions for public Health and recommended data elements. Atlanta (GA): Centers for Disease Control and Prevention; 2008.

5. Petersen A, Joseph J, Feit M. Committee on child maltreatment research policy and practice for the next decade phase II board on children youth and families Institute of Medicine National Research Council new directions in child abuse and neglect research. Washington, DC: National Academy of Sciences The National Academies Press; 2013.

6. GAO (Government Accountability Office). Child maltreatment: strengthening national data on child fatalities could aid in prevention. Washington, DC: GAO; 2011.

7. Sedlak AJ, Mettenburg J, Basena M, et al. Fourth national incidence study of children abuse and neglect (NIS-4): report to congress. Washington, DC: U.S. Department of Health and Human Services, Administration for Children and Families; 2010.

8. Gilbert R, Widom CP, Browne K, et al. Burden and consequences of child maltreatment in high-income countries. Lancet 2009;373:68–81.

9. Mandelli L, Petrelli C, Serretti A. The role of specific early trauma in adult depression: a meta-analysis of published literature. Childhood trauma and adult depression. Eur Psychiatry 2015;30:665–80.

10. Paul E, Eckenrode J. Childhood psychological maltreatment subtypes and adolescent depressive symptoms. Child Abuse Negl 2015;47:38–47.

11. Widom CS, DuMont K, Czaja SJ. A prospective investigation of major depressive disorder and comorbidity in abused and neglected children grown up. Arch Gen Psychiatry 2007;64(1):49–56.

12. Freeman AJ, Youngstrom EA, Youngstrom JK, et al. Disruptive mood dysregulation disorder in a community mental health clinic: prevalence, comorbidity and correlates. J Child Adolesc Psychopharmacol 2016;26(2):123–30.

13. Ford JD, Spinazzola J, van der Kolk B, et al. Toward an empirically based developmental trauma disorder diagnosis for children: factor structure, item characteristics, reliability, and validity of the developmental trauma disorder semi-structured interview. J Clin Psychiatry 2018;79(5):17m11675.

14. Weissman MM, Berry OO, Warner V, et al. A 30-year study of 3 generations at high risk and low risk for depression. JAMA Psychiatry 2016;73(9):970–7.

15. De Bellis M, Broussard E, Wexler S, et al. Psychiatric co-morbidity in caregivers and children involved in maltreatment: a pilot research study with policy implications. Child Abuse Negl 2001;25:923–44.

16. Rice F, Sellers R, Hammerton G, et al. Antecedents of new-onset major depressive disorder in children and adolescents at high familial risk. JAMA Psychiatry 2017;74(2):153–60.

17. Smith DK, Johnson AB, Pears KC, et al. Child maltreatment and foster care: unpacking the effects of prenatal and postnatal parental substance use. Child Maltreat 2007;12:150.

18. Birmaher B, Brent D, Bernet W, et al. Practice parameter for the assessment and treatment of children and adolescents with depressive disorders. J Am Acad Child Adolesc Psychiatry 2007;46(11):1503–26.

19. Nanni V, Uher R, Danese A. Childhood maltreatment predicts unfavorable course of illness and treatment outcome in depression: a meta-analysis. Am J Psychiatry 2012;169:141–51.

20. The TADS Team. The treatment for adolescents with depression study (TADS) long-term effectiveness and safety outcomes. Arch Gen Psychiatry 2007; 64(10):1132–44.

21. Lewis CC, Simons AD, Nguyen LJ, et al. Impact of childhood trauma on treatment outcome in the treatment for adolescents with depression study (TADS). J Am Acad Child Adolesc Psychiatry 2010;49(2):132–40.
22. Varigonda AL, Jakubovski E, Taylor MJ, et al. Systematic review and meta-analysis: early treatment responses of selective serotonin reuptake inhibitors in pediatric major depressive disorder. J Am Acad Child Adolesc Psychiatry 2015;54(7):557–64.
23. Cipriani A, Furukawa TA, Salanti G, et al. Comparative efficacy and acceptability of 21 antidepressant drugs for the acute treatment of adults with major depressive disorder: a systematic review and network meta-analysis. Lancet 2018; 391(10128):1357–66.
24. Brent D, Emslie G, Clarke G, et al. Switching to another SSRI or to venlafaxine with or without cognitive behavioral therapy for adolescents with SSRI-resistant depression: the TORDIA randomized controlled trial. JAMA 2008;299(8):901–13.
25. Hilton RC, Rengasamy M, Mansoor B, et al. Impact of treatments for depression on comorbid anxiety, attentional, and behavioral symptoms in adolescents with selective serotonin reuptake inhibitor-resistant depression. J Am Acad Child Adolesc Psychiatry 2013;52(5):482–92.
26. Rengasamy M, Mansoor BM, Hilton R, et al. The bi-directional relationship between parent-child conflict and treatment outcome in treatment-resistant adolescent depression. J Am Acad Child Adolesc Psychiatry 2013;52(4):370–7.
27. Shamseddeen W, Asarnow JR, Clarke G, et al. Impact of physical and sexual abuse on treatment response in the treatment of resistant depression in adolescent study (TORDIA). J Am Acad Child Adolesc Psychiatry 2011;50(3):293–301.
28. Weisz JR, McCarty CA, Valeri SM. Effects of psychotherapy for depression in children and adolescents: a meta-analysis. Psychol Bull 2006;132(1):132–49.
29. Ebert DD, Zarski AC, Christensen H, et al. Internet and computer-based cognitive behavioral therapy for anxiety and depression in youth: a meta-analysis of randomized controlled outcome trials. PLoS One 2015;10(3):e0119895.
30. Fang X, Brown DS, Florence CS, et al. The economic burden of child maltreatment in the United States and implications for prevention. Child Abuse Negl 2012;36(2):156–65.
31. De Bellis MD, Hooper SR, Chen SD, et al. Posterior structural brain volumes differ in maltreated youth with and without chronic posttraumatic stress disorder. Dev Psychopathol 2015;27:1555–76.
32. De Bellis MD, Zisk A. The biological effects of childhood trauma. In: Cozza SJ, Cohen JA, Dougherty JG, editors. Child and adolescent psychiatric clinics of North America: disaster and trauma, vol. 23. Philadelphia: Elsevier; 2014. p. 185–222.
33. Morey RA, Haswell CC, Hooper SR, et al. Amygdala, Hippocampus, and ventral medial prefrontal cortex volumes differ in maltreated youth with and without chronic posttraumatic stress disorder. Neuropsychopharmacology 2016;41: 791–801.
34. Leenarts LE, Diehle J, Doreleijers TA, et al. Evidence-based treatments for children with trauma-related psychopathology as a result of childhood maltreatment: a systematic review. Eur Child Adolesc Psychiatry 2013;22(5):269–83.
35. Cohen JA, Berliner L, Mannarino A. Trauma focused CBT for children with co-occurring trauma and behavior problems. Child Abuse Negl 2010;34(4):215–24.
36. Harned MS, Korslund KE, Linehan MM. A pilot randomized controlled trial of dialectical behavior therapy with and without the dialectical behavior therapy

prolonged exposure protocol for suicidal and self-injuring women with borderline personality disorder and PTSD. Behav Res Ther 2014;55:7–17.

37. Mehlum L, Tormoen AJ, Ramberg M, et al. Dialectical behavior therapy for adolescents with repeated suicidal and self-harming behavior: a randomized trial. J Am Acad Child Adolesc Psychiatry 2014;53(10):1082–91.

38. Curtis NM, Ronan KR, Borduin CM. Multisystemic treatment: a meta-analysis of outcome studies. J Fam Psychol 2004;18(3):411–9.

39. Dulcan M. Practice parameters for the assessment and treatment of children, adolescents, and adults with attention-deficit/hyperactivity disorder. American Academy of Child and Adolescent Psychiatry. J Am Acad Child Adolesc Psychiatry 1997;36(10 Suppl):85s–121s.

40. Steiner H. Practice parameters for the assessment and treatment of children and adolescents with conduct disorder. American Academy of Child and Adolescent Psychiatry. J Am Acad Child Adolesc Psychiatry 1997;36(10 Suppl):122s–39s.

41. Pringsheim T, Hirsch L, Gardner D, et al. The pharmacological management of oppositional behaviour, conduct problems, and aggression in children and adolescents with attention-deficit hyperactivity disorder, oppositional defiant disorder, and conduct disorder: a systematic review and meta-analysis. Part 1: psychostimulants, alpha-2 agonists, and atomoxetine. Can J Psychiatry 2015; 60(2):42–51.

42. Baweja R, Belin PJ, Humphrey HH, et al. The effectiveness and tolerability of central nervous system stimulants in school-age children with attention-deficit/hyperactivity disorder and disruptive mood dysregulation disorder across home and school. J Child Adolesc Psychopharmacol 2016;26(2):154–63.

43. Rosato N, Correll CU, Pappadopulos E, et al. Treatment of maladaptive aggression in youth: CERT guidelines II. Treatments and ongoing management. Pediatrics 2012;129(6):e1577–86.

44. Carliner H, Gary D, McLaughlin KA, et al. Trauma exposure and externalizing disorders in adolescents: results from the National Comorbidity Survey Adolescent Supplement. J Am Acad Child Adolesc Psychiatry 2017;56(9):755–64.

45. De Bellis MD. Developmental traumatology: a contributory mechanism for alcohol and substance use disorders. Psychoneuroendocrinology 2001;27:155–70.

46. Bukstein OG, Work Group on Quality Issues. Practice parameter for the assessment and treatment of children and adolescents with substance use disorders. J Am Acad Child Adolesc Psychiatry 2005;44(6):609–21.

47. Najavits LM, Hien D. Helping vulnerable populations: a comprehensive review of the treatment outcome literature on substance use disorder and PTSD. J Clin Psychol 2013;69(5):433–79.

48. Danielson CK, McCart M, Walsh K, et al. Reducing substance use risk and mental health problems among sexually assaulted adolescents: a pilot randomized controlled trial. J Fam Psychol 2012;26:628–35.

Depression in Medically Ill Children and Adolescents

Nasuh Malas, MD, MPH[a,b,]*, Sigita Plioplys, MD[c],
Maryland Pao, MD[d]

KEYWORDS

- Depression • Pediatrics • Child • Adolescent • Physically ill • Medically ill

KEY POINTS

- Clinicians should have early awareness of depression in medically ill youth.
- Developmental, psychological, biological, and familial risk factors contribute to the unique presentation of depression in medically ill youth.
- Depression in this population can result from a primary depressive disorder, poor adjustment to medical illness, and/or directly from the medical illness.
- Multidisciplinary collaboration across all care settings, with awareness of potential bidirectional interactions between physical and mental health, is important in the care of depression in medically ill youth.
- Depression treatment in medically ill youth requires understanding of other unique medical and psychiatric needs of a given patient and being flexible to adapt care based on an evolving medical course, adjustments in medical treatment, and response to psychotherapeutic and pharmacologic interventions.

INTRODUCTION

Pediatric medical illness is increasing in developed countries and affects more than 25% of youth in the United States.[1] The increase is multifactorial and influenced by environmental toxin exposure, changes in lifestyle, dietary practices, psychosocial stressors, and advances in medical technologies.[1–3] Although most medically ill youth

This article originally appeared in *Child and Adolescent Psychiatric Clinics*, Volume 28, Issue 3, July 2019.
[a] Department of Psychiatry, University of Michigan Medical School, Ann Arbor, MI, USA;
[b] Department of Pediatrics and Communicable Diseases, University of Michigan Medical School, Ann Arbor, MI, USA; [c] Department of Child and Adolescent Psychiatry, Ann and Robert H. Lurie Children's Hospital of Chicago, Feinberg School of Medicine, Northwestern University, 225 East Chicago Avenue Box# 10, Chicago, IL 60611, USA; [d] Intramural Research Program, National Institutes of Health, National Institute of Mental Health, Clinical Research Center, NIH Building 10, CRC East 6-5340, MSC 1276, Bethesda, MD 20892-1276, USA
* Corresponding author. C.S. Mott Children's Hospital, University of Michigan Health System, 1500 East Medical Center Drive, UH South, F6315, Ann Arbor, MI 48109.
E-mail address: nmalas@med.umich.edu

are resilient and function well, illness effects can worsen daily functioning, self-esteem, mood, and quality of life, with systemic impacts on family and schooling.[3–5] The relationship between medical illness and depression is bidirectional, with medical illness being a risk factor for depression.[4,5] Depression may increase treatment non-adherence, worsen physical disease, and lead to poor functioning, greater health care use, and increased school absenteeism.[3,6,7]

This article focuses on early identification, assessment, diagnosis, and management of medically ill youth with comorbid depression. It highlights specific considerations related to unique medical disease contributors to the presentation and management of depression with examples from common pediatric medical disorders in which depression is prevalent. The article highlights the importance of collaborative and integrative care while understanding the unique biopsychosocial factors influencing each child's presentation.

SPECIFIC RISKS FOR DEPRESSION IN MEDICALLY ILL YOUTH
Developmental Factors

The experience of medical illness and expression of depression is affected by the child's developmental stage (**Fig. 1**). Caution should be taken to not overidentify depressive symptoms in emotionally healthy youth with normative negative reactions to medical illness. However, vegetative symptoms accompanied by hopelessness,

Preschool Age:
- Limited understanding of illness, care, and environment
- Often misperceive physical disease as punishment
- Respond to medical treatment with behavioral changes, increased irritability, tantrums, and defiance that may be short-lived
  - Prolonged symptoms with associated changes in child's mood, may suggest emergence of depression

School Age:
- Understand physical factors result in generation of disease
- May worry about bodily harm, loss of control of either their body or their environment
- Chronic worry can result in feeling overwhelmed and may progress to depression

Adolescents:
- More abstract and nuanced understanding of physical disease and relationship between physical and emotional health
- Experience uncertainty around emerging physical symptoms while undergoing diagnostic assessment
  - Can result in hypervigilance, somatization and psychological distress
- Can be devastated by initial delivery of diagnosis with mixed emotions including disbelief, anger, sadness, anxiety and detachment

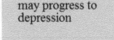

Fig. 1. Development factors influencing depression in medically ill youth.

guilt, and low self-esteem need to be thoroughly evaluated for possible subsyndromal depression or major depressive disorder.

Biological Factors

Most medical illnesses have clinical manifestations that can mimic, overlap, or exacerbate depressive illnesses. Medications, particularly immunomodulators, anticonvulsants, antibiotics, anticholinergics, opioids, and benzodiazepines, can all directly affect the presentation of depression and should be carefully reviewed. Depressive symptoms can be a harbinger of emerging medical illnesses such as hypothyroidism, autoimmune encephalitis, anemia, catatonia, or delirium. The severity of medical illnesses is directly correlated with depression risk.[8,9] Depression can also affect medical illness course through direct neuroendocrine and inflammatory pathways.[8,10,11]

Psychosocial Factors

Medically ill youth with preexisting maladaptive coping, anxious temperament, poor self-esteem, poor premorbid functioning, history of trauma, and limited social supports have increased risk of depression.[8] Missed school and illness-related social isolation can generate a sense of loss, loneliness, and feelings of guilt or hopelessness. Medical illness can result in youth perceiving themselves as different or deficient. This perception can lead to avoidant behavior that diminishes further risk of anticipated emotional, psychological, or physical harm, which may result in rejection and a poor self-concept. Medically ill youth are also more likely to be bullied because of their physical appearance, functional limitations, or psychological vulnerabilities, which can perpetuate further physical and emotional insult.[12]

Family Factors

Medical illness can have dramatic effects on family functioning and result in disruptions in family life, loss of relational and financial stability, and impaired parenting. Primary caregivers can be particularly vulnerable to the distress of observing their child impaired or in discomfort.[5] The child's helplessness and worry can engender a variety of responses from the primary caregiver, ranging from avoidance to hypervigilance and overprotection. However, parents may underestimate the impact of physical disease on the child, and underreport the presence of depression. Similarly, parents often overfocus on the medical illness management and do not recognize changes in the child's mood. These strong emotions, coupled with physical exhaustion and difficulty juggling multiple competing roles, can result in caregiver burnout and increased risk of parental depression or anxiety.[13] Parents of medically ill youth have a higher prevalence of depression that further affects their parenting and emotional availability.[5] Furthermore, sibling well-being can be neglected while focusing of the care of medically ill youth, leading to increased family and sibling conflict.[14]

IDENTIFICATION AND ASSESSMENT

Astute clinicians have a high index of suspicion for depressive symptoms early and often in medically ill youth.

- Detailed understanding of medical disease course, medication use, and past medical experiences should be thoroughly explored.
- Prudent assessment involves obtaining information from multiple sources longitudinally, and strategic use of screening instruments.
- Important to engage child's primary care provider (PCP) and other subspecialists to understand direct and indirect influences of medical illness on child's mood.

Parents of medically ill children can have strong biases and misattribute emerging mood symptoms to medical illness or its treatment. Medically ill youth with depression may show greater somatization, poor insight, maladaptive coping, and habituation to responding to emotional distress through physical symptoms.[3,6] Therefore, the child's general clinical presentation and diagnostic conceptualization should be regularly reviewed and revised while incorporating new, relevant medical information.

Screening

Medically ill youth may be naive to discussions of their emotional and behavioral health in the medical setting. Routine depression screening can normalize conversations regarding depressive symptoms. Screening can aid in monitoring depressive symptom evolution and response to intervention over time. Several professional pediatric organizations recommend routine screening for depression in medically ill youth, particularly adolescents, including the American Academy of Pediatrics, American Academy of Child and Adolescent Psychiatry, International Committee on Mental Health in Cystic Fibrosis, American Diabetes Association, American College of Gastroenterology, US Preventive Services Task Force, American Diabetes Association, and the Child Neurology Society.[15–21] Several depression screening instruments are available that are well suited for use with medically ill youth (**Table 1**).

Differential Diagnosis

Depressive symptoms in medically ill youth can originate from 3 causes, either in isolation or more commonly in combination:

- Poor adjustment to medical illness
- Primary depressive disorder
- Medical illness, and/or treatment, directly inducing depressive symptoms

Establishing the relative contribution of these 3 sources to a child's mood presentation is important to diagnosis and management. Maladjustment and depression stemming from persistent difficulty coping with medical illness can lead to behavioral regression characterized by separation anxiety, treatment nonadherence, frequent deference to family, withdrawal from normal activities and routines, social avoidance, and dramatic displays of emotion and behavior.[3,15] Grief and traumatic loss in the setting of lost functioning or terminal illness can compound depression in medically ill youth.[26]

It is important to recognize difficulty with illness-related adjustment early to prevent progression to a major depressive disorder. Differentiation between adjustment disorder and primary depression can be challenging, requiring an exploration of past psychiatric history and the timing of mood symptom development. Poor self-esteem, hopelessness, anhedonia, guilt, suicidal ideation/behavior, and the pervasiveness of mood symptoms over time are more typical of primary depression, particularly if they precede a medical illness.[27] Negative emotions and behavioral changes specific to a medical illness burden also distinguish adjustment disorder from depression. Youth experiencing difficulties adjusting generally do not have underlying issues with self-esteem.[26] Poor adjustment and potential progression to depression is influenced by disease burden, cognitive effects related to disease, psychosocial supports, bullying and psychological trauma, as well as the ability of the child and family to balance the competing and parallel processes of grief and survival in chronic illness.[26] Family history of depression may also suggest current primary depression.[3]

Table 1
Depression screening instruments

Name	Description	Content (%)	Cost
Patient Health Questionnaire-9	Most commonly used screening tool in the pediatric medical setting because of easy completion and scoring	Sensitivity: 89.5 Specificity: 77.5	Free
Patient Health Questionnaire-2	Very brief, 2-question screen with greater sensitivity and less specificity for busy practice	—	Free
Children's Depression Rating Scale Revised	Focuses on specific symptoms of depression, helps in distinguishing primary depressive disorder from depression related to medical illness	—	$2.50 per scale, $76.00 for manual
Children's Depression Inventory	Anhedonia subscale can be useful in early identification of depression, and subclinical manifestations in medical settings	Sensitivity: 83 Specificity: 83	$3–4 dollars per scale, $92.00 for manual
Abbreviated Children's Depression Inventory	10-item version	Sensitivity: 93 Specificity: 70	—
Hospital Anxiety and Depression Screen	14-item self-administered instrument designed to minimize the symptoms that might be ascribed to somatic disorders such as dizziness, insomnia, and fatigue	—	Not free

Data from Refs.[22–25]

Depressive symptoms can also arise from the direct pathophysiologic effects of medical illness and/or its treatment.[9,10] In these cases, depression onset is temporally associated with the medical illness development or its treatment.

SPECIFIC MEDICAL ILLNESS CONSIDERATIONS

Summarized in **Table 2** are epidemiologic and risk factors, disease-specific evaluation considerations, and evidence-based depression management strategies for youth with common pediatric medical illnesses.

TREATMENT
Non-pharmacologic Interventions

Education of the child, family, and within interdisciplinary teams is critical early and often in managing depression in medically ill youth (**Box 1**). Building off routine education and communication, psychotherapy is fundamental to the management of

Table 2
Specific considerations in the evaluation and management of depression in common pediatric medical illnesses

Disease	Prevalence of Depression (%)	Risk Factors	Evaluation and Management
Asthma	27–45[28,29]	• Need for regular asthma maintenance treatment, white race, tobacco smoke, poor family functioning, increased psychosocial stress associated with increased depression risk[29,33,34]	• SSRIs can alleviate depression and directly target asthma potentially through immunosuppression and anticholinergic regulation[35,36] • Asthma-related cholinergic dysregulation directly affects depression pathophysiology through downstream effects on neuronal nicotinic acetylcholine receptors[30,31] • Asthma and depression each independently associated with proinflammatory states with bidirectional impact[32]

Cystic fibrosis	8–29[13,37]	• 2–3 times greater depression risk than community with greatest risk in women, those with hemoptysis or pneumothorax in past 6 mo, comorbid anxiety, and parents with mental illness[13]
		• Depression associated with decreased lung function, lower body mass index, poor treatment adherence, worse quality of life, frequent hospitalizations, longer length of hospital stay, increased mortality following lung transplant, and increased health care costs[7,13,18]
			• Consensus statements for screening and treatment of depression published by The International Committee on Mental Health in Cystic Fibrosis, the Cystic Fibrosis Foundation, and European Cystic Fibrosis Society[18,38]
			  ○ Antidepressant medication, namely SSRIs, should be prescribed jointly with psychological interventions for moderate to severe depression
			  ○ To reduce drug-drug interactions, prescribers should be informed of all daily, cycled, or as-needed medications, including linezolid, an antibiotic that acts as a mild monoamine oxidase inhibitor and that should be used cautiously with SSRIs

Congenital heart disease	9–33[39,40]	• Depression risk increased with female gender, older age, poor social support, disease severity, lower IQ, low education level, presence of more than 1 cardiac defect, cyanotic disease, moderate to severe residual lesions, coexisting CNS abnormalities, and a history of more than 1 cardiac catheterization[39–42]	• Although there are no specific psychological interventions for this population, general psychotherapeutic intervention and SSRI use is safe and preferably provided in specialized, multidisciplinary service settings[43,44]
Epilepsy	22–35[45–47]	• Presence of depression results in more complicated epilepsy course[45–47] • Female gender, academic impairment, poor socialization, younger age at seizure onset and longer duration of epilepsy, unpredictability and high frequency of seizures, antiepileptic medications, and direct seizure effects on brain function[45,46] • Depressed youth with epilepsy have increased suicide risk compared with depressed physically healthy peers[45]	• SSRIs and SNRIs are safe and effective medications for treatment of depression[48] • Immediate-release bupropion has a higher risk for seizures (0.4%) than extended-release bupropion (0.1%) at total daily doses of 300–450 mg and should be avoided in this patient population[49]

(continued on next page)

Table 2
(continued)

Disease	Prevalence of Depression (%)	Risk Factors	Evaluation and Management
DM	30[50]	• Adolescents with type 2 DM may be at higher risk for depression compared with type 1 DM[51] • Increased depression risk with disease chronicity, dietary restrictions, stigma, DM management regimen, and need for close family involvement increases risk of psychosocial distress and depression[50,52] • Depression can lead to worse glycemic control, treatment nonadherence, increased frequency and duration of hospitalization, and higher rates of diabetic ketoacidosis[53]	• Clinical course of early DM can overlap with depression, including fatigue, irritability, poor concentration, and psychomotor agitation • Early depressive symptoms may be attributed to DM symptoms, so youth with DM should be screened and monitored for depression early and regularly, particularly because youth with DM are at increased risk of suicidal ideation and self-injurious behavior compared with physically healthy peers with depression[52,54] • Depression treatment positively affects mood, glycemic control, and DM course[55] • Psychosocial interventions, namely CBT and supportive therapy, are effective in improving depression and hemoglobin A1c levels in youth with diabetes compared with treatment as usual or psychoeducation alone[55,56] • Fluoxetine and sertraline show improvements in glycemic control and depression[57] • Bupropion is promising in addressing both depression and glycemic control[55] • Cost-effective stepped care and multimodal collaborative interventions, such as the Pathways Intervention and IMPACT are available for youth with diabetes[55]

| Obesity | >35[58,59] | • Sleep disturbance, fatigue, apathy, and sedentary behavior have synergistic and compounding effects on the progression of obesity and depression[60]
• Risk factors for depression are female gender, extent of body fat, HPA axis activation, increased cortisol level, and chronic stress[58,61,62]
• Both depression and obesity promote relative systemic proinflammatory state with release of interleukin-6 and effects on HPA[60]
• Obesity can result in lower quality of life, social difficulties and stigma, poor self-perception, suicidal thoughts and attempts, bullying, comorbid mental disorder, and depression in adulthood[61]
• Emotional eating to cope with negative emotions and depression affects development of obesity[63] | • No current formal recommendations for evaluation and treatment of depression in obese youth[64]
• National Institute of Mental Health 2009 report emphasizes need for increased study of associations and treatments in care of obese youth with depression[65]
• Most recent expert guidelines for pediatric obesity published in 1998 are directed at PCPs and recommend use of Primary Care Evaluation of Mental Disorders questionnaire and Children's Depression Inventory for screening[64]
  ○ Recommends screening for depression and psychological intervention if identified. Recommendations affirmed in 2011 Expert Panel on Integrated Guidelines for Cardiovascular Disease in Children and Adolescents[66]
• SSRIs can be effective in depression treatment but may increase abdominal obesity (OR = 1.4) and hypercholesterolemia (OR = 1.36) [67] |

(continued on next page)

Table 2
(continued)

Disease	Prevalence of Depression (%)	Risk Factors	Evaluation and Management

CA	Up to 33[68,69]	• Uncertainty in CA disease course and outcomes with lingering prospect of future morbidity and mortality increases risk for depression[70,71]
		
		• Depression leads to greater health care use, longer hospital stays, greater recidivism, and increased morbidity[11]
			• Both CA and depression can present with poor appetite, weight loss, fatigue, low energy, amotivation, irritability, and insomnia[68]
			
			• CA pathophysiology and treatments can have direct impact on depression development[68,69]
			
			• Regular screening for early depression symptoms is recommended with well-validated approaches, including the Distress Thermometer and the PAT[72]
			
			• Pediatric Preventive Psychosocial Health Model uses public health framework and uses PAT, which stratifies patients based on risk with matched treatment strategies[73]
			  ○ Most families have temporary distress and minimal risk with sufficient resources to cope and adapt to disease
			  ○ Smaller group of families are high risk and require multimodal, intensive, evidence-based treatments
			
			• Psychosocial, psychotherapeutic, and pharmacologic interventions are efficacious in depression treatment in patients with cancer[74]
			
			• Psychotherapy may be only therapeutic intervention needed for milder forms of depression
			  ○ Psychoeducation, CBT, relaxation strategies, and problem solving are efficacious[75]

o Supportive-expressive psychotherapy may aid in processing grief and loss in terminal illness[76]

o Other beneficial evidence-based therapies include meaning-centered group therapy, dignity therapy, mindfulness-based meditation[77–79]

• SSRIs are effective in moderate to severe depression, or for those who do not respond to psychotherapy alone[74]

o Depression treatment must be guided by limiting side effects and targeting comorbid somatic complaints such as poor appetite, disturbed sleep, fatigue, pain, and hot flashes

o Sertraline, escitalopram, and citalopram have fewest drug-drug interactions and a low potential side effect burden[80]

• Second-generation neuroleptics, such as quetiapine or olanzapine, may be used for symptom palliation; eg, sleep and nausea respectively, mitigating delirium risk, and adjunctive depression management[81]

o Requires caution because of potential adverse and long-term metabolic effects

• Mirtazapine can promote sleep regulation, reduce nausea, and improve appetite[81]

• Stimulants can be used in palliative setting, or in youth without enteral access but who can tolerate transdermal medication transmission, to address depressive symptoms given their rapid onset of action[74]

(continued on next page)

Table 2
(continued)

Disease	Prevalence of Depression (%)	Risk Factors	Evaluation and Management
IBD	10–25[8,82–85]	• Illness-related effects, such as lifelong IBD course with frequent relapses, colonic resection and diverting ostomies, abdominal pain, physical discomfort, worsening inflammation, and sleep disturbances are risk factors for depression[8,82–86] • Depression risk most significant after IBD onset, with 5-fold increase in first year of disease onset compared with general population[85,86] • Little differentiation in depression risk between ulcerative colitis, Crohn, or mixed disease[86] • Loss of control and poor self-perception can lead to stigma and increased risk for depression[85,86] • Youth with hopelessness, tearfulness, and suicidal ideation have longer IBD duration, more ostomies, and greater pain[83] • Depression, maladaptive coping and heightened somatization worsen visceral hypersensitivity, abdominal pain, IBD disease activity, and are more predictive of physical symptom development than many medical variables[82,87]	• Even after illness remission, depression risk is increased because of disruptions in daily life, family dysfunction, poor self-perception, disfigurement or disability, and worries about CA recurrence[71] • High risk of suicidal ideation and behavior with as many as 22% of subjects in 1 cohort endorsing lethality[82,83] • Treatment with steroids and immunosuppressants can worsen mood, increase fatigue, and disturb sleep, but can also improve depression through improvement in underlying medical illness[83,84] • Supportive therapy and CBT show significant reductions in depression and in IBD disease activity, leading to decreased hospital stay and use of intensive medical services and testing, with improved quality of life and adaptive coping, school attendance, and parental response to the child's physical symptoms[82,84] • SSRIs are safe in the treatment of depression[82]

| Chronic pain and pain-related disorders | 24[88,89] | • Particularly high risk in illnesses with prominent pain component (eg, SCD), in which prevalence of depression can be as high as 46%.[88,89]
　○ Youth with SCD and depression have more acute vasoocclusive pain crises, acute chest syndrome–related visits, end-organ complications, greater health care use with higher SCD-related costs[89]
• Pain causes considerable social and physical dysfunction, disruption to family interactions, and psychological distress leading to increased health use, disability, depression, and anxiety[90]
• Pain-related impairment is associated with older pediatric age, multiple locations of pain, increased hospitalization, and presence of depression[88]
• Level of pain acceptance, catastrophizing and other cognitive distortions, and functional disability all strongly correlate to manifestation of depression[91] | • Psychological therapies have moderate beneficial effects on reducing pain intensity, small benefit on pain-related disability, and variable benefit for depression, with particular benefits seen in youth with musculoskeletal pain and depression[90]
• CBT, acceptance and commitment therapy are efficacious for pediatric chronic pain and depression in which pain impairment beliefs and pain reactivity are mediating psychological factors affecting treatment outcomes[90,92]
• Dose-dependent psychotherapeutic improvements in headache are seen, whereas dose effects are not seen in other pain-related presentations[90]
• Youth with SCD often receive suboptimal treatment of comorbid depression, with up to 80% never receiving antidepressant medication[89]
　○ SSRIs more commonly used in this population, with SNRIs being used at an increasing rate for potential dual benefit in targeting neuropathic pain[89] |

(continued on next page)

Table 2
(continued)

Disease	Prevalence of Depression (%)	Risk Factors	Evaluation and Management

Transplant	35[93]	• Youth with liver transplant show worse total physical, emotional, social, and school functioning than healthy controls or peers with diabetes or cancer[94]
		• Poor medication adherence in solid organ transplant recipients associated with depression, anxiety, and posttraumatic stress[95,96]
		• Depression can worsen quality of life and adherence to immunosuppressive therapies, and result in youth engaging in high-risk behaviors directly affecting pretransplant and posttransplant course, including tobacco use, illicit drug use, poor adherence to dietary regimens, and poor exercise[97]
			• CBT, social support groups, exercise, and music therapy are all beneficial in youth with end-stage renal disease and transplant[98]
			• SSRIs are safe with cautious dosing because of absorption and end-organ effects[98,99]
			  ○ In liver failure, drug bioavailability may increase because of portosystemic shunting and doses may need to be decreased
			  ○ In peripheral edema with increased volume distribution, dosages may need to be increased
			  ○ Hepatic and renal metabolism may disrupt clearance of drugs, often requiring downward titration of dosing
			  ○ Citalopram and escitalopram have least risk of drug-drug interactions, but carry higher risk of QT prolongation[99,100]

Abbreviations: CA, cancer; CBT, cognitive behavior therapy; CNS, central nervous system; DM, diabetes mellitus; HPA, hypothalamic-pituitary-adrenal; IBD, inflammatory bowel disease; IMPACT, improving mood promoting access to collaborative treatment; IQ, intelligence quotient; OR, odds ratio; PAT, psychosocial assessment tool; SCD, sickle cell disease; SNRIs, serotonin norepinephrine reuptake inhibitors; SSRIs, selective serotonin reuptake inhibitors.

Box 1
Core components to effective education in care for medically ill youth with depression

Youth
- Developmentally informed
- Collaborative
- Consistent
- Include relevant medical and mental health providers
- Provided in time and setting when child comfortable and safe
- Use pictures, models, play, and toys to assist education delivery
- Language should be concrete, simple, succinct, familiar, nonthreatening

Families
- Can deliver simultaneously or independently to family depending on nature and complexity of communications
  - Avoid communications with significant uncertainty with patient alone because these communications often need to occur with the caregivers first before delivering to the patient and family
- Gear familial education to literacy level, language, culture, and level of understanding of the family
- Routinely check for caregiver understanding of child's physical disease and emotional state
  - Important to assess caregiver understanding of impact of disease on child's physical, social, and emotional functioning

Interdisciplinary team
- Highly important but often missed
- Many members of care team may have limited or differential understanding of interactions between child's mental health and medical illness
- Can be valuable to have routine multidisciplinary rounds or case conferences
- Education is an important component of mental health consultation to the primary medical team
- Highly encouraged to have regular interdisciplinary education to improve awareness of the complex interplay between medical and mental health needs

---

depression in medically ill youth. It is particularly important given the value of adaptive coping and the potential intolerance to psychiatric medications in this population.

Providing psychotherapies in medically ill youth can be challenging. Mental health clinicians must be able to tolerate frequent disruptions to psychotherapeutic interventions caused by fluctuations in medical illness course, particularly medical hospitalizations, which can be chaotic and potentially traumatic.[101] This ability requires strong collaborative communication between mental health and medical providers, as well as flexibility in mental health treatment structure, planning, and goals. The psychotherapeutic relationship may be especially important in reinforcing patient and family values in biopsychosocial treatments, as well as supporting end-of-life discussions when medical treatment is ineffective in stemming disease.[102]

Treatment recommendations for medically ill depressed youth need to be tailored to the individual child and family's needs. Clinicians first need to determine the depression severity and potential biopsychosocial contributors because these will inform the types of treatments recommended. Psychotherapeutic interventions should be provided early and often, even during diagnostic evaluations. Beyond the importance of psychotherapy for depression treatment in general, there is added importance in medically ill youth because psychopharmacologic interventions may not be indicated or tolerated because of young age, medical comorbidities, and/or serious drug-drug interactions.

In addition to addressing physical symptoms that may overlap with depression, stepwise psychotherapeutic approaches include supporting and building adaptive coping skills, psychoeducation, and recommending specific individual, familial, environmental, educational, and recreational supports. Nonpharmacologic interventions include teaching patients simple, concrete, and actionable behavioral strategies and coping skill activities targeting disease, pain, discomfort, and associated distorted cognitions, strong emotions, and maladaptive behaviors. This process usually involves challenging negative cognitive distortions that perpetuate pain or adverse experiences, thus promoting emotional self-regulation. These interventions can include deep breathing, muscle relaxation, and guided imagery.[103] Self-hypnosis and biofeedback to dampen aversive arousal can be particularly beneficial for youth with somatization and pain.[103,104] In medically ill youth, evidence is greatest for the use of supportive-expressive talk therapy and cognitive behavior therapies that include behavioral activation, problem solving, interpersonal therapy, and mindfulness-based therapy.[84,103,105,106]

Spirituality can be a powerful adaptive coping strategy in medically ill youth. Spiritual coping can be enhanced through hospital chaplaincy services or partnering with community-based spiritual resources.[107] Furthermore, family and marital therapy may be indicated given the nature of the chronic stress on the family system.[103] Addressing stressors, such as school difficulties, is an important component of depression management. Thoughtful, interdisciplinary, and collaborative communications between mental health providers, medical professionals, and school personnel can aid in limiting disruptions to schooling, easing transitions between school and health systems, and making strategic use of school-based and homebound instruction to enhance child autonomy, improve functionality, and preserve school engagement.[108] Psychotherapeutic interventions must comprehensively consider the whole person, family, school, and the community to mitigate the effects of physical disease on psychological health.

Pharmacologic and Somatic Treatments

There is a scarcity of randomized controlled depression treatment trials in medically ill youth because most studies exclude patients with medical illness. Psychiatric treatment is informed by standard depression treatment guidelines in children, evidence from the general pediatric population and medically ill adults, level 4 expert consensus publications, and clinical experience.[6,15–21,109]

Pharmacologic treatment: initiation, maintenance, and termination

Integrative primary care models for depressed medically ill youth have shown improvements in both physical and mental health outcomes.[110] Psychiatric care is needed when a patient shows recurrent or treatment-resistant depression; significant behavioral dysregulation, including life-threatening nonadherence; history of suicide attempts or ideations; substance abuse; other severe psychiatric comorbidities; or an unsafe family environment.

Approach to psychopharmacology in medically ill youth

- Careful evaluation of all home-prescribed medications, including over-the-counter, alternative, and dietary products.
- Polypharmacy should be avoided to reduce potential drug-drug interactions and mitigate risk for overdose.
- Barbiturates and benzodiazepines should be avoided, when possible, in severely depressed medically ill youth because of risk for serious respiratory and cardiovascular suppression.

- To monitor for drug-drug interactions, several pharmacologic resources and Web sites can be helpful in addition to individual medical institution–based drug databases and pharmacy consultation.
- Antidepressants should be started at low doses and slowly titrated to therapeutic effect.
  - Baseline laboratory tests are not routinely recommended before starting antidepressants but should be obtained when clinically relevant.
    - Common laboratory and diagnostic testing with a fasting lipid panel, complete blood count with differential, electrolyte studies, thyroid studies, renal and liver function tests, and electrocardiogram may be considered.
- Reassess tolerability, safety, and response to intervention no more than 2 weeks after starting medication with follow-up every 2 to 4 weeks.[111]
- If failure to show improvement, further dose increases should take place at small increments every 2 to 4 weeks.
  - Provide enough time to evaluate effectiveness of dose adjustments.
- Adherence and tolerability to antidepressant must be assessed regularly.
  - Medically ill youth often struggle with compliance because of competing medical needs, poor oral intake, or worsening physical disease.[112]
- In treatment-resistant depression, conduct thorough review of biopsychosocial factors and their changes, including a diagnostic assessment reevaluation.

Further genotyping of cytochrome P450 genes may be used as part of a broader assessment.[113]

Selective serotonin reuptake inhibitors (SSRIs) are considered first-line treatment of medically ill youth with depression.[112] Although generic antidepressants are safe and effective, the pharmacokinetic bioequivalence of generic compounds ranges from 80% to 125% compared with brand-name drugs.[111] Thus, switching between brand and generic medication can change the efficacy or produce side effects, particularly in medically ill youth who may be more sensitive to these changes. There are no specific recommendations for the first-choice antidepressant because the differences between the individual medications are small.[111] Antidepressant selection should involve understanding patient-specific psychiatric and medical needs, past antidepressant experience, potential drug interactions, and prescriber expertise (**Box 2**).

Box 2
Clinical pearls in psychopharmacologic management of depression in medically ill youth

- Patients with sleep disturbance may benefit from mirtazapine or trazodone, but beneficial sleep effects must be balanced against potential daytime sedation[111]
- Mirtazapine is frequently used in youth with cancer and cystic fibrosis because it can stimulate appetite, potentiate weight gain, has few drug-drug interactions, and is a 5-hydroxytryptamine receptor antagonist with antiemetic properties[81,114]
- In youth with pronounced pain, duloxetine or serotonin norepinephrine reuptake inhibitors (SNRIs) can be considered[81]
- Fluoxetine's long half-life and inhibition of cytochrome P450 2D6 make it less useful in medically ill youth[113]
- Stimulant medications, such as products based on methylphenidate or amphetamine, can improve motivation, energy, and appetite, especially in palliative care patients, because of their potentiation of opiate analgesics[81]

There are no specific guidelines for the duration of antidepressant treatment in medically ill youth after achieving symptomatic remission, therefore general population treatment guidelines are recommended.[6,109] Antidepressant discontinuation should be gradual unless required otherwise by unfavorable medical illness course or its treatment. Abrupt discontinuation of antidepressants with shorter duration of action, particularly paroxetine, may be associated with a withdrawal syndrome characterized by flulike symptoms, insomnia, dizziness, paresthesias, tiredness, nausea, visual disturbances, abnormal movements, and headaches.[115] These symptoms may be misinterpreted as worsening medical illness and lead to unnecessary interventions.

Neurostimulation treatment

Although rarely used, electroconvulsive therapy (ECT) can be an effective treatment of severe, life-threatening depression when more conservative treatments have been unsuccessful or when depression is associated with psychosis, unremitting suicidality, catatonia, neuroleptic malignant syndrome, intolerance of oral antidepressants, or rapidly deteriorating physical status.[128,129] ECT has been safely used in adults with medical illnesses, including central nervous system disease.[130] Pediatric data are still emerging but it seems promising as a potential treatment option in select cases.[129]

Repetitive transcranial magnetic stimulation has been effective in adults with epilepsy and stroke, but evidence-based data in medically ill youth are lacking.[131,132] Similarly, the evidence base regarding use of other neuromodulatory therapies, such as transcranial direct current stimulation, magnetic seizure therapy, vagus nerve stimulation, and deep brain stimulation, for depression in medically ill youth is just emerging.[133,134]

Special Considerations for Adverse Effects

Consultation with subspecialty pediatric providers may be warranted in youth at higher risk for specific side effects because of potential interaction between an antidepressant and medical illness or treatment (**Table 3**).

Serotonin syndrome/toxicity

Serotonin toxicity and adrenergic adverse effects have been reported in the concomitant use of SSRIs with other serotonergic drugs, including ondansetron, muscle relaxants, opioids, tricyclic antidepressants (commonly used for functional pain or headaches), and sumatriptan.[126] In particular, the antibiotic linezolid, a reversible monoamine oxidase inhibitor, is commonly used to treat patients with treatment-resistant gram-positive bacterial infections and leads to serotonin syndrome with concomitant SSRI use.[127]

LEVELS OF CARE

Integrated and collaborative care models provide opportunities for simultaneous care of medical and psychiatric concerns. The value of psychiatric consultation is significant and is associated with reductions in hospital length of stay and health care use in hospitalized medically ill youth.[135] Most medically ill youth with depression receive mental health care in outpatient settings. This care may be with their PCP, a mental health provider, or embedded as part of pediatric subspecialty care. The criteria for treatment of depression in medically ill youth in more intense outpatient treatment settings or inpatient psychiatric units are similar to those for youth without medical illness. In medically ill children, additional criteria that may warrant inpatient psychiatric admission include:

Table 3
Side effect considerations in antidepressant treatment of medically ill youth

Neurologic	• Seizure risk with antidepressant treatment very low (>0.1%)[116] • Seizure risk highest for clomipramine, then amitriptyline, venlafaxine, citalopram, sertraline, trazodone, mirtazapine, paroxetine, bupropion, and escitalopram[116] • Negligible seizure risk for fluoxetine and duloxetine[116] • Movement disorders, myoclonus, and extrapyramidal signs, particularly with abrupt discontinuation of treatment, reported with use of fluoxetine, paroxetine, fluvoxamine, and sertraline[117–119] • Dose-related, reversible frontal lobe–like amotivational syndrome, characterized by apathy, indifference, and disinhibition, has been reported in youth[120] • SSRIs can alter sleep architecture and quality[121] • Fluoxetine increases REM latency and suppresses REM sleep[121]
Hematologic	• SSRIs can inhibit platelet aggregation by altering platelet serotonin receptors, reduce platelet counts, and increase gastrointestinal bleeding risk[112] • Bupropion has least bleed risk, followed by SNRIs and SSRIs[122] • Bleed risk may be doubled with concomitant use of nonsteroidal antiinflammatory agents[123] • Antidepressants should be used cautiously with platelet disorders, thrombocytopenia, undergoing surgery, and in patients taking antiepileptic drugs • Recommended that platelet level be greater than 100,000 cubic milliliter of blood before initiating SSRI treatment[113]
Cardiovascular	• SSRI use, especially high doses of citalopram and escitalopram, should be carefully monitored in patients with arrhythmias, heart failure, and other cardiovascular disorders, because of dose-dependent QT prolongation and TdP[124] • TdP often idiosyncratic, and association with antidepressant dose and QTc prolongation remain unclear[125] • Sertraline has the least risk of QT prolongation of the SSRIs[100] • Caution should be taken in assessing for other agents that may prolong QT interval, electrolyte disturbances that may affect QT, and SSRI dose escalation in youth with history of prolonged QT
Metabolic	• Weight changes and fluid shifts affect serum drug concentrations, especially in patients with hepatic and renal insufficiency • Dosing adjusted according to patient's evolving weight and volume to prevent drug toxicity and subtherapeutic treatment[81]

Abbreviations: REM, rapid eye movement; TdP, torsades de pointes.

• Somatization resulting in severe impairment and decompensation in functioning
• Severe treatment nonadherence posing high risk of imminent harm
• Further diagnostic assessment for complex presentations with significant medical and psychiatric overlay

Care of medically ill children in the inpatient psychiatric unit requires access to medical staffing and acute medical support when needed, close communication with involved medical providers, and routine review of potential drug-drug and medical-psychiatric disease interactions.

The transition from higher levels of psychiatric care to less restrictive outpatient environments is equally important. Careful disposition planning is important to prevent recidivism and to coordinate care with multiple outpatient providers. PCPs, key pediatric subspecialists, and outpatient mental health providers should be contacted early during inpatient psychiatric admission and provided a summary report of the patient's stay. Partial hospital day treatment models, particularly with a family-based focus, allow for intensive intervention in complex pediatric illness in which clinicians can address family illness beliefs and relationships to improve health outcomes.[136]

OUTCOMES AND PROGNOSIS

Pediatric medical illness increases the risk of adult depression.[137] In a large systematic review and meta-analysis of 34 studies of 45,358 patients, there was an association of childhood chronic physical illness and adult depression (odds ratio, 1.31; 95% confidence interval, 1.12–1.54).[138] When separately assessing childhood medical illness by disease type, cancer, more than asthma or type 1 diabetes mellitus, is significantly associated with adult depression.[138] This finding is particularly relevant given increasing cancer survival in youth. Adult depression in the setting of previous childhood medical illness often presents with more intense symptoms and is more impairing than in the general population.[139] Psychosocial adjustment can also be impaired in adults who experience chronic medical illness in youth.[139] This impairment is compounded by missed developmental, academic, social, and work-related opportunities in youth with medical illness, which can cause increased purposelessness and lower functionality at the critical transitional period to adulthood.[140,141] Childhood depression also increases the risk of physical disease in adulthood, increasing risk of both physical morbidity and mortality.[137,142,143] Therefore, early identification and management of depression in medically ill youth, along with effective medical treatment, is important for future adult physical and emotional health.

SUMMARY

Medically ill youth are at higher risk of developing depression because of complex interactions between biological, psychosocial, developmental, and environmental factors. Early identification and prevention of depression require a proactive approach with early awareness, interdisciplinary collaboration, and a thoughtful diagnostic evaluation. Depression management is driven by a sound diagnostic formulation routinely revised based on emerging information regarding both medical illness and psychiatric symptoms. With a coordinated approach and an understanding of the delicate interface of physical disease and depressive illness, clinicians can ameliorate physical and emotional difficulties, enhance patient functioning, and improve quality of life during a critical period in their patients' lives and futures.

REFERENCES

1. Van Cleave J, Gortmaker SL, Perrin JM. Dynamics of obesity and chronic health conditions among children and youth. JAMA 2010;303(7):623–30.
2. Russell CJ, Simon TD. Care of children with medical complexity in the hospital setting. Pediatr Ann 2014;43(7):e157–62.
3. Maneta E, DeMaso D. Depression in medically ill children. In: Barsky A, Silbersweig D, editors. Depression in medical illness. New York: McGraw Hill Education; 2017. p. 325–34.
4. Pinquart M, Shen Y. Depressive symptoms in children and adolescents with chronic physical illness: an updated meta-analysis. J Pediatr Psychol 2011; 36(4):375–84.

5. Popp JM, Robinson JL, Britner PA, et al. Parent adaptation and family functioning in relation to narratives of children with chronic illness. J Pediatr Nurs 2014;29:58–64.
6. Birmaher B, Brent D, AACAP Work Group on Quality Issues. Practice parameter for the assessment and treatment of children and adolescents with depressive disorders. J Am Acad Child Adolesc Psychiatry 2007;46(11):1503–26.
7. Snell C, Fernandes S, Bujoreanu IS, et al. Depression, illness severity, and healthcare utilization in cystic fibrosis. Pediatr Pulmonol 2014;49(12):1177–81.
8. Clark JG, Srinath AI, Youk AO, et al. Predictors of depression in youth with Crohn disease. J Pediatr Gastroenterol Nutr 2014;58(5):569–73.
9. Kim J, Szigethy EM, Melhem NM, et al. Inflammatory markers and the pathogenesis of pediatric depression and suicide: a systematic review of the literature. J Clin Psychiatry 2014;75(11):1242–53.
10. Brzozowski B, Mazur-Bialy A, Pajdo R, et al. Mechanisms by which stress affects the experimental and clinical inflammatory bowel disease (IBD): role of brain-gut Axis. Curr Neuropharmacol 2016;14(8):892–900.
11. Smith HR. Depression in cancer patients: pathogenesis, implications and treatment (Review). Oncol Lett 2015;9(4):1509–14.
12. Pinquart M. Systematic review: bullying involvement of children with and without chronic physical illness and/or physical/sensory disability- a meta-analytic comparison with health/nondisabled peers. J Pediatr Psychol 2017;42(3):245–59.
13. Quittner AL, Goldbeck L, Abbott J, et al. Prevalence of depression and anxiety in patients with cystic fibrosis and parent caregivers: results of the International Depression Epidemiological Study across nine countries. Thorax 2014;69: 1090–7.
14. Incledon E, Williams L, Hazell T, et al. A review of factors associated with mental health in siblings of children with chronic illness. J Child Health Care 2015;19(2): 182–94.
15. DeMaso DR, Martini DR, Cahen LA. Practice parameter for the psychiatric assessment and management of physically ill children and adolescents. J Am Acad Child Adolesc Psychiatry 2009;48(2):213–33.
16. Forman-Hoffman V, McClure E, McKeeman J, et al. Screening for major depressive disorder in children and adolescents: a systematic review for the U.S. Preventive services Task Force. Ann Intern Med 2016;164(5):342–9.
17. Farraye FA, Melmed GY, Lichtenstein GR, et al. ACG clinical guideline: preventative care in inflammatory bowel disease. Am J Gastroenterol 2017;112(2): 241–58.
18. Quittner AL, Abbott J, Georgiopoulos AM, et al. International committee on mental health in cystic fibrosis: cystic fibrosis foundation and European cystic fibrosis society consensus statements for screening and treating depression and anxiety. Thorax 2016;71(1):26–34.
19. Siu AL. Screening for depression in children and adolescents: US Preventative services Task Force recommendation statement. Pediatrics 2016;137:1–8.
20. American Diabetes Association. Standards of medical care in diabetes 2016. Diabetes Care 2016;39(supplement 1):S1–12.
21. Hauser W, Moser G, Klose P, et al. Psychosocial issues in evidence-based guidelines on inflammatory bowel diseases: a review. World J Gastroenterol 2014;20:3663.
22. Richardson LP, McCauley E, Grossman DC, et al. Evaluation of the Patient Health Questionairre-9 Item for detecting major depression among adolescents. Pediatrics 2010;126(6):1117–23.

23. Nomura Y, Wickramaratne PJ, Warner V, et al. Family discord, parental depression, and psychopathology in offspring: ten-year follow-up. J Am Acad Child Adolesc Psychiatry 2002;41(4):402–9.

24. Allgaier A, Fruhe B, Pietsch K, et al. Is the Children's Depression Inventory Short version a valid screening tool in pediatric care? A comparison to its full-length version. J Psychosom Res 2012;73:369–74.

25. White D, Leach C, Sims R, et al. Validation of the hospital anxiety and depression scale for use with adolescents. Br J Psychiatry 1999;175:452–4.

26. Russell CE, Bouffet E, Beaton J, et al. Balancing grief and survival: experiences of children with brain tumors and their parents. J Psychosoc Oncol 2016;34(5):376–99.

27. Benton T, Staab J, Evans DL. Medical co-morbidity in depressive disorders. Ann Clin Psychiatry 2007;19(4):289–303.

28. Safa M, Boroujerdi FG, Talischi F, et al. Relationship of coping styles with suicidal behavior in hospitalized asthma and chronic obstructive pulmonary disease patients: substance abusers versus non-substance abusers. Tanaffos 2014;13(3):23–30.

29. Lu Y, Mak KK, van Bever HP, et al. Prevalence of anxiety and depressive symptoms in adolescents with asthma: a meta-analysis and meta-regression. Pediatr Allergy Immunol 2012;23(8):707–15.

30. Van Lieshout RJ, MacQueen GM. Relations between asthma and psychological distress: an old idea revisted. Chem Immunol Allergy 2012;98:1–13.

31. Mineur YS, Picciotto MR. Nicotine receptors and depression: revisiting and revising the cholinergic hypothesis. Trends Pharmacol Sci 2010;31(12):580–6.

32. Shanahan L, Copeland WE, Worthman CM, et al. Children with both asthma and depression are at risk for heightened inflammation. J Pediatr 2013;163(5):1443–7.

33. Ferro MA, Van Lieshout RJ, Scott JG, et al. Condition-specific associations of symptoms of depression and anxiety in adolescents and young adults with asthma and food allergy. J Asthma 2016;53(3):282–8.

34. Booster GD, Oland AA, Bender BG. Psychosocial factors in severe pediatric asthma. Immunol Allergy Clin North Am 2016;36(3):449–60.

35. Gobin V, Van Steendam K, Denys D, et al. Selective serotonin reuptake inhibitors as a novel class of immunosuppressants. Int Immunopharmacol 2014;20(1):148–56.

36. Brown ES, Sayed N, Van Enkevort E, et al. A randomized, double-blind, placebo-controlled trial of escitalopram in patients with asthma and major depressive disorder. J Allergy Clin Immunol Pract 2018. https://doi.org/10.1016/j.jaip.2018.01.010.

37. Garcia G, Snell C, Sawicki G, et al. Mental health screening of medically-admitted patients with cystic fibrosis. Psychosomatics 2018;59(2):158–68.

38. Iturralde E, Adams RN, Barley RC, et al. Implementation of depression screening and global health assessment in pediatric subspecialty clinics. J Adolesc Health 2017;61(5):591–8.

39. Awaad MI, Darahim KE. Depression and anxiety in adolescents with congenital heart disease. Middle East Current Psychiatry 2015;22(1):2–8.

40. Areias ME, Pinto CI, Vieira PF, et al. Long term psychosocial outcomes of congenital heart disease (CHD) in adolescents and young adults. Transl Pediatr 2013;2(3):90–8.

41. DeMaso DR, Calderon J, Taylor GA, et al. Psychiatric disorders in adolescents with single ventricle congenital heart disease. Pediatrics 2017;139(3): e20162241.
42. Jackson JL, Misiti B, Bridge JA, et al. Emotional functioning of adolescents and adults with congenital heart disease: a meta-analysis. Congenit Heart Dis 2015; 10(1):2–12.
43. Karsdorp PA, Everaerd W, Kindt M. Psychological and cognitive functioning in children and adolescents with congenital heart disease: a meta-analysis. J Pediatr Psychol 2007;32(5):527–41.
44. Lane DA, Millane TA, Lip GY. Psychological interventions for depression in adolescents and adults with congenital heart disease. Cochrane Database Syst Rev 2013;(10):CD004372.
45. Dunn DW, Besag F, Caplan R, et al. Psychiatric and behavioral disorders in children with epilepsy (ILAE Task Force Report): anxiety, depression and childhood epilepsy. Epileptic Disord 2016. https://doi.org/10.1684/epd.2016.0813.
46. Kwong KL, Lam D, Tsui S, et al. Anxiety and depression in adolescents with epilepsy. J Child Neurol 2016;31(2):203–10.
47. Camfield P, Camfield C. Incidence, prevalence and aetiology of seizures and epilepsy in children. Epileptic Disord 2015;17(2):117–23.
48. Kanner AM. Most antidepressant drugs are safe for patients with epilepsy at therapeutic doses: a review of the evidence. Epilepsy Behav 2016;61:282–6.
49. Brown KM, Crouch BI. Bupropion overdose: significant toxicity in pediatrics. Clin Pediatr Emerg Med 2017;18(3):212–7.
50. Buchberger B, Huppertz H, Krabbe L, et al. Symptoms of depression and anxiety in youth with type 1 diabetes: a systematic review and meta-analysis. Psychoneuroendocrinology 2016;70:70–84.
51. Hood KK, Beavers DP, Yi_Frazier J, et al. Psychosocial burden and glycemic control during the first 6 years of diabetes: results from the SEARCH for Diabetes in Youth study. J Adolesc Health 2014;55(4):498–504.
52. Butwicka A, Frisen L, Almqvist C, et al. Risks of psychiatric disorders and suicide attempts in children and adolescents with type 1 diabetes: a population-based cohort study. Diabetes Care 2015;38(3):453–9.
53. Plener PL, Molz E, Berger G, et al. Depression, metabolic control, and antidepressant medication in young patients with type 1 diabetes. Pediatr Diabetes 2015;16(1):58–66.
54. Sarkar S, Balhara YPS. Diabetes mellitus and suicide. Indian J Endocrinol Metab 2014;18(4):468–74.
55. Markowitz S, Gonzalez JS, Wilkinson JL, et al. Treating depression in diabetes: emerging findings. Psychosomatics 2011;52(1):1–18.
56. Georgiades A, Zucker N, Friedman KE, et al. Changes in depressive symptoms and glycemic control in diabetes mellitus. Psychosom Med 2007;69:235–41.
57. Goodnick PJ. Use of antidepressants in treatment of comorbid diabetes mellitus and depression as well as in diabetic neuropathy. Ann Clin Psychiatry 2001; 13:31–4.
58. Morrison KM, Shin S, Tarnopolsky M, et al. Association of depression and health related quality of life with body composition in children and youth with obesity. J Affect Disord 2015;172:18–23.
59. Quek Y, Tam WW, Zhang MWB, et al. Exploring the association between childhood and adolescent obesity and depression: a meta-analysis. Obes Rev 2017; 18(7):742–54.

60. Reeves GM, Postolache TT, Snitker S. Childhood obesity and depression: connection between these growing problems in growing children. Int J Child Health Hum Dev 2008;1(2):103–14.

61. Anderson SE, Cohen P, Naumova EN, et al. Adolescent obesity and risk for subsequent major depressive disorder and anxiety disorder: prospective evidence. Psychosom Med 2007;69:740–7.

62. Dockray S, Susman EJ, Dorn LD. Depression, cortisol reactivity, and obesity in childhood and adolescence. J Adolesc Health 2009;45:344–50.

63. Goosens L, Braet C, Van Vlierberghe L, et al. Loss of control over eating in overweight youngsters: the role of anxiety, depression and emotional eating. Eur Eat Disord Rev 2009;17(1):68–78.

64. Mihalopoulos NL, Spigarelli MG. Comanagement of pediatric depression and obesity: a clear need for evidence. Clin Ther 2015;37(9):1933–7.

65. Allison DB, Newcomer JW, Dunn AL, et al. Obesity among those with mental disorders: a National Institute of Mental Health meeting report. Am J Prev Med 2009;36:341–50.

66. ·Expert Panel on Integrated Guidelines for Cardiovascular Health and Risk Reduction in Children and Adolescents, National Heart, Lung, and Blood Institute. Expert panel on integrated guidelines for cardiovascular health and risk reduction in children and adolescents: summary report. Pediatrics 2011; 128(Suppl 5):S213–56.

67. Raeder MB, Bjelland I, Emil Vollset S, et al. Obesity, dyslipidemia, and diabetes with selective serotonin reuptake inhibitors: the Hordaland Health Study. J Clin Psychiatry 2006;67:1974–82.

68. Mavrides N, Pao M. Updates in paediatric psycho-oncology. Int Rev Psychiatry 2014;26(1):63–73.

69. Coughtrey A, Millington A, Bennett S, et al. The effectiveness of psychosocial interventions for psychological outcomes in pediatric oncology: a systematic review. J Pain Symptom Manage 2018;55(3):1004–17.

70. Kurtz BP, Abrams AN. Psychiatric aspects of pediatric cancer. Child Adolesc Psychiatr Clin N Am 2010;19:401–21.

71. Kaye EC, Brinkman TM, Baker JN. Development of depression in survivors of childhood and adolescent cancer: a multi-level life course conceptual framework. Support Care Cancer 2017;25(6):2009–17.

72. Kazak AE, Brier M, Alderfer MA, et al. Screening for psychosocial risk in pediatric cancer. Pediatr Blood Cancer 2012;59(5):822–7.

73. Kazak AE. Pediatric Psychosocial Preventative Health Model (PPPHM): research, practice and collaboration in pediatric family systems medicine. Fam Syst Health 2006;24:381–95.

74. Li M, Fitzgerald P, Rodin G. Evidence-based treatment of depression in patients with cancer. J Clin Oncol 2012;30:1187–96.

75. Strong VR, Waters R, Hibberd C, et al. Management of depression for people with cancer (SMaRT oncology 1): a randomised trial. Lancet 2008;372:40–8.

76. Kissane DW, Levin T, Hales S, et al. Psychotherapy for depression in cancer and palliative care. In: Kissane DW, Maj M, Sartorius N, editors. Depression and cancer. Chichester (United Kingdom): Wiley-Blackwell; 2011. p. 177–206.

77. Breitbart W, Rosenfeld B, Gibson C, et al. Meaning-centered group psychotherapy for patients with advanced cancer: a pilot randomized controlled trial. Psychooncology 2010;19:21–8.

78. Chochinov HM, Hack T, Hassard T, et al. Dignity therapy: a novel psychotherapeutic intervention for patients near the end of life. J Clin Oncol 2005;23:5520–5.

79. Ando MT, Morita T, Akechi T, et al. The efficacy of mindfulness-based meditation therapy on anxiety, depression, and spirituality in Japanese patients with cancer. J Palliat Med 2009;12:1091–4.
80. Hemeryck A, Belpaire FM. Selective serotonin reuptake inhibitors and cytochrome P-450 mediated drug-drug interactions: an update. Curr Drug Metab 2002;3:13–37.
81. Rackley S, Bostwick JM. Depression in medically ill patients. Psychiatr Clin North Am 2012;35:231–47.
82. Keethy D, Mrakotsky C, Szigethy E. Pediatric IBD and depression: treatment implications. Curr Opin Pediatr 2014;26(5):561–7.
83. Szigethy EM, Youk AO, Benhayon D, et al. Depression subtypes in pediatric inflammatory bowel disease. J Pediatr Gastroenterol Nutr 2014;58(5):574–81.
84. Szigethy E, Bujoreanu SI, Youk AO, et al. Randomized efficacy trial of two psychotherapies for depression in youth with inflammatory bowel disease. J Am Acad Child Adolesc Psychiatry 2014;53(7):726–35.
85. Loftus EV, Guerin A, Yu AP, et al. Increased risks of developing anxiety and depression in young patient with Crohn's disease. Am J Gastroenterol 2011; 106:1670–7.
86. Mikocka-Walus A, Knowles SR, Keefer L, et al. Controversies revisited: a systematic review of the comorbidity of depression and anxiety with inflammatory bowel diseases. Inflamm Bowel Dis 2016;22:752–62.
87. McLafferty L, Craig A, Levine A, et al. Thematic analysis of physical illness perceptions in depressed youth with inflammatory bowel disease. Inflamm Bowel Dis 2011;17(supplement 1):S54.
88. Zernikow B, Wager J, Hechler T. Characteristics of highly impaired children with severe chronic pain: a 5-year retrospective study on 2249 pediatric pain patients. BMC Pediatr 2012;12:54.
89. Jerrell JM, Tripathi A, McIntyre RS. Prevalence and treatment of depression in children and adolescents with sickle Cell disease: a retrospective cohort study. Prim Care Companion CNS Disord 2011;13(2). https://doi.org/10.40088/PCC. 10m01063.
90. Fisher E, Heathcote L, Palermo TM, et al. Systematic review and meta-analysis of psychological therapies for children with chronic pain. J Pediatr Psychol 2014;39(8):763–82.
91. Weiss KE, Hahn A, Wallace DP, et al. Acceptance of pain: associations with depression, Catastrophizing, and functional disability among children and adolescents in an interdisciplinary chronic pain rehabilitation program. J Pediatr Psychol 2013;38(7):756–65.
92. Wicksell RK, Olsson GL, Hayes SC. Mediators of change in acceptance and commitment therapy for pediatric chronic pain. Pain 2011;152(12):2792–801.
93. Kirk AD, Knechtle SJ, Larsen CP, et al. Textbook of organ transplantation. West Sussex, UK: Wiley; 2014. p. 1482.
94. Fredricks EM, Lopez MJ, Magee JC, et al. Psychological functioning, nonadherence and health outcomes after pediatric liver transplantation. Am J Transplant 2007;7(8):1974–83.
95. McCormick King ML, Mee LL, Gutierrez-Colina AM, et al. Adherence in pediatric transplant recipients. J Pediatr Psychol 2014;39(3):283–93.
96. Killian MO, Schuman DL, Mayersohn GS, et al. Psychosocial predictors of medication non-adherence in pediatric organ transplantation: a systematic review. Pediatr Transplant 2018;22(4):e13188.

97. Dobbels F, Decorte A, Roskams A, et al. Health-related quality of life, treatment adherence, symptom experience and depression in adolescent renal transplant patients. Pediatr Transplant 2010;14:216–23.

98. Cohen SD, Norris L, Acquaviva K, et al. Screening, diagnosis, and treatment of depression in patients with end-stage renal disease. Clin J Am Soc Nephrol 2007;2(6):1332–42.

99. Crone CC, Gabriel GM. Treatment of anxiety and depression in transplant patients: pharmacokinetic considerations. Clin Pharmacokinet 2004;43(6):361–94.

100. Beach SR, Celano CM, Sugrue AM, et al. QT prolongation, torsades de pointes, and psychiatric medication medications: a 5-year update. Psychosomatics 2018;59(2):105–22.

101. Pao M, Ballard ED, Rosenstein DL. Growing up in the hospital. JAMA 2007; 297(24):2752–5.

102. Pao M, Mahoney MR. "Will you remember me?": talking with adolescents about death and dying. Child Adolesc Psychiatr Clin N Am 2018;27(4):511–26.

103. Balon R. Cognitive-behavioral therapy, psychotherapy and psychosocial interventions in the medically ill. Psychother Psychosom 2009;78(5):261–4.

104. Thrabrew H, Ruppeldt P, Sollers JJ. Systematic review of biofeedback interventions for addressing anxiety and depression in children and adolescents with long-term physical conditions. Appl Psychophysiol Biofeedback 2018;43(3): 179–92.

105. Eccleston C, Palermo TM, Fisher E, et al. Psychological interventions for parents of children and adolescents with chronic illness. Cochrane Database Syst Rev 2012;(8):CD009660.

106. Schwab A, Rusconi-Serpa S, Schechter DR. Psychodynamic approaches to medically ill children and their traumatically stressed parents. Child Adolesc Psychiatr Clin N Am 2013;22(1):119–39.

107. Reynolds N, Mrug S, Hensler M, et al. Spiritual coping and adjustment in adolescents with chronic illness: a 2-year prospective study. J Pediatr Psychol 2014;39(5):542–51.

108. Shaw SR, McCabe PC. Hospital-to-school transition for children with chronic illness: meeting the new challenges of an evolving health care system. Psychol Sch 2008;45(1):74–87.

109. Cheung AH, Zuckerbrot RA, Jensen PS, et al. Guidelines for adolescent depression in primary care (GLAD-PC): II. Treatment and ongoing m5rttanagement. Pediatrics 2007;120(5):e1313–26.

110. Woltmann E, Grogan-Kaylor A, Perron B, et al. Comparative effectiveness of collaborative chronic care models for mental health conditions across primary, specialty, and behavioral health care settings: systematic review and meta-analysis. Am J Psychiatry 2012;169(8):790–804.

111. Kennedy SH, Lam RW, McIntyre RS, et al. Canadian Network for Mood and Anxiety Treatments (CANMAT) 2016 clinical guidelines for the management of adults with major depressive disorder: section 3. Pharmacological treatments. Can J Psychiatry 2016;61(9):540–60.

112. Bursch B, Forgey M. Psychopharmacology for medically ill adolescents. Curr Psychiatry Rep 2013;15:395.

113. Boland JR, Duffy B, Myer NM. Clinical utility of pharmacogenetics-guided treatment of depression and anxiety. Pers Med Psychiatry 2018;7-8:7–13.

114. Kast RE, Foley KF. Cancer chemotherapy and cachexia: mirtazapine and olanzapine are 5-HT3 antagonists with good anti-nausea effects. Department Medical Laboratory and Radiation Sciences, University of Vermont, Burlington, VT,

USASearch for more papers by this author. Eur J Cancer Care 2007;16(4): 351–4.

115. Renoir T. Selective serotonin reuptake inhibitor antidepressant treatment discontinuation syndrome: a review of the clinical evidence and the possible mechanisms involved. Front Pharmacol 2013;4:45.

116. Steinert T, Fröscher W. Epileptic seizures under antidepressive drug treatment: systematic review. Pharmacopsychiatry 2018;51:121–35.

117. Hamilton MS, Opler LA. Akathisia, suicidality, and fluoxetine. J Clin Psychiatry 1992;53(11):401–6.

118. Nicholson SD. Extra pyramidal side effects associated with paroxetine. West Engl Med J 1992;107(3):90–1.

119. Opler LA. Sertraline and akathisia. Am J Psychiatry 1994;151(4):620–1.

120. Opler LA, Ramirez PM, Lee SK. Serotonergic agents and frontal lobe syndrome. J Clin Psychiatry 1994;55(8):362–3.

121. Rush AJ, Armitage R, Gillin JC, et al. Comparative effects of nefazadone and fluoxetine on sleep in outpatients with major depressive disorder. Biol Psychiatry 1998;44(1):3–14.

122. Bixby AL, Vandenberg A, Bostwick JR. Clinical management of bleeding risk with antidepressants. Ann Pharmacother 2018. https://doi.org/10.1177/1060028018794005.

123. Anglin R, Yuan Y, Moayyedi P, et al. Risk of upper gastrointestinal bleeding with selective serotonin reuptake inhibitors with or without concurrent nonsteroidal anti-inflammatory use: a systematic review and meta – analysis. Am J Gastroenterol 2014;109:811–9.

124. Waring WS, Graham A, Gray J, et al. Evaluation of a QT nomogram for risk assessment after antidepressant overdose. Br J Clin Pharmacol 2010;70(6): 881–5.

125. Viewing WV, Hasnain M, Howland RH, et al. Citalopram, QTc interval prolongation, and torsade de pointes. How should we apply the recent FDA ruling? Am J Med 2012;125(9):859–68.

126. Kawai Y, DeMonbrun AG, Chambers RS, et al. A previously healthy adolescent with acute encephalopathy and decorticate posturing. Pediatrics 2017;139(1): e20153779.

127. Ramsey TD, Lau TT, Ensom MH. Serotonergic and adrenergic drug interactions associated with linezolid: a critical review and practical management approach. Ann Pharmacother 2013;47(4):543–60.

128. Ghaziuddin N, Kutcher SP, Knapp P, The Work Group on Quality Issues. Practice parameter for use of electroconvulsive therapy with adolescents. J Am Acad Child Adolesc Psychiatry 2004;43(12):1521–39.

129. Shoirah H, Hamoda HM. Electroconvulsive therapy in children and adolescents. Expert Rev Neurother 2011;11(1):127–37.

130. Rasmussen KG, Rummans TA, Richardson JW. Electroconvulsive therapy in the medically ill. Psychiatr Clin North Am 2002;25(1):177–93.

131. Fregni F, Pascual-Leone A. Transcranial magnetic stimulation for the treatment of depression in neurologic disorders. Curr Psychiatry Rep 2005;7(5):381–90.

132. Muszkat D, Polanczyk GV, Costa Dias TG, et al. Transcranial direct current stimulation in child and adolescent psychiatry. J Child Adolesc Psychopharmacol 2016;26(7):590–7.

133. Croarkin PE, Rotenberg A, Wall CA, et al. Magnetic resonance imaging-guided, open –label, high frequency repetitive transcranial magnetic stimulation for

adolescents with major depressive disorder. J Child Adolesc Psychopharmacol 2016;26(7):582–9.

134. Croarkin PE, Rotenberg A. Pediatric neuromodulation comes of age. J child Adolesc Psychopharmacol 2016;26(7):578–81.

135. Bujoreanu S, White MT, Gerber B, et al. Effect of timing of psychiatry consultation on length of pediatric hospitalization and hospital charges. Hosp Pediatr 2015;5(5):269–75.

136. Rickerby ML, DerMarderosian D, Nassau J, et al. Family-based integrated care (FBIC) in a partial hospital program for complex pediatric illness: fostering shifts in family illness beliefs and relationships. Child Adolesc Psychiatr Clin N Am 2017;26(4):733–59.

137. Fryers T, Brugha T. Childhood determinants of adult psychiatric disorder. Clin Pract Epidemiol Ment Health 2013;9:1–50.

138. Secinti E, Thompson EJ, Richards M, et al. Research review: childhood chronic physical illness and adult emotional health- a systematic review and meta-analysis. J Child Psychol Psychiatry 2017;58(7):753–69.

139. LeBlanc LA, Goldsmith T, Patel DR. Behavioral aspects of chronic illness in children and adolescents. Pediatr Clin North Am 2003;50(4):859–78.

140. Nathan PC, Henderson TO, Kirchhoff AC, et al. Financial hardship and the economic effect of childhood cancer survivorship. J Clin Oncol 2018;36(21): 2198–205.

141. Stabile M, Allin S. The economic costs of childhood disability. Future Child 2012; 22(1):65–96.

142. Archer G, Kuh D, Hotopf M, et al. Adolescent affective symptoms and mortality. Br J Psychiatry 2018;213(1):419–24.

143. Hayes BD, Klein-Schwartz W, Clark RF, et al. Comparison of toxicity of acute overdoses with citalopram and escitalopram. J Emerg Med 2010;39(1):44–8.

Perinatal Mixed Affective State
Wherefore Art Thou?

Alexia Emilia Koukopoulos, MD, PhD[a,b,c,]*,
Gloria Angeletti, MD[b,c,d], Gabriele Sani, MD[e,f,1],
Delfina Janiri, MD[b,c,d], Giovanni Manfredi, MD, PhD[b,c,d],
Georgios D. Kotzalidis, MD, PhD[b,c,d], Lavinia De Chiara, MD[b,c,d]

KEYWORDS

- Perinatal period • Postpartum • Peripartum • Pregnancy • Mixed affective state
- Mixed depression • Bipolar disorder • Women

KEY POINTS

- The mixed affective state during the perinatal period is the least studied affective mood state.
- The perinatal period is most vulnerable for the emergence of mood episodes in women.
- Depression with symptoms of an excitatory nature is common in clinical practice.
- Women present higher rates then men of mixed episodes during their life span; the perinatal period could be a time of particularly high risk for mixed episodes.

It is known to every clinician that at about the fifth or sixth day of the lying in period many women get nervous, irritable, depressed and demanding. This mood is somewhat similar to premenstrual tension.

—S. Haas, 1952[1]

…the phrase thinking too much ("kufungisisa") was also identified as both a cause and a symptom of depression by new mothers of the Shona people in Zimbabwe
—Thandi Davies et al., 2016[2]

This article originally appeared in *Psychiatric Clinics*, Volume 43, Issue 1, March 2020.
[a] SPDC, Azienda Ospedaliera Universitaria Policlinico Umberto I, Sapienza School of Medicine and Dentistry, Rome, Italy; [b] Centro Lucio Bini, Rome, Italy; [c] Azienda Ospedaliera Sant'Andrea, UOC di Psichiatria, Via di Grottarossa 1035, CAP 00189, Rome 00185, Italy; [d] NESMOS Department, Sapienza School of Medicine and Psychology, Sant'Andrea University Hospital, Rome, Italy; [e] Institute of Psychiatry, Università Cattolica del Sacro Cuore, Roma, Italy; [f] Department of Psychiatry, Fondazione Policlinico Universitario "Agostino Gemelli" IRCCS, Roma, Italy
[1] Present address: Institute of Psychiatry, Largo Francesco Vito 1, 00168 Roma
* Corresponding author. Viale dell'Università 30, Rome 00185, Italy.
E-mail address: alexiakoukopoulos@gmail.com

Abbreviations	
BD	Bipolar disorder
BPII	Bipolar disorder type II
DSM	Diagnostic and Statistical Manual of Mental Disorders, 5th edition
EPDS	Edinburgh Postnatal Depression Scale
HCL-32	32-Item Hypomania Checklist
MxD	Mixed depression

INTRODUCTION

The perinatal period is the time frame in childbearing women's lives that includes the whole duration of pregnancy and the first 4 weeks (*Diagnostic and Statistical Manual of Mental Disorders*, 5th edition [DSM-5] criteria) or up to the first year (commonly used in research and clinical practice) postpartum. This loosely defined window is universally considered the most vulnerable time for emergence of psychiatric disturbances in women.

The literature regarding perinatal psychiatric disorders has focused primarily on typical postpartum depression and on postpartum psychosis. The excitatory symptoms that often accompany depressive states has received less attention. The least studied affective mood state during the perinatal period is certainly the mixed affective state. However, major depression with symptoms of an excitatory nature is common in clinical practice.[3–5] The most striking difference is found between depressive syndromes characterized by inhibitory symptoms and those marked by disinhibition, which are of an opposite polarity. Symptoms like irritable mood, mood lability, inner tension, distractibility, psychomotor agitation, impulsivity, aggressiveness, racing or crowded thoughts, talkativeness, early insomnia, dramatic description of suffering, or weeping spells are frequently observed among patients diagnosed with a major depressive episode[6,7]; they are, in our view, symptoms of nervous excitability and constitute the essence of a mixed affective episode. In contrast, hypomanic symptoms of euphoria, grandiosity, and hypersexuality have been found less frequently.[8–12]

Compared with nonmixed depression, mixed depression (MxD) is considered to be more severe and worse in its clinical presentation, is more common in bipolar disorders (BD) and is more frequently associated with a family history of BD, younger age at onset, longer duration, higher prevalence of suicide attempts, and comorbidities, worse outcome, poorer response to treatments,[5,6,8,10] and higher switch rates with antidepressant treatment.[9,11–14]

Unlike unipolar disorder, where depression is twice as common in women, gender distribution in BD is more balanced; however, women have an increased risk of BD type II (BDII)/hypomania, rapid cycling, and mixed episodes.[15] Compared with men, women have higher rates of depressive mixed episodes,[16] mixed hypomania,[17] mixed episodes,[18–20] rapid cycling,[21] and atypical depressive features,[22] despite differences in applied criteria. Between 5% and 7% of men and 6.7% and 18.2% women show such symptoms.[20] Among patients with MxD, female gender has been associated with BDII diagnosis and hyperthymic temperament.[7]

Women with mood episodes during reproductive-related events (ie, premenstrual, perinatal, and menopausal transition) may be particularly sensitive to intense hormonal fluctuations,[23] which could influence neurochemical pathways linked to depression.[24,25] Early recognition and clinical diagnosis of perinatal excitatory symptoms is an important prerequisite to offer adequate treatment and to prevent the possible negative impact on child development.[26] Given the high rates of mixed affective states in women[7,22] and the high rates of mood recurrences during the perinatal period,[27,28] we hypothesized that the perinatal period would be a critical time for the onset of mixed affective states.

METHODS

We conducted a PubMed search (1974–2019) on July 3, 2019, using the following Boolean search strategy: (depressive[ti] OR depression[ti] OR "bipolar disorder"[ti] OR "mood disorder*"[ti] OR "affective disorder*"[ti] OR Psychosis[ti] OR Psychotic [ti]) AND (puerperal[ti] OR pregnan*[ti] OR postpartum[ti] OR perinatal[ti] OR child-birth[ti] OR postnatal[ti] OR peripartum[ti] OR delivery[ti]) AND (hyperactivity OR rest-lessness OR "mood lability" OR Irritability OR "racing thoughts" OR "inner tension" OR suicid* OR Impulsiv* OR dysphori* OR anger OR "increased libido" OR "mixed feature*" OR "mixed state*" OR "mixed symptom*" OR "mixed episode*" OR Insomnia OR hypomani* OR euphori* OR highs OR agitat*).

All authors viewed the search output and examined eligibility independently. Eligibility was determined through Delphi rounds, until complete consensus was reached. Eligible were studies focusing on depressive episodes in the perinatal period including pregnancy up to 1 year postpartum and/or detailing affective symptomatology in which the simultaneous presence of excitatory and inhibitory mood symptoms was reported. Excluded were studies reporting on perinatal nonmixed mood episodes without describing symptoms, and any unfocused or unrelated study. We excluded single case reports, reviews/meta-analyses, opinion papers without data such as letters and editorials, nonclinical studies, and animal studies. However, we used reviews for possibly identifying additional relevant studies from their reference lists.

We did not use the DSM-5 MxD mixed symptoms definition, but rather the psychopathology-oriented diagnostic definition (**Box 1**).[4,6,7,29–31] According to the DSM-5, at least 3 hypomanic or manic symptoms that do not overlap with major depression symptoms are needed to apply the "with mixed features" specifier to an major depressive episode case. In case of mania or hypomania, the presence of at least 3 depressive symptoms is required during the hypomanic or manic episodes to apply the specifier. In our clinical practice, we have seen the third and fourth criteria (namely, more talkative than usual or pressure to keep talking, and flight of ideas or subjective experience that thoughts are racing) frequently in MxD, but the other 5 criteria are extremely rare, if ever present. Furthermore, these criteria are closer to the research-based diagnostic criteria, which proved to be more reliable than the DSM-5 in a large sample.[32]

Box 1
Koukopoulos' diagnostic criteria for mixed depression

Major depressive episode plus at least 3 of the following 8 items:
  Psychic agitation or inner tension
  Racing or crowded thoughts
  Irritability or unprovoked rage
  Absence of retardation
  Talkativeness
  Dramatic description of suffering or frequent spells of weeping
  Mood lability or marked reactivity
  Early insomnia

Adapted from Sani G, Vöhringer PA, Napoletano F, et al. Koukopoulos' diagnostic criteria for mixed depression: a validation study. J Affect Disord 2014;164:15; with permission.

RESULTS
Mixed Affective States in the Perinatal Period

In contrast with the lack of data examining a relationship with the menstrual cycle or the menopause,[15] there is consistent evidence of a strong temporal relationship between depressive,[33] manic, or mixed episodes of BD[34–39] and childbirth,[28,40–42] particularly in the first postpartum month.[43] Women with BD are at particular risk for developing mood symptoms postpartum.[44]

A mood episode during the perinatal period has been suggested as an indicator for BD.[45–47] Unlike depression, which can occur anytime postpartum, manic or mixed episodes are more likely to occur soon after delivery.[36,46,48]

The postpartum period also seems to be a time of high risk for a conversion from major depressive disorder to BD, which is more than 6%,[3,36] considerably higher than the about 1% per year in the general population, which fades away during longer follow-ups.[49] Furthermore, women at their first delivery are at a higher risk for BD diagnosis than women at their second or higher parity.[36]

Retrospective as well as prospective studies indicate that approximately 60% to 70% of women with BD experienced a mood episode during pregnancy and the postpartum period.[28,33,50] Rates as high as 67% were found for postpartum depression,[50] and between 25% and 50% for postpartum mania and psychosis.[39,41] Women in nonclinical populations who show hypo/manic symptoms immediately after delivery range from 9.6% to 20.4% across studies.[51–56]

Mixed episodes may occur during the perinatal period either in women with previously diagnosed BD or in those without a previous history of mood disorder, the 4-week criteria allowed by the DSM-5 seems to be insufficient.[57] Furthermore, depressive or dysphoric-mixed episodes seem to be more prevalent in pregnant than nonpregnant bipolar women.[58]

A hallmark study by Viguera and collegues[28] estimated the risk of recurrence of mood episodes in BD women who continued or discontinued treatment with mood stabilizers during pregnancy in a prospective observational clinical cohort study. Most recurrences were depressive or dysphoric/mixed (74%), especially early in pregnancy, and exceeded by far manic-hypomanic episodes. The depressive-dysphoric versus manic-hypomanic prevalence became even more prominent after discontinuation of mood stabilizer treatment, compared with continued treatment. Predictors of recurrence included BDII disorder diagnosis, earlier onset, more recurrences/y, recent illness, use of antidepressants, and use of anticonvulsants rather than lithium.[28] The authors confirmed Marcé's 1858 original observations that pregnancy predisposed vulnerable patients to depressive-dysphoric recurrences.[59]

Within the international BRIDGE study,[60] higher BD rates in first episode postpartum depression were shown compared with first episode nonpostpartum depression. Women with first episode postpartum depression showed significantly more psychotic symptoms, atypical features, and MxD. They had younger age at onset, more prior episodes, episodes of short duration, first-degree relatives with BD, switches while on antidepressants, and seasonality of mood episodes.[60] Furthermore, first episode postpartum depression women scored significantly higher on the active/elated subscore of the 32-item self-rated Hypomania Checklist (HCL-32).[60]

Data from 276 BD women untreated during pregnancy showed 75.0% of them developing psychiatric episodes after delivery, with depressive episodes being the most frequent (79.7%), followed by DSM-IV-TR manic (13.5%), mixed (3.9%), and hypomanic episodes (2.9%). A history of psychotic symptoms during postpartum was associated with depression in 22.4% of patients, with mania in 67.8%, and with mixed episodes in 87.5%.[43] Younger age at onset, type I disorder, MDI cycle, and psychotic symptoms were associated with (hypo)manic or mixed postpartum episodes.[43,61]

In a recent study focusing on the prevalence of MxD during the postpartum period, Çelik and colleagues[62] included 63 postpartum women. The participants were administered the Beck Depression Inventory, the Edinburgh Postnatal Depression Scale (EPDS), the Mood Disorders Questionnaire, and the Modified HCL-32. The Mood Disorder Questionnaire scores of women "depressive" according to the EPDS cut-off scores, were significantly higher than those of women with EPDS scores lower than the cut-off. The modified hypomania scores were significantly higher in the women with higher depression scores compared with those scoring under the EPDS cut-off. According to the Modified HCL-32 results, 79.4% of women had at least 1 symptom, 71.4% of women had at least 3 symptoms, and 68.3% of women had at least 5 symptoms of MxD.[62] In other words, hypomanic symptoms were more prevalent in severe depression, which suggests that MxD is a more severe type of depression, in line with Koukopoulos, Sani, Ghaemi, and their colleagues.[29,30]

Clinical Characteristics

There is no consensus in the literature on what the typical clinical presentation of perinatal depressive episodes is. Some authors support that perinatal depression is indistinguishable from depressive episodes occurring at other times in a woman's life span,[63,64] whereas others point to particular symptom clusters in perinatal depressive episodes.[65] We sought studies describing perinatal episode symptomatology to highlight the importance and frequency of symptoms that would pertain to mixed affective episodes according to these broader criteria (see **Box 1**).[7] Overlapping manic symptoms as psychomotor agitation, irritability and mood lability were reported to be the most prevalent symptoms in MxD in nonperinatal populations, despite being all excluded from the DSM-5 specifier.[7,29,30]

Unfortunately, the great majority of studies in the perinatal research area uses the EPDS as the sole instrument both as screening and as diagnostic tool. Although the EPDS is valid and useful for the detection of depressive symptomatology, it is not designed to capture mixed or atypical symptomatology. At this time, there is no specific validated screening method to confirm the presence of postpartum mania or postpartum mixed episodes; hence, we review here studies that used instruments able to detect a broader spectrum of symptoms that included symptoms typically present in mixed affective states. The most common symptoms reported were dysphoria, irritability, anger, agitation, mood lability, early insomnia, racing thoughts, and impulsivity; we discuss these symptoms in detail.

Mood lability

Several studies reported that excitatory symptoms are common in women in the early postpartum period,[52,54,55,66–69] with an 8-fold increase in hypomanic symptoms soon after delivery, compared with pregnancy.[56] The emergence of these symptoms should not be confused with the physiologic happiness usually surrounding the arrival of a baby; a strong correlation has in fact been frequently observed between hypomanic symptoms in the early postpartum and depressive symptoms.[33,51,52,66,70–72] The prevalence rates of postpartum hypomanic symptoms ranged from 9.6% to 29% across studies 2 to 4 days after delivery.[33,51,73] In a South African sample, 17.5% of women met both cut-off scores for depression and hypomania on postpartum day 3. This subgroup had significantly higher depression scores at week 6 postpartum than the rest of the sample. The lability of mood, typically observed in women after birth, has been described as follows: they were "giggly," "excited," "oversensitive," "cried at nothing," "laughed at nothing," or were "up and down."[68]

Although detecting mood lability in the early postpartum period may require expert observation and interviewing, it has important implications for clinical management and longitudinal diagnosis.[74] In fact, a striking 83% of women with combined postpartum depression and postpartum hypomania on the Highs Scale had an BD diagnosis based on the Structured Clinical Interview for DSM-IV in 1 study.[75]

Irritability and anger

Irritability is the single mixed symptom most commonly reported in perinatal depressive episodes by these reviewed reports.[71,76] A depressive episode characterized by irritability or anger or aggressiveness could be defined as dysphoric depression.[77] Feelings of anger are reported in 75% of women meeting the criteria for postpartum depression.[78] High anger scores were reported both in the antenatal and in the postnatal periods, and anger was directed both inward (manifesting itself as self-denigration or suicidality) or outward (manifesting as anger attacks).[79] In the perinatal population, irritability that is manifested outwards has especially important consequences because it is mainly directed on children and/or partner, thus creating a negative familial environment.[80] A study of the effects of prenatal depression of the mother on the neonate noted many more correlations between prenatal anger than prenatal depression and neonatal outcomes.[81,82] Irritability, which may be considered as a proxy to anger, could be a hallmark of perinatal depressive episodes,[83,84] although, being excluded from DSM-5 criteria for depression and not being considered in the EPDS, it is not assessed routinely.

Agitation

The few studies we found that assessed agitation during perinatal episodes found higher rates of agitation in these episodes as compared with nonperinatal depressive episodes,[65] especially in patients with BD.[85] Lack of psychomotor retardation is also reported in depressive postpartum episodes, which should be considered a clue for mixicity.[86,87] Agitation is frequently correlated with suicidal ideation and thoughts of self-harm and should therefore always be taken into serious consideration.[88,89]

Early insomnia

Sleep disturbances are characteristic of the perinatal period for most women in the general population. Sleep is usually impaired during the last part of pregnancy owing to physical discomfort and even more so after delivery owing to neonate care, which is usually performed by the new mother, whether breastfeeding or not. Postpartum sleep, especially in patients with BD, may protect from perinatal episodes and its derangement may constitute a trigger for such episodes.[90] Insomnia is defined as difficulty falling asleep or returning to sleep in the absence of physical discomfort or environmental disturbances (eg, noise or demands from the infant). Insomnia is present in more than 50% of women seeking psychiatric help in the perinatal period and severe insomnia is present in 12%.[91] Early insomnia or difficulty falling asleep is in particular highly correlated with postpartum depressive symptoms,[92] which is a distinctive trait of atypical depressive episodes and may herald psychosis in women with BD.[90]

Suicidality

Suicide is the second leading cause of death in postpartum women, accounting for approximately 20% of postpartum mortality.[93,94] A prospective study found that 16.97% of women with major depressive disorder or BDII had thoughts of self-harm and 6.16% reported suicidal ideation during the first year postpartum.[95] Interestingly, women with thoughts of self-harm or suicidal ideation also reported higher levels of depression and hypomanic symptoms. High suicidality in depressed mothers has been associated with more sleep and eating problems, more anxiety, and more emotional lability compared with depressed mothers with low suicidality; the former also scored significantly higher on psychoticism scales.[96] Importantly, those who made actual attempts to take their lives used more violent and lethal methods (eg, jumping from a building, self-incineration, or intentional traffic accidents), indicating high intent.[97–99]

Racing or crowded thoughts

Even though racing or crowded thoughts are frequently observed in clinical practice among women during the perinatal period, it is a symptom that is scarcely reported in the literature. Interesting descriptions are given in a study by Davies and colleagues,[2] who examined experiences and explanations of depression among Xhosa-speaking pregnant women, mothers, and health workers in an urban township in Cape Town, South Africa. Interestingly, many of the expressions used by the women are descriptive of what we would label MxD. Here follow some of their descriptions:

- "It's when your brain is, is cramped … It's not focused on who I'm talking to, the brain is busy, it's under suffocation, and everything can just blow up right now."
- They are angry, and when they talk about their problems they cry.
- Thinking too much, and when she is thinking, it's like she is going to go mad, and lose control. For example, when she thinks, she can even scream thinking about committing suicide.
- Interestingly, the phrase thinking too much ("kufungisisa") was also identified as both a cause and a symptom of depression by the Shona people in Zimbabwe.
- One mother said that she knew she was depressed because she thinks until her "brain is tired."[2]

This example makes clear that racing thoughts are present across cultures and are perceived as part of a not better specified "depression."

Screening

Screening for the presence of mixed episodes in the perinatal period is currently performed with classical clinical interviews when there are suspicions for their presence. Routine mood assessments during the perinatal period focuses on depression and the sole instrument used is the EPDS,[100] yet many an investigator calls for careful screening for BD in women with their first onset of depression in the postpartum period, in cases of recurrence of depression immediately after delivery,[39] in treatment-resistant postpartum depression,[33] in depression with psychotic features, or in cases of a positive family history for BD.[27,75] To avoid missing the diagnosis of postpartum MxD, appropriate diagnostic tools should be used.

For the time being, several instruments validated in nonperinatal populations have been used and proved useful. The HCL-32 can be helpful in detecting hypomania and proved to be reliable and easy to administer, with measurement properties largely invariant across cultures.[101] The Highs Scale[51] addresses cognitive and affective symptoms of hypomania assessing feeling elated, being more active and/or more talkative than usual, racing thoughts, feeling like an especially important person, decreased sleep requirement, and difficult concentration. The Mood Disorder Questionnaire is a 15-item self-report inventory that assesses the lifetime prevalence of hypomanic or manic symptoms based on DSM-IV criteria.[102] The Koukopoulos Mixed Depression Rating Scale is the first rating scale specifically designed to assess

MxD. It was developed to enable clinicians and research investigators to collect data assessing the presence and severity of symptoms of excitatory or mixed nature in people with a DSM-IV major depressive episode. It consists of 14 clinician-rated items and recently received validation.[103]

The conjoint application of these assessment tools may be useful in completing our knowledge of patients who all too often suffer undiagnosed BD and whose mixed states are missed, with deleterious consequences on their optimal treatment.

Limitations

Because this is not a systematic review, caveats of nonsystematic reviews such as the lack of exhaustive review of the literature and formal data extraction apply.

SUMMARY AND FUTURE PERSPECTIVES

Mixed symptoms seem to be common in the perinatal period, even though they are scarcely noted in the literature. The neglect of modern psychiatry on mixed affective states is probably rooted in our current nosologic approach and this holds true, especially in the perinatal area where the term postpartum depression has encompassed all types depressive episodes and the term postpartum psychosis all types of manic episodes with a clear cut distinction between the two.

It is not easy to resolve the puzzle why the perinatal period is a vulnerable one, beginning with the third trimester of pregnancy, for the expression of MxD, but it could be related to excitability changes in the stress system and in particular, in GABAergic activity, which is influenced by neurosteroids. This has been shown in the mouse[104,105] and may occur also in the human; recent data point to the efficacy of the allopregnanolone analog, brexanolone, in treating postpartum depression.[1] Future studies should address whether GABAergic instability in late pregnancy and puerperium is related with a higher rate of mixed symptoms.

In our view, the diagnostic evaluation, even for women who present for depression should include questions on manic, hypomanic, and mixed symptoms to differentiate MxD from the classic melancholic states. We propose to carefully evaluate any case of perinatal depression that raises clinical suspicions for bipolarity and to consider the Koukopoulos' scale, or other similar criteria, for identifying mixed states. This should impact the treatment of women with MxD, because commonly prescribed antidepressants, which are associated with cycle acceleration and switch to opposite polarity, would not be the optimal treatment for this condition.

REFERENCES

1. Haas S. Psychiatric complications in gynecology and obstetrics. In: Bellack L, editor. Psychology of physical illness: psychiatry applied to medicine, surgery and the specialties. New York: Grune & Stratton; 1952.
2. Davies T, Schneider M, Nyatsanza M, et al. The sun has set even though it is morning": experiences and explanations of perinatal depression in an urban township, Cape Town. Transcult Psychiatry 2016;53(3):286–312.
3. Sharma V, Xie B, Campbell MK, et al. A prospective study of diagnostic conversion of major depressive disorder to bipolar disorder in pregnancy and postpartum. Bipolar Disord 2014;16(1):16–21.
4. Koukopoulos A, Sani G, Koukopoulos AE, et al. Melancholia agitata and mixed depression. Acta Psychiatr Scand 2007;115(Suppl. 433):50–7.
5. Maj M, Pirozzi R, Magliano L, et al. Agitated depression in bipolar I disorder: prevalence, phenomenology, and outcome. Am J Psychiatry 2003;160:2134–40.

6. Koukopoulos A, Albert MJ, Sani G, et al. Mixed depressive states: nosologic and therapeutic issues. Int Rev Psychiatry 2005;17:21–37.
7. Sani G, Vöhringer PA, Napoletano F, et al. Koukopoulos diagnostic criteria for mixed depression: a validation study. J Affect Disord 2014;164:14–8.
8. Akiskal HS, Benazzi F. Family history validation of the bipolar nature of depressive mixed states. J Affect Disord 2003;73:113–22.
9. Sato T, Bottlender R, Schröter A, et al. Frequency of manic symptoms during a depressive episode and unipolar 'depressive mixed state' as bipolar spectrum. Acta Psychiatr Scand 2003;107(4):268–74.
10. Maj M, Pirozzi R, Magliano L, et al. Agitated "unipolar" major depression: prevalence, phenomenology, and outcome. J Clin Psychiatry 2006;67(5):712–9.
11. Goldberg JF, Perlis RH, Bowden CL, et al. Manic symptoms during depressive episodes in 1,380 patients with bipolar disorder: findings from the STEP-BD. Am J Psychiatry 2009;166(2):173–81.
12. Perugi G, Angst J, Azorin JM, et al, BRIDGE-II-Mix Study Group. Mixed features in patients with a major depressive episode: the BRIDGE-II-MIX study. J Clin Psychiatry 2015;76(3):e351–8.
13. Bottlender R, Sato T, Kleindienst N, et al. Mixed depressive features predict maniform switch during treatment of depression in bipolar I disorder. J Affect Disord 2004;78(2):149–52.
14. Vieta E, Grunze H, Azorin JM, et al. Phenomenology of manic episodes according to the presence or absence of depressive features as defined in DSM-5: results from the IMPACT self-reported online survey. J Affect Disord 2014;156: 206–13.
15. Diflorio A, Jones I. Is sex important? Gender differences in bipolar disorder. Int Rev Psychiatry 2010;22(5):437–52.
16. Cassidy F, Carroll BJ. The clinical epidemiology of pure and mixed manic episodes. Bipolar Disord 2001;3:35–40.
17. Suppes T, Mintz J, McElroy SL, et al. Mixed hypomania in 908 patients with bipolar disorder evaluated prospectively in the Stanley Foundation Bipolar Treatment Network: a sex-specific phenomenon. Arch Gen Psychiatry 2005;62: 1089–96.
18. Grant BF, Stinson FS, Hasin DS, et al. Prevalence, correlates, and comorbidity of bipolar I disorder and axis I and II disorders: results from the National Epidemiologic Survey on alcohol and related conditions. J Clin Psychiatry 2005;66: 1205–15.
19. Kessing LV. Gender differences in the phenomenology of bipolar disorder. Bipolar Disord 2004;6:421–5.
20. Kessing LV. The prevalence of mixed episodes during the course of illness in bipolar disorder. Acta Psychiatr Scand 2008;117:216–24.
21. Robb JC, Young LT, Cooke RG, et al. Gender differences in patients with bipolar disorder influence outcome in the medical outcomes survey (SF-20) subscale scores. J Affect Disord 1998;49:189–93.
22. Benazzi F. The role of gender in depressive mixed state. Psychopathology 2003; 36:213–7.
23. Soares CN, Zitek B. Reproductive hormone sensitivity and risk for depression across the female life cycle: a continuum of vulnerability? J Psychiatry Neurosci 2008;33:331–43.
24. Schmidt PJ, Nieman LK, Danaceau MA, et al. Differential behavioral effects of gonadal steroids in women with and in those without premenstrual syndrome. N Engl J Med 1998;338:209–16.

25. Bloch M, Schmidt PJ, Danaceau M, et al. Effects of gonadal steroids in women with a history of postpartum depression. Am J Psychiatry 2000;157:924–30.

26. Rusner M, Berg M, Begley C. Bipolar disorder in pregnancy and childbirth: a systematic review of outcomes. BMC Pregnancy Childbirth 2016;16(1):331.

27. Sharma V, Khan M, Corpse C, et al. Missed bipolarity and psychiatric comorbidity in women with postpartum depression. Bipolar Disord 2008;10:742–7.

28. Viguera AC, Whitfield T, Baldessarini RJ, et al. Risk of recurrence in women with bipolar disorder during pregnancy: prospective study of mood stabilizer discontinuation. Am J Psychiatry 2007;164:1817–24.

29. Koukopoulos A, Sani G, Ghaemi SN. Mixed features of depression: why DSM-5 is wrong (and so was DSM-IV). Br J Psychiatry 2013;203(1):3–5.

30. Koukopoulos A, Sani G. DSM-5 criteria for depression with mixed features: a farewell to mixed depression. Acta Psychiatr Scand 2014;129(1):4–16.

31. Sani G, Tondo L, Koukopoulos A, et al. Suicide in a large population of former psychiatric inpatients. Psychiatry Clin Neurosci 2011;65(3):286–95.

32. Mazzarini L, Kotzalidis GD, Piacentino D, et al, BRIDGE-II-Mix Study Group. Is recurrence in major depressive disorder related to bipolarity and mixed features? Results from the BRIDGE-II-Mix study. J Affect Disord 2018;229:164–70.

33. Sharma V, Khan M. Identification of bipolar disorder in women with postpartum depression. Bipolar Disord 2010;12:335–40.

34. Kendell RE, Chalmers JC, Platz C. Epidemiology of puerperal psychosis. Br J Psychiatry 1987;150:662–73.

35. Kadrmas A, Winokur G, Crowe R. Postpartum mania. Br J Psychiatry 1979;135:551–4.

36. Munk-Olsen T, Jones I, Laursen TM. Birth order and postpartum psychiatric disorders. Bipolar Disord 2014;16(3):300–7.

37. Hunt N, Silverstone T. Does puerperal illness distinguish a subgroup of bipolar patients? J Affect Disord 1995;34:101–7.

38. Valdimarsdottir U, Hultman CM, Harlow B, et al. Psychotic illness in first-time mothers with no previous psychiatric hospitalizations: a population-based study. PLoS Med 2009;6:e13.

39. Brockington I, Margison F, Schofield E, et al. The clinical picture of the depressed form of puerperal psychosis. J Affect Disord 1998;15:29–37.

40. Heron J, Robertson Blackmore E, McGuinness M, et al. No 'latent period' in the onset of bipolar affective puerperal psychosis. Arch Womens Ment Health 2007;10(2):79–81.

41. Jones I, Craddock N. Bipolar disorder and childbirth: the importance of recognising risk. Br J Psychiatry 2005;186:453–4.

42. Viguera AC, Nonacs R, Cohen LS, et al. Risk of recurrence of bipolar disorder in pregnant and nonpregnant women after discontinuing lithium maintenance. Am J Psychiatry 2000;157:179–84.

43. Maina G, Rosso G, Aguglia A, et al. Recurrence rates of bipolar disorder during the postpartum period: a study on 276 medication-free Italian women. Arch Womens Ment Health 2014;17(5):367–72.

44. Viguera AC, Tondo L, Koukopoulos AE, et al. Episodes of mood disorders in 2,252 pregnancies and postpartum periods. Am J Psychiatry 2011;168(11):1179–85.

45. Howard LM, Molyneaux E, Dennis C-L, et al. Non-psychotic mental disorders in the perinatal period. Lancet 2014;384:1775–88.

46. Jones I, Chandra PS, Dazzan P, et al. Bipolar disorder, affective psychosis, and schizophrenia in pregnancy and the postpartum period. Lancet 2014;384: 1789–99.
47. Khan M, Sharma V. Post-partum depressive episodes and bipolar disorder. Lancet 2015;385:771–2.
48. Wesseloo R, Kamperman AM, Munk-Olsen T, et al. Risk of postpartum relapse in bipolar disorder and postpartum psychosis: a systematic review and meta-analysis. Am J Psychiatry 2016;173(2):117–27.
49. Musliner KL, Østergaard SD. Patterns and predictors of conversion to bipolar disorder in 91 587 individuals diagnosed with unipolar depression. Acta Psychiatr Scand 2018;137(5):422–32.
50. Freeman MP, Smith KW, Freeman SA, et al. The impact of reproductive events on the course of bipolar disorder in women. J Clin Psychiatry 2002;63(4):284–7.
51. Glover V, Liddle P, Taylor A, et al. Mild hypomania (the highs) can be a feature of the first postpartum week: association with later depression. Br J Psychiatry 1994;164:517–21.
52. Lane A, Keville R, Morris M, et al. Postnatal depression and elation among mothers and their partners: prevalence and predictors. Br J Psychiatry 1997; 171:550–5.
53. Hasegawa M. Mild hypomania phenomenon in Japanese puerperal women. Nurs Health Sci 2000;2:231–5.
54. Webster J, Pritchard MA, Creedy D, et al. A simplified predictive index for the detection of women at risk for postnatal depression. Birth 2003;30:101–8.
55. Farias ME, Wenk E, Cordero M. Adaptacion de la escala highs para la deteccion de sintomatologia hipomaniaca en el puerperio. Trastornos Del Animo 2007;3: 27–36.
56. Heron J, Haque S, Oyebode F, et al. A longitudinal study of hypomania and depression symptoms in pregnancy and the postpartum period. Bipolar Disord 2009;11:410–7.
57. Sharma V, Mazmanian D. The DSM-5 peripartum specifier: prospects and pitfalls. Arch Womens Ment Health 2014;17(2):171–3.
58. Viguera AC, Baldessarini RJ, Tondo L. Response to lithium maintenance treatment in bipolar disorders: comparison of women and men. Bipolar Disord 2001;3(5):245–52.
59. Marcé LV. Traité de la Folie des Femmes Enceintes: Des Nouvelles Accouchés et des Nourrices. Paris: Baillière et Fils; 1858.
60. Azorin JM, Angst J, Gamma A, et al. Identifying features of bipolarity in patients with first-episode postpartum depression: findings from the international BRIDGE study. J Affect Disord 2012;136(3):710–5.
61. Rybakowski JK, Suwalska A, Lojko D, et al. Types of depression more frequent in bipolar than in unipolar affective illness: results of the Polish DEP-BI study. Psychopathology 2007;40(3):153–8.
62. Çelik SB, Bucaktepe GE, Uludağ A, et al. Screening mixed depression and bipolarity in the postpartum period at a primary health care center. Compr Psychiatry 2016;71:57–62.
63. Colom F, Cruz N, Pacchiarotti I, et al. Postpartum bipolar episodes are not distinct from spontaneous episodes: implications for DSM-V. J Affect Disord 2010;126(1–2):61–4.
64. Whiffen VE, Gotlib IH. Comparison of postpartum and nonpostpartum depression: clinical presentation, psychiatric history, and psychosocial functioning. J Consult Clin Psychol 1993;61(3):485–94.

65. Bernstein IH, Rush AJ, Yonkers K, et al. Symptom features of postpartum depression: are they distinct? Depress Anxiety 2008;25(1):20–6.
66. Sharma V, Burt VK, Ritchie HL. Bipolar II postpartum depression: detection, diagnosis, and treatment. Am J Psychiatry 2009;166(11):1217–21.
67. Smith S, Heron J, Haque S, et al. Measuring hypomania in the postpartum: a comparison of the Highs Scale and the Altman Mania Rating Scale. Arch Womens Ment Health 2009;12(5):323–7.
68. Pingo J, van den Heuvel LL, Vythylingum B, et al. Probable postpartum hypomania and depression in a South African cohort. Arch Womens Ment Health 2017; 20(3):427–37.
69. Leight KL, Fitelson EM, Weston CA, et al. Childbirth and mental disorders. Int Rev Psychiatry 2010;22:453–71.
70. O'Hara MW. Postpartum depression: what we know. J Clin Psychol 2009;65: 1258–69.
71. Pitt B. Atypical depression following childbirth. Br J Psychiatry 1968;114: 1325–35.
72. McCoy SJG, Beal JM, Payton ME, et al. Correlations of visual analog scales with Edinburgh Postnatal Depression Scale. J Affect Disord 2005;86(2–3):295–7.
73. Ballinger CB, Kay DS, Naylor GJ, et al. Some biochemical findings during pregnancy and after delivery in relation to mood change. Psychol Med 1982;12: 549–56.
74. Robin AA. The psychological changes of normal parturition. Psychiatr Q 1962; 36:129–50.
75. Sharma V. Management of bipolar II disorder during pregnancy and the postpartum period–Motherisk Update 2008. Can J Clin Pharmacol 2009;16(1): e33–41.
76. Andrews-Fike C. A review of postpartum depression. Prim Care Companion J Clin Psychiatry 1999;1(1):9–14.
77. Maloni JA, Park S, Anthony MK, et al. Measurement of antepartum depressive symptoms during high-risk pregnancy. Res Nurs Health 2005;28(1):16–26.
78. Shlomi Polachek I, Huller Harari L, Baum M, et al. Postpartum anxiety in a cohort of women from the general population: risk factors and association with depression during last week of pregnancy, postpartum depression and postpartum PTSD. Isr J Psychiatry Relat Sci 2014;51(2):128–34.
79. Field T, Diego M, Hernandez-Reif M, et al. Pregnancy anxiety and comorbid depression and anger: effects on the fetus and neonate. Depress Anxiety 2003;17(3):140–51.
80. Ou CH, Hall WA. Anger in the context of postnatal depression: an integrative review. Birth 2018;45(4):336–46.
81. Field T, Diego M, Hernandez-Reif M, et al. Prenatal anger effects on the fetus and neonate. J Obstet Gynaecol 2002;22(3):260–6.
82. Slomian J, Honvo G, Emonts P, et al. Consequences of maternal postpartum depression: a systematic review of maternal and infant outcomes. Womens Health (Lond) 2019;15. 1745506519844044. [Erratum appears in Womens Health (Lond) 2019;15:1745506519854864].
83. Williamson JA, O'Hara MW, Stuart S, et al. Assessment of postpartum depressive symptoms: the importance of somatic symptoms and irritability. Assessment 2015;22(3):309–18.
84. Kettunen P, Koistinen E, Hintikka J. Is postpartum depression a homogenous disorder: time of onset, severity, symptoms and hopelessness in relation to the course of depression. BMC Pregnancy Childbirth 2014;14:402.

85. Fisher SD, Wisner KL, Clark CT, et al. Factors associated with onset timing, symptoms, and severity of depression identified in the postpartum period. J Affect Disord 2016;203:111–20.

86. Fox M, Sandman CA, Davis EP, et al. A longitudinal study of women's depression symptom profiles during and after the postpartum phase. Depress Anxiety 2018;35(4):292–304.

87. Hoertel N, López S, Peyre H, et al. Are symptom features of depression during pregnancy, the postpartum period and outside the peripartum period distinct? Results from a nationally representative sample using item response theory (IRT). Depress Anxiety 2015;32(2):129–40.

88. Serra F, Gordon-Smith K, Perry A, et al. Agitated depression in bipolar disorder. Bipolar Disord 2019. https://doi.org/10.1111/bdi.12778.

89. Kamperman AM, Veldman-Hoek MJ, Wesseloo R, et al. Phenotypical characteristics of postpartum psychosis: a clinical cohort study. Bipolar Disord 2017; 19(6):450–7.

90. Sharma V, Mazmanian D. Sleep loss and postpartum psychosis. Bipolar Disord 2003;5(2):98–105.

91. Swanson LM, Pickett SM, Flynn H, et al. Relationships among depression, anxiety, and insomnia symptoms in perinatal women seeking mental health treatment. J Womens Health (Larchmt) 2011;20(4):553–8.

92. Goyal D, Gay C, Lee K. Fragmented maternal sleep is more strongly correlated with depressive symptoms than infant temperament at three months postpartum. Arch Womens Ment Health 2009;12(4):229–37.

93. Lindahl V, Pearson JL, Colpe L. Prevalence of suicidality during pregnancy and the postpartum. Arch Womens Ment Health 2005;8(2):77–87.

94. Cantwell R, Clutton-Brock T, Cooper G, et al. Saving Mothers' Lives: reviewing maternal deaths to make motherhood safer: 2006-2008. The Eighth Report of the Confidential Enquiries into Maternal Deaths in the United Kingdom. BJOG 2011;118(Suppl 1):1–203 [Erratum appears in BJOG. 2015;122(5):e1].

95. Dudek D, Jaeschke R, Siwek M, et al. Postpartum depression: identifying associations with bipolarity and personality traits. Preliminary results from a cross-sectional study in Poland. Psychiatry Res 2014;215(1):69–74.

96. Paris R, Bolton RE, Weinberg MK. Postpartum depression, suicidality, and mother-infant interactions. Arch Womens Ment Health 2009;12(5):309–21.

97. Henshaw C. Maternal suicide. In: Cockburn J, Pawson M, editors. Psychological challenges in obstetrics and gynecology: the clinical Management. New York: Springer; 2007. p. 157–64.

98. Högberg U, Innala E, Sandström A. Maternal mortality in Sweden, 1980–1988. Obstet Gynecol 1994;84:240–4.

99. Appleby L. Suicide after pregnancy and the first postnatal year. Br Med J 1991; 302:137–40.

100. Cox JL, Holden JM, Sagovsky R. Detection of postnatal depression. Development of the 10-item Edinburgh Postnatal Depression Scale. Br J Psychiatry 1987;150:782–6.

101. Angst J, Meyer TD, Adolfsson R, et al. Hypomania: a transcultural perspective. World Psychiatry 2010;9(1):41–9.

102. Hirschfeld RM, Williams JB, Spitzer RL, et al. Development and validation of a screening instrument for bipolar spectrum disorder: the Mood Disorder Questionnaire. Am J Psychiatry 2000;157(11):1873–5.

103. Sani G, Vöhringer PA, Barroilhet SA, et al. The Koukopoulos Mixed Depression Rating Scale (KMDRS): an International Mood Network (IMN) validation study of a new mixed mood rating scale. J Affect Disord 2018;232:9–16.
104. Maguire J, Ferando I, Simonsen C, et al. Excitability changes related to GABAA receptor plasticity during pregnancy. J Neurosci 2009;29(30):9592–601.
105. Zheng W, Cai DB, Zheng W, et al. Brexanolone for postpartum depression: a meta-analysis of randomized controlled studies. Psychiatry Res 2019;279:83–9.

Postpartum Depression
Identification and Treatment in the Clinic Setting

Emily B. Kroska, PhD[a], Zachary N. Stowe, MD[b],*

KEYWORDS

- Postpartum depression • Diagnosis • Prevalence • Antidepressants
- Psychotherapy

KEY POINTS

- Postpartum depression (PPD) is a common disorder that if left untreated may have adverse consequences for women, children, and families.
- A variety of risk factors have been reliably characterized, enabling clinicians to identify women at risk and develop treatment plans for prevention and intervention.
- Use of a screening tool, such as the Edinburgh Postnatal Depression Scale (10-item, self-rated), will improve early identification in the primary care setting.
- Antidepressants and psychotherapies are effective in the treatment of PPD.
- The selective serotonin reuptake inhibitors have a large database for use during pregnancy and breast-feeding.

INTRODUCTION

Postpartum depression (PPD) is broadly defined as an episode of major depression occurring during the perinatal period. PPD affects about 10% to 15% of women in developed countries following childbirth. PPD is the leading cause of nonobstetric hospitalization among childbearing women in the United States.[1] PPD confers a substantial risk to the mother, family, and offspring across several domains. As such, recent initiatives to increase screening and preventive care have been released by the US Preventive Services Task Force.[2,3] The current review addresses the *diagnosis, prevalence, predictors, consequences, and treatment* of PPD.

This article originally appeared in Obstetrics and Gynecology Clinics, Volume 47, Issue 3, September 2020.
a Department of Psychological and Brain Sciences, University of Iowa, W311 Seashore Hall, Iowa City, IA 52242, USA; b Department of Psychiatry, University of Wisconsin-Madison, 6001 Research Park Boulevard, Madison, WI 53719, USA
* Corresponding author. 6001 Research Park Drive, Madison, WI 63719.
E-mail address: zstowe@wisc.edu

Diagnosis

PPD is not defined as a unique diagnostic code by the *Diagnostic and Statistical Manual (DSM-5)*.[4] Instead, a diagnosis of major depressive disorder is given with the specifier "with peripartum onset," which indicates that onset of symptoms is during pregnancy or in the first 4 weeks after delivery.[4] Criteria include 5 of 9 symptoms for most of 2 weeks, clinical impairment, and elimination of alternative causes. In research contexts, the postpartum period is less rigidly defined, with the World Health Organization classifying PPD as occurring during pregnancy or within the 12 months following delivery.

It is clinically important to distinguish from PPD the postpartum blues, which include mood symptoms (eg, tearfulness, lability) in the first 4 to 10 days following delivery. Postpartum blues are considered mild in severity and limited in duration, and most importantly, do not impair functioning.[5] Estimates indicate that most women experience postpartum blues symptoms following childbirth. Furthermore, PPD is also distinct from postpartum psychosis, characterized by severe mood disturbances and psychotic symptoms, and often requiring inpatient hospitalization.[6] Symptoms of anxiety are frequently comorbid with PPD, with some studies suggesting that nearly half of symptoms in late pregnancy and 40% of symptoms in the postpartum were related to anxiety (as measured by the Edinburgh Postnatal Depression Scale [EPDS]).[7] Also observed in this study were elevated obsessive-compulsive symptoms in the perinatal and postpartum assessments as compared with nonpregnant women.[7] Miller and O'Hara[8] found that about 30% of women reported clinically significant obsessive-compulsive symptoms at 2 –weeks' postpartum, and 11% at 12 –weeks' postpartum. Furthermore, intrusive thoughts and compulsive behaviors were associated with worsened depressive symptoms at both 2 and 12 weeks' postpartum.[8]

Prevalence

Given variability in the time course of measurement, assessment methodology, and study sample, prevalence estimates for PPD vary substantially. Frequently, studies use self-report screening instruments to estimate prevalence, which creates substantial variability in estimates across studies and samples. Estimates of prevalence are also impacted by the time interval specified by the investigators as to what constitutes or defines the postpartum period.

A seminal metaanalysis published in 1996 identified a prevalence of 13%[9]; this was followed by a meta-analysis that only included studies that used interview assessments, rather than self-report measures, finding a prevalence of minor or major depression of 19.2% (7.1% for major depression) in the 3 months following delivery.[10] One metaanalysis specifically examined prevalence of PPD symptoms among mothers who were healthy before pregnancy, finding a prevalence of 17%.[11] A recent metaanalysis comparing prevalence across nations found substantial variability among a global pooled prevalence of 17.7%.[12] Importantly, 73% of the variability in prevalence was accounted for by economic and health variability, suggesting the importance of socioeconomic and health disparities in determining risk for PPD.[12]

A question of particular interest that has continued to generate investigation has been whether the prevalence of depression in the postpartum period is elevated relative to the risk for non-postpartum women in the childbearing years. Methods undertaken to study this phenomenon have included pairing pregnant women and closely matched nonpregnant acquaintances through pregnancy and postpartum, finding that risk for depression diagnosis was not elevated among the pregnant women, but higher depressive symptoms were observed late in pregnancy and in the early postpartum.[13] A large population-based study in Sweden calculated relative risk of depression following childbirth as compared with a computer-generated random date unrelated to childbirth, finding that depression was no more likely to occur following childbirth.[14] In contrast, there have been several longitudinal studies indicating that the postpartum period is a time of elevated risk for both depression[15-17] and psychiatric hospital admission.[18] One study examined both trait (susceptibility to develop depression) and state (episodic depressive symptoms) depression across 10 years, finding that when controlling for trait depression, the risk for depression in the postpartum period is elevated, with the highest risk in the first months postpartum.[19] Finally, heritability research has indicated that one-third of the genetic variability in PPD was unique, unshared with nonperinatal depression.[20] Future research should continue to examine relative risk for depression postpartum and account for variables that may compound risk, including perinatal complications.

Predictors of Risk for Postpartum Depression

Substantial research has focused on identification of factors that increase individual risk for development of PPD. A limitation of much of this research is that factors are not often considered in conjunction given small sample sizes within particular categories of risk, limiting statistical power. A recent population-based study addressed such limitations by comparing mothers with and without a history of depression, and as such, identified risk factors within this context.[21] This study identified that a history of depression increased risk for PPD 20-fold.[21] When accounting for history of depression, maternal age conferred increased risk for PPD, both for adolescents with no history of depression and for women 35 years of age and older with a history of depression.[21] Furthermore, a recent metaanalysis indicated an increase in risk for PPD among women with gestational diabetes.[22] Silverman and colleagues[21] found that among those with a history of depression, the risk for PPD increased 1.5-fold. Emotional symptoms in the early postpartum period, such as postpartum blues,[23] as well as high negative affect and low positive affect,[24] predict PPD symptoms longitudinally. **Box 1** summarizes the replicated predictors identified through metaanalysis.

Screening

The US Preventive Services Task Force recommended screening of pregnant and postpartum women to encourage early identification of symptoms, appropriate referral, and treatment.[25] The American College of Obstetricians and Gynecologists recommends use of the EPDS[26] for screening. The scale considers both depressive and anxiety symptoms and measures mood-related symptoms rather than somatic symptoms that may be associated with pregnancy and delivery (eg, lack of sleep, fatigue). Elevated scores ($\geq$10) indicate *possible* PPD and warrant further evaluation. A large study in Ireland found when using a score of greater than 12 on the EPDS, 15.8% of women demonstrated *probable* depression, with higher symptoms later in pregnancy.[27] The final item assesses suicidal ideation and should be given consideration independent of the total score. Suicide contributes significantly to postpartum maternal mortality. Consistent screening for depression during the prenatal and the early postpartum period and with follow-up for women who screen positive could substantially reduce maternal mortality related to suicide. Other scales commonly used for screening include the Patient Health Questionnaire-9[28] and the Beck Depression Inventory.[29]

Another widely used method includes screening for dysphoric mood or anhedonia, and if positive, administration of a depression questionnaire. The US Agency for

> **Box 1**
> **Risk factors for postpartum depression**
>
> History of depression[21,68,69]
>
> Higher maternal age[21]
>
> Shorter gestational age[21]
>
> Gestational diabetes[21,22]
>
> Depression or anxiety symptoms during pregnancy[9,68]
>
> Postpartum blues symptoms[69]
>
> Stressful life events[9,68,69]
>
> Poor quality of marital relationship[9,69]
>
> Poor social support[9,68,69]
>
> Low socioeconomic status[9,12,69]
>
> Low self-esteem[69]
>
> Difficult infant temperament[69]
>
> Unplanned or unwanted pregnancy[69]

Healthcare Research and Quality and the United Kingdom's National Institute for Health and Care Excellence both recommend serial testing methodology. The use of this method has proved both sensitive and specific.

Screening with self-report questionnaires should be followed with formal diagnostic assessment and intervention. Evaluation should include assessment of symptoms, duration of symptoms, and clinical impairment. Alternative causes should be ruled out via both clinical interview and laboratory measures (eg, thyroid levels). Symptoms of mania and psychosis should be thoroughly evaluated in order to rule out postpartum psychosis and bipolar disorder. A complete personal and family history should be ascertained. Suicidal ideation, intent, means, and plan should be evaluated, as well as personal and family history of suicidality. Identification of imminent risk requires immediate psychiatric attention, which likely includes hospitalization and subsequent outpatient treatment. Finally, comorbid symptoms, including anxiety, obsessive-compulsive, panic, and substance use symptoms, should be assessed. Appropriate follow-up should be scheduled to monitor symptoms and treatment response.

Consequences

PPD is known to have a broad array of adverse effects on the mother, infant, and family. Although depression is associated with substantial disease burden and disability, PPD may be particularly consequential given the additional demands of child care. Studies indicate that PPD symptoms were the strongest predictor of poorer maternal responsiveness to the infant when including comorbid obsessive-compulsive symptoms and baseline depressive symptoms in the model.[8] Other studies have linked maternal PPD to insecure attachment and poor interaction between mother and child.[30] Poor interactions can impact long-term emotion regulation and distress tolerance, and several studies have conceptualized these abilities as ego-resilience.[31] Children of mothers with PPD had lower cognitive performance at 18 months, and boys were most adversely affected.[32] Child cognitive,[33] social,[31] and behavioral[33,34] functioning also has been shown to be adversely impacted by maternal PPD.

Beyond the impact on the child, PPD is associated with increased risk for psychiatric hospitalization.[18,35] Furthermore, PPD increases risk for maternal suicide if left undiagnosed, or if diagnosed but without follow-up and treatment.[36,37] Among parenting behaviors, PPD has been shown to impact breast-feeding, sleep, health care utilization, and infant vaccinations.[38] PPD also affects the partner of the mother, with increased paternal depression and parenting stress.[39] PPD is also associated with social isolation and marital discord.[40] As such, PPD has a significant impact on the mother but also on family dynamics, which can have long-term consequences.

Treatment

A review of the literature suggested that education about PPD can encourage help-seeking behavior and promote early recognition of symptoms.[41] Several treatments have been identified through randomized trials as effective for reducing PPD symptoms, including both psychotherapy and medications (Table 1).

Psychotherapy

Cognitive behavioral therapy (CBT) has demonstrated the most short- and long-term effectiveness when compared with treatment-as-usual interventions in reducing PPD symptoms in a recent metaanalysis.[42] CBT approaches may include strategies to address dysfunctional patterns of thoughts or promote behavioral engagement. Mindfulness- or acceptance-based CBT approaches may also emphasize changing the way one relates or responds to thoughts or emotions, rather than trying to alter the experience itself.[43]

Interpersonal psychotherapy (IPT) has garnered strong evidence of effectiveness in treating PPD in both individual and group formats.[44,45] IPT is a time-limited approach that contextualizes depression within the woman's relationships, aiming to reduce symptoms, expand interpersonal functioning, and increase social support. One metaanalysis found that when compared with control conditions, IPT had greater effect sizes than CBT.[46]

Other studies investigating supportive counseling approaches have found reductions in PPD.[47] Also based in a client-centered approach are listening visits, an intervention developed in the United Kingdom to be delivered by home visiting nurses.[48] The listening visits intervention has demonstrated effectiveness in treating depression in the United Kingdom, Sweden, and United States.[48–50] It is feasible that these listening interventions could be further facilitated through telemedicine or other media, if available.

Table 1 Treatment of postpartum depression	
Psychotherapy	**Medication**
Cognitive-behavioral therapy[a]	Sertraline[a]
Interpersonal psychotherapy[a]	Fluoxetine[a]
Listening visits[a]	Paroxetine[a]
Supportive counseling	Escitalopram
	Fluvoxamine
	Venlafaxine
	Nortriptyline
	Bupropion
	Nefazodone
	Brexanolone[a]

[a] Indicates support by at least 1 randomized controlled trial.

Medication

Typically, the first-line medication treatments for PPD are selective serotonin reuptake inhibitors (SSRI),[51] which carry low toxicity risk with regard to potential overdose and are less commonly associated with severe side effects. The SSRIs with the most randomized controlled trials to treat PPD are sertraline[52–54] and fluoxetine.[55] Fluoxetine was superior to placebo and comparable to psychotherapy.[55] Also identified as appropriate for PPD are paroxetine,[56,57] fluvoxamine,[58] and escitalopram.[59] A serotonin-norepinephrine reuptake inhibitor, venlafaxine,[60] is supported for treatment of PPD. As a class, antidepressants, particularly the SSRIs, have the largest database in breast-feeding and appear largely devoid of adverse effects. The most detailed data on nursing infant exposure through human breast milk rest with sertraline.[61]

Tricyclic antidepressants are not a first-line treatment and are considered high risk for potential overdose. In this class, nortriptyline has demonstrated preliminary indications of treating PPD.[51] Other medications that have been used in treating PPD include buproprion[62] and nefazodone.[63] Nortriptyline, bupropion, and nefazodone have not been examined in randomized trials, and thus, conclusions regarding effectiveness cannot be drawn.

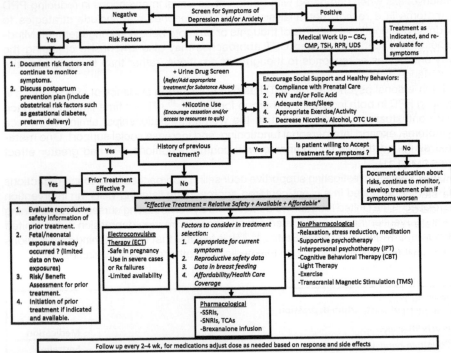

Fig. 1. Guidelines for identification and treatment planning for women during the perinatal period, modified from www.angelsguidelines.com. CBC, complete blood count; CMP, comprehensive metabolic panel; OTC, over the counter; Rx, prescription; TCAs, tricyclic antidepressants; TSH, thyroid stimulating hormone; PNV, prenatal vitamin; RPR, rapid plasma regain; UDS, urine drug screen; SSRI, selective serotonin re-uptake inhibitors; SNRI, serotonin / norepinephrine re-uptake inhibitors. (*Adapted from* The Antenatal and Neonatal Guidelines, Education and Learning System (ANGELS). Treatment of depression in pregnancy and postpartum period. ANGELS was established by two major state agencies, the University of Arkansas College of Medicine and the Arkansas Department of Human. www. angelsguidelines.com.)

It is important to educate patients that all aforementioned medication treatments for PPD often require several adherent weeks to be beneficial. As such, it is important to have follow-up to determine effectiveness of the treatment regimen in improving symptoms as the mother is attempting to navigate the many challenges that might present in the first months following childbirth. This follow-up is especially important for the mother who has given birth to a preterm infant, the mother who has given birth to an infant with a birth defect, or the mother who has given birth to a child with physical or emotional needs. A new treatment offering a solution to this limitation of other treatments is allopregnanolone (Brexanolone), which modulates GABA type A receptors. Recent trials indicated reductions in depressive symptoms in as early as 60 hours.[64,65] The major limitation of this medication is the considerable time and monitoring required for administration (ie, 60 hours of intravenous infusion). However, this drug is the first drug approved by the Food and Drug Administration (March 2019) specifically for treatment of PPD.

It is important for clinicians to consider treatment planning for preventing PPD in high-risk populations. A recent review[66] provided a summary of the available literature, including a randomized trial of sertraline that demonstrated dramatic efficacy in the prevention of PPD.[67] Identification of at-risk populations and incorporation of additional risk factors over the course of pregnancy and childbirth can better determine those women who are candidates for preventative treatment.

Several information sites are available to support clinicians in the identification and treatment planning for women during the perinatal period, such as www.angelsguidelines.com. **Fig. 1** provides a modification of such guidelines (see the Web site for additional information).

SUMMARY

In summary, PPD is a common, debilitating illness that has demonstrated distinction from major depression in research, despite categorization under major depression in the *DSM-5*. The risk factors associated with PPD span demographic, obstetric, psychiatric, and psychosocial variables. Predictors of PPD have been replicated in multiple studies and examined in multiple metaanalyses. As recommended by national standards, screening is of utmost importance in early detection of PPD in order to facilitate referral for treatment and ongoing monitoring. Consequences of untreated PPD for the mother range from social isolation to suicide, and consequences for the infant and family unit persist throughout child development. Treatment of PPD may include psychotherapy approaches, such as CBT, IPT, or listening visits. Medication treatment of PPD may include SSRI or newly approved brexanolone. Although PPD poses substantial risk for a mother and infant, early identification of risk for development of PPD, ongoing screening, and appropriate referrals for treatment may limit the adverse sequelae of the syndrome and thus promote lifelong maternal and familial health.

System recommendations include the following:
1. Ensure that all women are screened at least once for depression during both pregnancy and the postpartum period,
2. Educate providers on risk factors and screening tools,
3. Optimize detection of risk factors and symptoms,
4. Expedite referral and treatment,
5. Promptly identify suicidal behavior and refer for psychiatric intervention,
6. Discuss the impact of pregnancy on preexisting mental health conditions, including prior PPD, during preconception and prenatal care.

DISCLOSURE

E.B. Kroska has no competing interests to report. Z.N. Stowe has received research support and consultation honorarium from GlaxoSmithKline, Pfizer, and Wyeth Corporations and received speakers honoraria from these companies and Eli Lilly and Forest Corporations, but none of these relationships since 2008. He has received clinical trial support from Janssen Pharmaceuticals and Sage Therapeutics in the past 24 months and has received salary and research support from the National Institutes of Health and the Centers for Disease Control and Prevention.

REFERENCES

1. O'Hara MW. Postpartum depression: what we know. J Clin Psychol 2009;65: 1258–69.
2. O'Connor E, Senger CA, Henninger ML, et al. Interventions to prevent perinatal depression. JAMA 2019;321(6):588.
3. Curry SJ, Krist AH, Owens DK, et al. Interventions to prevent perinatal depression. JAMA 2019;321(6):580.
4. American Psychiatric Association. Diagnostic and statistical manual of mental disorders. 5th edition. Arlington (VA): American Psychiatric Association; 2013.
5. O'Hara MW, Schlechte JA, Lewis DA, et al. Prospective study of postpartum blues: biologic and psychosocial factors. Arch Gen Psychiatry 1991;48(9):801–6.
6. Heron J, McGuinness M, Blackmore ER, et al. Early postpartum symptoms in puerperal psychosis. BJOG 2008;115(3):348–53.
7. Ross LE, Gilbert Evans SE, Sellers EM, et al. Measurement issues in postpartum depression part 1: anxiety as a feature of postpartum depression. Arch Womens Ment Health 2003;6:51–7.
8. Miller ML, O'Hara MW. Obsessive-compulsive symptoms, intrusive thoughts and depressive symptoms: a longitudinal study examining relation to maternal responsiveness. J Reprod Infant Psychol 2019. https://doi.org/10.1080/02646838.2019.1652255.
9. O'Hara MW, Swain AM. Rates and risk of postpartum depression—a meta-analysis. Int Rev Psychiatry 1996;8(1):37–54.
10. Gavin NI, Gaynes BN, Lohr KN, et al. Perinatal depression: a systematic review of prevalence and incidence. Obstet Gynecol 2005;106(5, Part 1):1071–83.
11. Shorey S, Yin C, Chee I, et al. Prevalence and incidence of postpartum depression among healthy mothers: a systematic review and meta-analysis. J Psychiatr Res 2018;104:235–48.
12. Hahn-Holbrook J, Cornwell-Hinrichs T, Anaya I. Economic and health predictors of national postpartum depression prevalence: a systematic review, meta-analysis, and meta-regression of 291 studies from 56 countries. Front Psychiatry 2018;8. https://doi.org/10.3389/fpsyt.2017.00248.
13. O'Hara MW, Zekoski EM, Philipps LH, et al. Controlled prospective study of postpartum mood disorders: comparison of childbearing and nonchildbearing women. J Abnorm Psychol 1990;99(1):3–15.
14. Silverman ME, Reichenberg A, Lichtenstein P, et al. Is depression more likely following childbirth? A population-based study. Arch Womens Ment Health 2019;22(2):253–8.
15. Vesga-López O, Blanco C, Keyes K, et al. Psychiatric disorders in pregnant and postpartum women in the United States. Arch Gen Psychiatry 2008;65(7):805–15.

16. Eberhard-Gran M, Eskild A, Tambs K, et al. Depression in postpartum and non-postpartum women: prevalence and risk factors. Acta Psychiatr Scand 2002; 106(6):426–33.
17. Davé S, Petersen I, Sherr L, et al. Incidence of maternal and paternal depression in primary care: a cohort study using a primary care database. Arch Pediatr Adolesc Med 2010;164(11):1038–44.
18. Munk-Olsen T, Laursen TM, Pedersen CB, et al. New parents and mental disorders: a population-based register study. J Am Med Assoc 2006;296(21):2582–9.
19. Merkitch KG, Jonas KG, O'Hara MW. Modeling trait depression amplifies the effect of childbearing on postpartum depression. J Affect Disord 2017;223:69–75.
20. Viktorin A, Meltzer-Brody S, Kuja-Halkola R, et al. Heritability of perinatal depression and genetic overlap with nonperinatal depression. Am J Psychiatry 2016; 173:158–65.
21. Silverman ME, Reichenberg A, Savitz DA, et al. The risk factors for postpartum depression: a population-based study. Depress Anxiety 2017;34(2):178–87.
22. Azami M, Badfar G, Soleymani A, et al. The association between gestational diabetes and postpartum depression: a systematic review and meta-analysis. Diabetes Res Clin Pract 2019;149:147–55.
23. Hannah P, Adams D, Lee A, et al. Links between early post-partum mood and post-natal depression. Br J Psychiatry 1992;160:777–80.
24. Miller ML, Kroska EB, Grekin R. Immediate postpartum mood assessment and postpartum depressive symptoms. J Affect Disord 2017;207:69–75.
25. Siu AL, Bibbins-Domingo K, Grossman DC, et al. Screening for depression in adults: US preventive services task force recommendation statement. JAMA 2016;315(4):380–7.
26. Cox JL, Holden JM, Sagovsky R. Detection of postnatal depression: development of the 10-item Edinburgh postnatal depression scale. Br J Psychiatry 1987; 150(6):782–6.
27. Jairaj C, Fitzsimons CM, McAuliffe FM, et al. A population survey of prevalence rates of antenatal depression in the Irish obstetric services using the Edinburgh Postnatal Depression Scale (EPDS). Arch Womens Ment Health 2019;22(3): 349–55.
28. Kroenke K, Spitzer RL, Williams JBW. The PHQ-9: validity of a brief depression severity measure. J Gen Intern Med 2001;16(9):606–13.
29. Beck AT, Steer RA, Carbin MG. Psychometric properties of the Beck Depression Inventory: twenty-five years of evaluation. Clin Psychol Rev 1988;8(1):77–100.
30. Goodman SH, Gotlib IH. Risk for psychopathology in the children of depressed mothers: a developmental model for understanding mechanisms of transmission. Psychol Rev 1999;106(3):458–90.
31. Kersten-Alvarez LE, Hosman CMH, Riksen-Walraven JM, et al. Early school outcomes for children of postpartum depressed mothers: comparison with a community sample. Child Psychiatry Hum Dev 2012;43(2):201–18.
32. Murray L. The impact of postnatal depression on infant development. J Child Psychol Psychiatry 1992;33(3):543–61.
33. Grace SL, Evindar A, Stewart DE. The effect of postpartum depression on child cognitive development and behavior: a review and critical analysis of the literature. Arch Womens Ment Health 2003;6(4):263–74.
34. Sinclair D, Murray L. Effects of postnatal depression on children's adjustment to school: teacher's reports. Br J Psychiatry 1998;172:58–63.
35. Wisner KL, Chambers C, Sit DKY. Postpartum depression: a major public health problem. JAMA 2006;296(21):2616.

36. Meltzer-Brody S, Stuebe A. The long-term psychiatric and medical prognosis of perinatal mental illness. Best Pract Res Clin Obstet Gynaecol 2014;28(1):49–60.
37. Lindahl V, Pearson JL, Colpe L. Prevalence of suicidality during pregnancy and the postpartum. Arch Womens Ment Health 2005;8(2):77–87.
38. Field T. Postpartum depression effects on early interactions, parenting, and safety practices: a review. Infant Behav Dev 2010;33(1):1–6.
39. Goodman JH. Influences of maternal postpartum depression on fathers and on father-infant interaction. Infant Ment Health J 2008;29(6):624–43.
40. Letourneau NL, Dennis C-L, Benzies K, et al. Postpartum depression is a family affair: addressing the impact on mothers, fathers, and children. Issues Ment Health Nurs 2012;33(7):445–57.
41. Dennis C-L, Chung-Lee L. Postpartum depression help-seeking barriers and maternal treatment preferences: a qualitative systematic review. Birth 2006; 33(4):323–31.
42. Huang L, Zhao Y, Qiang C, et al. Is cognitive behavioral therapy a better choice for women with postnatal depression? A systematic review and meta-analysis. PLoS One 2018;13(10):e0205243.
43. Hayes SC. Acceptance and commitment therapy, relational frame theory, and the third wave of behavioral and cognitive therapies. Behav Ther 2004;35(4):639–65.
44. O'Hara MW, Stuart S, Gorman LL, et al. Efficacy of interpersonal psychotherapy for postpartum depression. Arch Gen Psychiatry 2000;57(11):1039–45.
45. Klier CM, Muzik M, Rosenblum KL, et al. Interpersonal psychotherapy adapted for the group setting in the treatment of postpartum depression. J Psychother Pract Res 2001;10(2):124–31.
46. Sockol LE, Epperson CN, Barber JP. Preventing postpartum depression: a meta-analytic review. Clin Psychol Rev 2013;33:1205–17.
47. Glavin K, Smith L, Sørum R, et al. Supportive counselling by public health nurses for women with postpartum depression. J Adv Nurs 2010;66(6):1317–27.
48. Holden JM, Sagovsky R, Cox JL. Counselling in a general practice setting: controlled study of home visitor intervention in treatment of postnatal depression. BMJ 1989;298:223–6.
49. Morrell CJ, Ricketts T, Tudor K, et al. Training health visitors in cognitive behavioural and person-centred approaches for depression in postnatal women as part of a cluster randomised trial and economic evaluation in primary care: the PoNDER trial. Prim Health Care Res Dev 2011;11–20. https://doi.org/10.1017/S1463423610000344.
50. Segre LS, Stasik SM, O'hara MW, et al. Listening visits: an evaluation of the effectiveness and acceptability of a home-based depression treatment. Psychother Res 2010;20(6):712–21.
51. Wisner KL, Peindl KS, Gigliotti TV. Tricyclics vs SSRIs for postpartum depression. Arch Womens Ment Health 1998;1(4):189–91.
52. Stowe ZN, Casarella J, Landry J, et al. Sertraline in the treatment of women with postpartum major depression. Depression 1995;3(1–2):49–55.
53. Hantsoo L, Ward-O'Brien D, Czarkowski KA, et al. A randomized, placebo-controlled, double-blind trial of sertraline for postpartum depression. Psychopharmacology (Berl) 2014;231(5):939–48.
54. Milgrom J, Gemmill AW, Ericksen J, et al. Treatment of postnatal depression with cognitive behavioural therapy, sertraline and combination therapy: a randomised controlled trial. Aust N Z J Psychiatry 2015;49(3):236–45.
55. Appleby L, Warner R, Whitton A, et al. A controlled study of fluoxetine and cognitive-behavioural counselling in the treatment of postnatal depression. Br Med J 1997;314(7085):932–6.

56. Misri S, Reebye P, Corral M, et al. The use of paroxetine and cognitive-behavioral therapy in postpartum depression and anxiety. J Clin Psychiatry 2004;65(9): 1236–41.
57. Yonkers KA, Lin H, Howell HB, et al. Pharmacologic treatment of postpartum women with new-onset major depressive disorder: a randomized controlled trial with paroxetine. J Clin Psychiatry 2008;69(4):659–65.
58. Suri R, Burt VK, Altshuler LL, et al. Fluvoxamine for postpartum depression. Am J Psychiatry 2001;158(10):1739–40. https://doi.org/10.1176/appi.ajp.158.10.1739.
59. Misri S, Abizadeh J, Albert G, et al. Restoration of functionality in postpartum depressed mothers. J Clin Psychopharmacol 2012;32(5):729–32.
60. Cohen LS, Viguera AC, Bouffard SM, et al. Venlafaxine in the treatment of postpartum depression. J Clin Psychiatry 2001;62(8):592–6.
61. Stowe ZN, Hostetter AL, Owens MJ, et al. The pharmacokinetics of sertraline excretion into human breast milk: determinants of infant serum concentrations. J Clin Psychiatry 2003;64(1):73–80.
62. Nonacs RM, Soares CN, Viguera AC, et al. Bupropion SR for the treatment of postpartum depression: a pilot study. Int J Neuropsychopharmacol 2005;8(3): 445–9.
63. Suri R, Burt VK, Altshuler LL. Nefazodone for the treatment of postpartum depression. Arch Womens Ment Health 2005;8:55–6.
64. Meltzer-Brody S, Colquhoun H, Riesenberg R, et al. Brexanolone injection in postpartum depression: two multicentre, double-blind, randomised, placebo-controlled, phase 3 trials. Lancet 2018;392(1058–1070):1058–70.
65. Kanes S, Colquhoun H, Gunduz-Bruce H, et al. Brexanolone (SAGE-547 injection) in post-partum depression: a randomised controlled trial. Lancet 2017; 390(10093):480–9.
66. Werner E, Miller M, Osborne LM, et al. Preventing postpartum depression: review and recommendations. Arch Womens Ment Health 2015;18(1):41–60.
67. Wisner KL, Perel JM, Peindl KS, et al. Prevention of postpartum depression: a pilot randomized clinical trial. Am J Psychiatry 2004;161(7):1290–2.
68. Robertson E, Grace S, Wallington T, et al. Antenatal risk factors for postpartum depression: a synthesis of recent literature. Gen Hosp Psychiatry 2004;26(4): 289–95.
69. Beck CT. Predictors of postpartum depression: an update. Nurs Res 2001;50(5): 275–85.

Depression and Menopause
An Update on Current Knowledge and Clinical Management for this Critical Window

Claudio N. Soares, MD, PhD, FRCPC, MBA[a,b,*]

KEYWORDS

- Depression • Menopause • Hot flashes • Anxiety • Sleep
- Estrogen therapy and mood regulation • Nonhormonal interventions

KEY POINTS

- Depression is a disabling condition, which often leads to significant personal, societal, and economic costs.
- Windows of vulnerability for depression likely are associated with an increased sensitivity to changes in the hormonal milieu experienced by some (but not all) women during the luteal phase of their cycles, the postpartum period, and/or during the menopause transition.
- An increased awareness of those windows of vulnerability has resulted in greater adoption of screening tools for mood and behavioral changes and tailored therapies for postpartum-related depressive episodes.
- Therapies uniquely designed for menopause-related depression are still debated. Part of the controversy has derived from conflicting methodologies to characterize reproductive staging or assess psychiatric conditions, and different targeted populations identified and assessed for the efficacy and tolerability of various antidepressant treatments, hormone therapies, or other interventions.

This article originally appeared in *Medical Clinics*, Volume 103, Issue 4, July 2019.
This is an update of an article that first appeared in the *Psychiatric Clinics of North America*, Volume 40, Issue 2, June 2017.
Disclosure: Dr C.N. Soares has received research and educational grants from the Ontario Brain Institute (OBI) and the Ontario Research Funds–Research Excellence (ORF-RE). He has served as a consultant for Pfizer, Sunovion, Merck, Otsuka, Servier, and Lundbeck.
[a] Department of Psychiatry, Queen's University School of Medicine, 752 King Street West, Kingston, Ontario K7L 4X3, Canada; [b] Research and Innovation, Providence Care Hospital, Kingston, Ontario, Canada
* Department of Psychiatry, Queen's University School of Medicine, 752 King Street West, Kingston, Ontario K7L 4X3, Canada.
E-mail address: c.soares@queensu.ca

2352-7986/21/© 2020 Elsevier Inc. All rights reserved.

INTRODUCTION

Depression is a disabling condition that affects more than 300 million people worldwide and often leads to significant personal, societal, and economic costs. It affects 1 in every 5 adults in North America, with women being disproportionately more affected than men. Such an increased risk (2-fold on average) has been the subject of debate and research over the years and from different viewpoints, including epidemiology, genetics, socioeconomic determinants of health, coping strategies, and hormone variations.[1,2]

Several researchers have been instrumental in proposing a paradigm to examine why some (but not all) women would be more likely to experience greater vulnerability for depression at certain stages (or windows) across the lifespan.[3–7] Based on this paradigm, the notion of windows of vulnerability for depression, also known as reproductive-related depressive episodes, was postulated to describe an increased sensitivity experienced by some women to changes in the hormonal milieu that occur during the luteal phase of their cycles, during the postpartum period, and/or during the menopause transition.

There has been an increased awareness of those windows of vulnerability, which is reflected in greater adoption of screening tools for mood and behavioral changes in the postpartum period, as well as the recognition by the American Psychiatric Association of the severity and functional impairment associated with the occurrence of premenstrual dysphoric disorder (PMDD). This has led to the inclusion of PMDD as a diagnostic category in the *Diagnostic and Statistical Manual of Mental Disorders, 5th edition*. Likewise, researchers and clinicians have developed therapeutic strategies tailored to reproductive-related mood events such as postpartum depression.[8]

The existence of a menopause-associated depression has been a more controversial point, despite undeniable evidence that this stage in life might be accompanied by other medical conditions, cardiovascular issues, vasomotor symptoms, sleep problems, and stressful life events, just to name a few.[9] The controversy has been fueled by conflicting methodologies used to characterize reproductive staging or assess psychiatric conditions in various studies, and by the scarcity of trials in which this targeted population (midlife women with depression and well-characterized menopause staging) was properly ascertained and assessed for the efficacy and tolerability of various antidepressant treatments, hormone therapies, or other interventions.

Depression and Menopause: Some Facts and Guiding Principles

The heightened burden associated with a major depressive disorder (MDD) is undeniable at any given point in the life cycle. However, the occurrence and persistence of depressive symptoms (not fully meeting criteria for clinical depression) may also lead to psychosocial impairment and adversely affect overall health.[10,11] Therefore, it is important that clinicians keep a closer monitoring and periodically reassess the need for therapies to address bothersome depressive symptoms (eg, low mood, reduced motivation and enjoyment with usual activities, disrupted sleep) through the use of pharmacologic agents, behavioral or lifestyle changes, or other treatments.

Cross-sectional and prospective studies have now investigated a potential association between menopause staging and the risks for depressive symptoms or MDD (new onset or recurrent).[12] Overall, data from cross-sectional studies indicate that depressive symptoms might be endorsed by up to 70% of women during perimenopause compared with around 30% in premenopausal years. Longitudinal studies, perhaps representing a better strategy for the assessment of this potential association, have suggested an increased risk of 1.5-fold to 3.0-fold for the occurrence of depressive symptoms during the menopause transition.[13,14] Importantly, such increased risk was identified even among women with no previous episodes; that is, new onset of symptoms. Finally, cohort studies have documented an increased risk for clinical depression (MDD, 2-fold to 4-fold increased risk) throughout the menopause transition and early postmenopausal years.

Risk factors for depression associated with the menopausal years can be grouped into 2 categories:

1. Continuum of risk factors: Longitudinal studies have identified risk factors for the occurrence of midlife depression that seem pervasive throughout the lifespan; these constitute a continuum of risk for depression and most likely act as moderating factors. These factors could be characterized as demographic or socioeconomic (ie, unemployment, low education, being black or Hispanic), health-related (eg, greater body mass index, being a smoker, reporting poor health and impaired functioning due to chronic medical conditions), and psychosocial (eg, poor social support, history of anxiety, 1 or more stressful life events). Importantly, a previous depressive episode is the strongest predictor for depression during midlife years, whereas a history of mood symptoms with a hormone-related context (ie, history of premenstrual syndrome, PMDD, or postpartum depression) has been moderately linked to depressive symptoms during the menopause transition and early postmenopausal years.
2. Window of risk–related factors: Researchers have also investigated the role of timing-related, context-related factors. Again, data from cross-sectional and longitudinal studies were valuable sources and helped identify mediating or precipitating factors associated with menopause-related depression. These factors include hormone variations (ie, the experience of wider fluctuations in follicle-stimulating hormone [FSH] and estradiol [E2] levels over time), menopause-related symptoms (eg, the presence and severity of vasomotor symptoms, sleep problems), overall health (current poor health, low functioning due to chronic medical conditions), and psychosocial stressors (including poor social support and stressful life events). The latter is characterized not only by the magnitude and number of events but also based on the temporal proximity (ie, timing of their occurrence in relation to the menopause transition per se).

Long-term trajectories

More recent studies have taken a closer look at prospective data to determine mediators for distinct trajectories of depressive symptoms throughout the menopause transition and beyond. The Study of Women's Health Across the Nation (SWAN) used data from a 13-year follow-up period to examine the course of clinical depression. The SWAN investigators determined that about 30% of those who developed depression at some point during the study ultimately experienced evolution into a persistent or recurrent condition. This was true even among those with new-onset cases of depression. Sleep problems and recent upsetting life events were among contributing factors to more persistent and/or recurrent depressive outcomes.[15,16] The Australian Longitudinal Study on Women's Health, on the other hand, identified 4 distinct patterns for depressive symptoms over a 15-year follow-up based on changes in the Center for Epidemiologic Studies Depression Scale (CES-D) scores over time: stable low (80.0%), increasing scores (9.0%), decreasing scores (8.5%), and stable high (2.5%). Those exhibiting stable high or increasing depressive symptoms over time (around 10%) were likely to experience continuum of risk factors such as previous diagnosis or treatment of depression and socioeconomic challenges. There were also context-related risk factors such as the exposure to a prolonged perimenopause or a surgically induced menopause.[17]

The role of anxiety and sleep

Anxiety and sleep problems are often identified as contributing factors to greater psychiatric morbidity among midlife women. Anxiety disorders constitute a heterogeneous group in which comorbid conditions are quite common and symptoms may overlap considerably. SWAN investigators attempted to explore 4 components or symptoms of anxiety (irritability, nervousness or tension, feeling fearful for no reason, and heart pounding or racing) and categorized their occurrence as high or low anxiety based on their scoring on the General Anxiety Disorder-7 scale.[18] They also examined whether anxiety symptoms at study entry would be more likely or less likely to occur during or after the menopausal transition than in their premenopausal years, regardless of the presence of vasomotor symptoms, health factors, or psychosocial stressors. Overall, women with high anxiety symptoms at study entry maintained significant rates of anxiety (16%–21%) throughout the 10-year follow-up period. Interestingly, the percentage of documented high anxiety visits declined from 71.4% (occurring during premenopausal years) to 30.0% (in the postmenopausal period). Moreover, those who reported high anxiety at baseline experienced a peak in symptoms during late perimenopausal years (13.5%), which is a much higher percentage than those observed in premenopausal years (4.6%), suggesting a possible window of vulnerability for increased anxiety in some women during midlife years.

More recently, Freeman and Sammel[19] (2016) examined the association between anxiety and severity of hot flashes over a 14-year follow-up interval (Penn Ovarian Aging Cohort). Somatic anxiety was strongly associated with hot flashes in the menopause transition, even after adjusting for important factors such as age, menopausal staging, reproductive hormone levels, history of depression, and others. Importantly, rather than cooccurring with vasomotor symptoms, somatic anxiety actually predicted the risk of further developing moderate or severe hot flashes.

Clinicians and patients often question whether sleep problems in midlife years represent a primary condition or an expression of an underlying problem (eg, presence of vasomotor symptoms or depression). Kravitz and colleagues[20] investigated possible interactions between menopause changes and sleep, and found an association between changes in bleeding patterns during the menopause transition and the emergence of sleep disturbances. Others indicated that women experiencing depression and vasomotor symptoms are likely to report poorer perceived sleep quality despite the lack of objective measures of sleep disruption; that is, an actual increase in number of awakenings or night sweats, or even significant changes in wakefulness after sleep onset (WASO) time.[21,22]

Joffe and colleagues[23] submitted 39 healthy, premenopausal women to gonadal hormone suppression by administering leuprolide to examine the independent contribution of hot flashes and sleep disturbances to the emergence of depressive symptoms among estrogen-deprived women. After 4 weeks of leuprolide use, 20 women (69%) developed hot flushes, whereas only 1 subject developed clinical depression. The increase in depressive symptoms (Montgomery-Åsberg Depression Rating Scale [MADRS] scores) was associated with objective and subjective changes in sleep patterns. However, only nocturnal hot flashes (and not daytime vasomotor symptoms) seemed to be significantly associated with an increase in depressive symptoms, even after adjusting for changes on sleep, suggesting that disturbed sleep does not fully explain the association of nocturnal hot flashes and mood disturbance in women experiencing estrogen depletion due to surgical or natural menopause.

Lampio and colleagues[24] (2016) examined the effects of aging and menopausal hormonal changes on sleep architecture during the menopause transition (6-year follow-up). The investigators collected overnight polysomnography recordings at baseline and at the follow-up visit, as well as FSH levels over time. Both aging and increased FSH concentration had an impact on sleep architecture. The age-related changes included shorter total sleep time, lower sleep efficiency, and greater sleep fragmentation; for example, increased WASO. Clinical characteristics and increased FSH levels (a marker of transition from premenopause to postmenopause) were associated with higher proportion of slow wave sleep and increased WASO.

WHAT ABOUT THE ESTROGEN CONNECTION?
Estrogen and Mood Regulation

The mediating effects of estrogen on monoaminergic systems, namely serotonin (5-hydroxytryptamine [5-HT]) and noradrenaline (NE) neurotransmission, may contribute to the development of depressive symptoms in women.[25–27] The presence and wide distribution of estrogen receptors in the brain and the estrogen activity found in regions known to be involved in mood and cognitive regulation (eg, prefrontal cortex, hippocampus) are contributing arguments to the notion that estrogen exerts mediating effects (and possibly therapeutic effects) on mood.[25,28,29]

Overall, the effects of E on 5-HT and NE could be characterized as beneficial to mood.[30] E2 administration limits the activity of monoamine oxidases (MAOs) A and B, which are enzymes involved in 5-HT degradation.[31] It also increases both isoforms of tryptophan hydroxylase, the rate-limiting enzyme of serotonin synthesis.[32,33] Thus, E2 administration results in an overall net increase in 5-HT synthesis and availability. Moreover, estrogens increased 5-HT receptor density in brain regions containing E receptors, such as the hypothalamus, the preoptic area, and the amygdala.[34–37] E2 downregulates $5HT_{1a}$ auto-receptors and upregulates $5HT_{2a}$ receptors, increasing the amount of serotonin found in the synapse and consequently the amount available for postsynaptic transmission. Estrogen effects also promote NE availability by decreasing the expression of MAOs and increasing the activity of tyrosine hydroxylase, the rate-limiting enzyme in the synthesis of catecholamine.[38,39] Acute E2 administration increases dopamine β-hydroxylase (DBH) gene transcription; DBH catalyzes the hydroxylation of dopamine to form NE. In sum, estrogen works via distinct pathways to regulate synthesis, metabolism, and receptor density or activity of the classical neurotransmitters implicated in mood regulation.[40,41] Finally, estrogen may also have mood-enhancing (or antidepressant-like) properties due to its stimulating effect on brain-derived neurotrophic factor, an important neuroprotective agent at multiple levels.[42]

Estrogen Therapy for Depression: Level I Evidence of a Critical Window

Despite some evidence of E2 antidepressant properties, particularly among depressed, perimenopausal women, the acceptability of estrogen therapy (ET) as part of the therapeutic armamentarium for depression remains limited. A recent, comprehensive systematic review examined the efficacy of estrogen-based interventions for depression.[30] Potentially relevant studies were selected based on the following criteria: (1) clinical administration of estrogen-based, hormone therapy and (2) assessment of mood symptoms or depression with standardized instruments.

Surprisingly, only a few randomized controlled trials (RCTs) have examined the benefits of ET on clinically depressed women. Most studies included women who were either asymptomatic or mildly affected at study entry, again making it more difficult to generalize and/or compare their findings. Thus, given the scarce number of RCTs with estrogen-based therapies for menopause depression, the author has expanded the review conducted by Rubinow and colleagues and included open-label, single-blind, and double-blind interventions.

The author also recognizes that clinical trials have not been the only source of information for a better understanding of the effects of estrogen on mood. Some have explored the brain-related effects of estrogen in longitudinal observational studies; for example, by comparing women who underwent oophorectomy before the onset of menopause (average follow-up 25 years) to an aged-matched sample from the same community; a particular study demonstrated that those who underwent surgery had a significant increased risk for developing depressive and anxiety symptoms when compared with the referent group.[43] The risks were even greater among those who underwent surgery at younger age, leading the author to speculate a potential association of these findings with an early loss of neuroprotective effects of estrogen during reproductive years.

Mood Regulation: Estrogen Therapies in Nondepressed Women

Perimenopausal women

A single RCT assessed mood in strictly nondepressed, perimenopausal women (N = 83, aged 40–52 years).[44] Menopausal staging was based on menstrual patterns and the presence of vasomotor symptoms, whereas depressive symptoms were assessed via a standardized instrument: the Zung Self Rating Depression Scale. This was a 6-month, crossover study comparing a hormone treatment (estrogen-progestin therapy [EPT]) with 2 weeks of conjugated equine estrogen (CEE) followed by 2 weeks of CEE plus medroxyprogesterone acetate (MPA). No significant effects on mood were observed when the order of treatment allocation was ignored. Study limitations included the lack of a calibration or run-in period, and the treatment duration.

In a recent pilot study of perimenopausal women (N = 38, aged 38–52 years) who were predominantly nondepressed, the investigators compared the effects of levonorgestrel-containing intrauterine system (LNG-IUS) plus low-dose transdermal E2 (gel 0.06% containing 0.75 mg E2 per 1.25 g metered dose) to LNG-IUS alone (plus inactive gel) for 50 days. The study assessed depressive symptoms using the CES-D, the impact of hot flashes using the Hot Flash–Related Daily Interference Scale, fatigue using the Fatigue Severity Scale, and sleep characteristics via the Pittsburgh Sleep Quality Index. Although most women were symptomatic with respect to hot flashes (61%) and poor sleep (71%), only a small number reported significant depressive symptoms (CES-D scores >16, n = 5 or 13%) or fatigue (n = 5, 13%) at study entry. Overall, the study revealed beneficial effects of LNG-IUS plus TDE for the improvement of hot flashes and daytime fatigue, with minimal or nonsignificant effects on sleep and no significant changes in mood (improvement or worsening).[45]

To date, only 1 randomized trial has investigated the efficacy of estrogen in preventing the onset of significant depressive symptoms in perimenopausal and early postmenopausal women. Euthymic perimenopausal or early postmenopausal women (n = 172) were assigned to receive either transdermal E2 (0.1 mg/d) plus intermittent oral micronized progesterone (200 mg/d for 12 days every 3 months) or placebo patches plus pills. After 12 months, women receiving active HT were significantly less likely to develop depressive symptoms compared with women receiving placebo (32.3% vs 17.3%). Those in the early perimenopausal stage (but not late perimenopausal or early postmenopausal stages) benefited the most from estrogen as a preventive strategy. The benefits were also modified by stressful life events, with greater benefits for women who had experienced stressful life events in the preceding

6 months of the intervention. Vasomotor symptoms and prior history of MDD did not modify the effect of HT on depressive symptoms. These findings, if further replicated, highlight the importance of a careful clinical interview to facilitate personalized interventions for midlife women.

Postmenopausal women
The effects of HT on mood have been assessed in clinical studies in younger, postmenopausal women (ie, up to 10 years postmenopause and aged <70 years). In most studies, the presence of menopause-related symptoms (ie, vasomotor, sleep, pain) was documented at study entry, making the alleviation of these symptoms with hormone interventions an important factor (mediating and/or confounding) to be considered. Haines and colleagues[46] (2003) studied 152 postmenopausal women (posthysterectomy, aged 48 ± 5 years) in a randomized, double-blind placebo-controlled trial of 1 or 2 mg of oral E2 or placebo for 12 months (primary outcome: prevention of bone loss, ie, reduced risk for osteoporosis). Women had their depressive symptoms assessed via the Hospital Anxiety and Depression Scale and their psychological wellbeing and quality of life (QOL) using the World Health Organization QOL questionnaire. Over a 12-month follow-up period, menopausal symptoms were significantly reduced in the 2 mg arm (not among those using 1 mg or placebo), whereas no significant changes in mood or QOL were observed (from mild or no significant impairment observed at baseline).

Fifty-four asymptomatic postmenopausal women (average age 52 ± 4 years) were randomized to receive oral ET (CEE 0.625 mg/d), EPT (CEE + MPA, 10 mg/d), or placebo in a 6-month trial. Subjects were recruited based on the absence of psychiatric symptoms (HAM-D and HAM-A scales) and assessed at baseline and endpoint for psychological symptoms using the Beck Depression Inventory (BDI) and the Profile of Moods States. Hormone treatment did not lead to a significant change in mood over time when compared with placebo.[47]

In another trial (3-month duration), 183 postmenopausal women (average age 48 years, postmenopausal for at least 1 year) were recruited based on the presence of severe menopausal symptoms and randomized into 3 treatment groups: (1) transdermal E2 plus oral norethisterone acetate, (2) oral continuous combination of norethisterone and E2 hemihydrate, or (3) placebo. Menopausal, depressive, and anxiety symptoms were assessed using the Kupperman scale, the Hamilton Depression Rating Scale (HDRS), and the Beck Anxiety Inventory (BAI), respectively. Compared with placebo, the use of transdermal E2 (alone or in combination with norethisterone) led to a significant improvement of menopausal symptoms, as well as reduction in HDRS and BAI scores depression and anxiety symptoms.[48]

Almeida and colleagues[49] examined the benefits of ET (oral E2, 2 mg/d) for cognition, mood, and QOL in older postmenopausal women (n = 115, average age 73 years) in a 20-week randomized double-blind placebo-controlled trial. Outcome measures included changes in the BDI, changes in QOL scores (SF-36), and cognitive function (CAMCOG, Block Design, Memory for Faces, California Verbal Learning Test, and verbal fluency). After 20 weeks of treatment, unopposed estrogen administered orally was not associated with significant changes in cognitive function, mood, or QOL.

In another placebo-controlled trial, 412 postmenopausal women (average age 71 years) were allocated into 4 different treatment groups: ET with 0.625 of CEE, CEE plus 2.5 mg of MPA, calcitriol 0.25 g twice a day alone, and a combination of HT and calcitriol. Depression symptoms were assessed via the Geriatric Depression Scale (GDS) at baseline and at the end of the 36-month trial. GDS scores suggested that about 12% of the sample was depressed at study entry. No significant effects of hormone treatment on mood were observed at endpoint, and the percentage of depressed women (based on GDS scores) decreased across all treatment groups.[50]

In sum, these results suggest a lack of significant beneficial effects of estrogen on mood (ie, mood improvement) when administered to nondepressed women, particularly in their postmenopausal years. Preliminary but promising results suggest a potential role for estrogen in mitigating the risk for developing depressive symptoms among specific at-risk subpopulations transitioning to menopause.

Additional information has been derived from large trials such as the Heart and Estrogen/Progestin Replacement Study (HERS),[51] the Women's Health Initiative Study of Cognitive Aging (WHISCA)[52,53] and the Women's International Study of long Duration Estrogen after the Menopause (WISDOM).[54,55] These studies offered additional opportunities to examine the effects of hormone therapies on mood and QOL among both younger and older nondepressed postmenopausal women. Altogether, these studies failed to demonstrate a significant impact of hormone therapies on mood and reiterate the notion that estrogen-based therapies should not be considered as a strategy for prevention or alleviation of mood symptoms in otherwise nondepressed, asymptomatic perimenopausal, or postmenopausal women.[30] Recent data from the Kronos Early Estrogen Prevention Study (KEEPS) examined the effects of estrogen-based therapies on mood symptoms among nondepressed, early postmenopausal women.[56,57] Contrary to other studies, the investigators identified a positive impact on mood with the use of oral CEEs but not with transdermal E2.

Mood Improvement: The Use of Estrogen Therapies in Depressed Women

Perimenopausal women

At least 4 small studies, including 2 RCTs, have demonstrated the efficacy of E2 for the management of depressive disorders during perimenopause.[58–61] The 2 RCTS (Soares and Schmidt) had similar designs and are considered of high quality due to the utilization of standardized tools to confirm the diagnosis of depression and the characterization of menopausal staging using FSH levels and history of menstrual irregularity. In addition, treatment compliance was monitored by serum E2 measurements in both studies. Antidepressant effects were well-documented (reduction in CES-D, HDRS, and MADRS scores) and significant mood improvement was observed among those suffering from new-onset or recurrent MDD in the presence or absence of concomitant vasomotor symptoms. Moreover, the antidepressant effects of E2 persisted after a 4-week washout period, even after reemergence of hot flashes and night sweats.[61]

Estrogen has also been used as an augmentation strategy for women with unsatisfactory response to antidepressants. Most studies suggest that estrogen might augment clinical response to antidepressants, including selective serotonin reuptake inhibitors (SSRIs) and serotonin-norepinephrine reuptake inhibitor (SNRIs).[62–68]

Postmenopausal women

Two RCTs have assessed the use of hormone therapy in postmenopausal women with depressive disorders. Morrison and colleagues (2004) examined the efficacy of transdermal E2 (0.1 mg) compared with placebo in late postmenopausal women (N = 57; average age 67 years, postmenopausal for about 16 years) suffering from mild-to-moderate depression. After 8 weeks of treatment, both groups showed similar decrease in depressive symptoms based on changes in HDRS scores or self-assessed CES-D scores from baseline. The study also suggested that a subgroup of depressed postmenopausal women (ie, those with a past history of major depression) could be particularly responsive to placebo.

In another RCT, Rudolph and colleagues (2004) examined the effects of oral HT (a continuous combination of E2 valerate 2 mg and dienogest 2 mg/d) in a 24-week trial of 129 postmenopausal women. In this study, women were considerably younger (average age 55 years) and the use of HT led to significant improvements in depressive scores (reduction in HDRS scores). These findings, however, should be examined with caution given the unusually high dropout rates observed among treatment users (33%) and placebo users (58%).

Finally, an RCT included 72 women with depression and was confirmed by the Structured Clinical Interview for Axis I Disorders of mild to moderate severity (ie, MADRS) scores of 15 to 31 at study entry. Women were perimenopausal and post-menopausal (mean age 51.1 ± 5.0 years), experiencing sleep disturbances (insomnia syndrome) that affected their functioning and reporting 3 or more nights per week with significant hot flashes. Subjects were randomly assigned to transdermal 17β-E2 0.05 mg/d, zolpidem 10 mg/d, or placebo for 8 weeks. All groups showed improvement in depressive symptoms (MADRS scores); that is, the study failed to demonstrate meaningful differences between active treatment groups and placebo. Interestingly, overall improvement in mood was significantly correlated with an increase in serum E2 over time and improvement in perceived quality. It is plausible that an increase in E2 levels occurred due to ET use in 1 treatment arm and/or to naturally occurring fluctuations among study participants. Mood improvement, however, was not significantly correlated with suppression of hot flashes or changes in objectively measures of sleep.[69]

Schmidt and colleagues[70] tested the estrogen withdrawal theory (previously examined in premenstrual and postnatal populations) in asymptomatic postmenopausal women (N = 56) with history of perimenopausal depression. After 3 weeks of open-label administration of transdermal E2 (100 μg/d), study participants were randomized to receive either E2 or matched placebo skin patches for 3 additional weeks in a double-blind fashion. There were no reports of depressive symptoms during the open-label phase with E2. Women with history of perimenopausal depression who were crossed over from E2 to placebo reported an increase in depressive symptoms (assessed by the CES-D and HDRS), whereas those (also with past history of perimenopausal depression) who remained on E2 therapy continued to be asymptomatic. Of note, both groups had similar hot-flush severity and plasma E2 levels while on placebo. The study by Schmidt and colleagues[70] elegantly demonstrated that some midlife women could be particularly susceptible to developing behavioral or mood changes when exposed to changes in estrogen levels or secretion. These findings corroborate the notion of a critical timing to consider estrogen's role as a contributing and/or mitigating factor for depression in midlife women.

In sum, ET, particularly transdermal E2, has shown antidepressant effects of similar magnitude to that observed with classic antidepressant agents when administered to perimenopausal women suffering from clinical depression, whereas it seems to be ineffective as a mood enhancer among depression-free (asymptomatic) women. Transdermal 17β-E2 seems to lead to a greater antidepressant effect size (ie, drug-placebo difference) and could therefore constitute a potential treatment of depressed mood in this population.[71,72] On the other hand, the same hormone intervention formulation (E2) and route of administration (transdermally) was not effective in treating depressed postmenopausal women.[73,74] This particular finding suggests that the menopausal transition might not only be a critical window of risk for depression but also a window of opportunity for the effective use of estrogen therapies for depression in midlife years.[9] However, existing data on estrogen-based therapies for depressed perimenopausal and postmenopausal women are limited in terms of number of randomized trials, sample sizes recruited, and number of study completers (**Table 1**), making the interpretation and generalization or applicability of some of these findings more challenging.

FINAL CONSIDERATIONS AND RECOMMENDATIONS REGARDING ESTROGEN THERAPIES

There are indicators of windows of vulnerability for cardiovascular, mood, and cognitive conditions in midlife women; at the same time, the critical window hypothesis suggests the existence of a window of opportunity for the administration of E2 to symptomatic women across different systems or domains. Further investigation is needed to disentangle common underlying mechanisms.[77]

Clinicians should always consider the various treatment strategies available and determine the extent to which they can be tailored to address the multiple symptom domains for each patient. For example, based on the author's review and accumulated clinical experience, an argument can be made that perimenopausal women presenting with significant, bothersome menopausal symptoms (significant VMS) and concurrent depressive symptoms could benefit from an initial, brief trial (2–4 weeks) with transdermal E2 as a monotherapy to determine the benefits and tolerability of hormone treatment for the alleviation of both mood and menopausal symptoms. After that, the need for antidepressant use (monotherapy or concomitant use) could be reassessed. Obviously, women who experienced multiple depressive episodes in the past (not necessarily hormone-related), and women presenting with severe depressive symptoms and/or expressing suicidal ideation should always be evaluated and treated with more intensive, widely used antidepressant strategies.

The type of hormone treatment and route of administration should be carefully considered if alleviation of depression is an important goal. Different HT formulations (eg, transdermal E2 vs oral conjugated estrogens, E alone vs estrogen plus progestin therapies) should take into consideration not only the risks or benefits for bone and cardiovascular health but also for cognitive and mood functioning. So far, the evidence for the use of transdermal E2 for depression is more robust and reinforced by its absorption process (no hepatic first-pass effects) and overall safety profile.

WHAT ABOUT NONHORMONAL INTERVENTIONS?

Antidepressants remain the first-line treatment of depression during midlife years, particularly for those who experienced multiple depressive episodes in the past (not necessarily hormone-related), reporting severe symptoms or significant functional impairment, and/or expressing suicidal ideation. For recurrent episodes, a previous response to a specific antidepressant (agent, class) should guide the primary decision on what to try first. For those experiencing depression for the first time, those who are treatment-naïve, or those presenting with history of partial or no response to antidepressants past, existing data support the efficacy and tolerability of various SSRIs and SNRIs at usual doses. There are studies on fluoxetine, sertraline, venlafaxine, citalopram, escitalopram, duloxetine, desvenlafaxine, and vortioxetine.[78–86]

Existing data do not support superior efficacy of a particular antidepressant agent or class over the others for the management of midlife depression. Still, a few important points should be taken into consideration when choosing an antidepressant for this population. First, despite small numbers and methodological limitations, data on efficacy and tolerability of various agents for this particular population could inform and guide some of the preliminary discussions with midlife women suffering from depression. Second, data on tolerability and adverse events (and how they seem to affect

Table 1
Randomized trials on estrogen therapies for symptomatic or depressed perimenopausal and postmenopausal women

Authors	Population Studied (Type, n)	Design	Intervention	Outcome Measures	Key Findings
Schmidt et al,[60] 2001	Perimenopause-related depression (n = 31)	DB, PL Parallel study followed by crossover, PL-controlled	ET (transdermal E2), followed by MPA	HDRS, CES-D scores	ET led to significant improvements in depressive symptoms (HDRS and CES-D scores)
Soares et al,[61] 2001	Perimenopause-related depression (n = 45)	DB, PL Parallel study	ET (transdermal E2)	MADRS scores	ET led to significant improvements in depressive symptoms (MADRS scores)
Rudolph et al,[75] 2004; Santoro,[76] 2005	Postmenopausal women with mild or moderate depressive symptoms (n = 129)	DB, PL Parallel study	EPT (oral E2 valerate + progestin [dienogest])	HDRS scores	EPT led to improvements in HDRS scores; high attrition rates in both groups
Morrison et al,[73] 2004	Postmenopausal women with depressive disorders (n = 57)	DB, PL Parallel study	ET (transdermal E2) followed by MPA	HDRS, CES-D scores	No differences with active treatment (both groups showed improvement)
Joffe et al,[69] 2011	Mixed perimenopausal and postmenopausal women with depressive symptoms, VMS and insomnia (n = 72)	DB, PL Parallel study	ET (transdermal E2), Zolpidem	MADRS, BDI, PSQI scores	No significant differences with respect to mood changes between treatment and PL groups

Abbreviations: DB, double-blind; PL, placebo; PSQI, Pittsburgh Sleep Quality Index.

treatment adherence) should be carefully examined, particularly when issues such as sexual dysfunction and changes in metabolism are already part of the clinical scenario or reported as important concerns. Conversely, look for data supporting the efficacy of some of the antidepressants for the relief of menopause-related symptoms (eg, hot flashes, pain, disrupted sleep) and QOL improvement. Finally, data available on drug safety (eg, drug-drug interactions) should always be considered because multiple medications that are often prescribed to this population.[87]

SUMMARY

Evidence-based psychotherapies, particularly behavioral-based interventions, should have a place in the treatment armamentarium to ultimately reduce the overall burden and functional impairment associated with depression in this population.[88] Nonpharmacologic or hormonal strategies (eg, exercise, balanced diet, dietary supplements) need to be better examined as additional tools to help improve QOL and reduce functional impairment during the menopause transition and beyond.

REFERENCES

1. Steiner M. Female-specific mood disorders. Clin Obstet Gynecol 1992;35(3): 599–611.
2. Thurston RC, Joffe H, Soares CN, et al. Physical activity and risk of vasomotor symptoms in women with and without a history of depression: results from the Harvard Study of Moods and Cycles. Menopause 2006;13(4):553–60.
3. Bloch M, Schmidt PJ, Danaceau M, et al. Effects of gonadal steroids in women with a history of postpartum depression. Am J Psychiatry 2000;157(6):924–30.
4. Bloch M, Rotenberg N, Koren D, et al. Risk factors for early postpartum depressive symptoms. Gen Hosp Psychiatry 2006;28(1):3–8.
5. Boyle GJ, Murrihy R. A preliminary study of hormone replacement therapy and psychological mood states in perimenopausal women. Psychol Rep 2001; 88(1):160–70.
6. Bromberger JT, Harlow S, Avis N, et al. Racial/ethnic differences in the prevalence of depressive symptoms among middle-aged women: the Study of Women's Health Across the Nation (SWAN). Am J Public Health 2004;94(8): 1378–85.
7. Rubinow DR, Schmidt PJ, Roca CA. Estrogen-serotonin interactions: implications for affective regulation. Biol Psychiatry 1998;44(9):839–50.
8. Kanes S, Colquhoun H, Gunduz-Bruce H, et al. Brexanolone (SAGE-547 injection) in post-partum depression: a randomised controlled trial. Lancet 2017; 390(10093):480–9.
9. Soares CN. Mood disorders in midlife women: understanding the critical window and its clinical implications. Menopause 2014;21(2):198–206.
10. Pietrzak RH, Kinley J, Afifi TO, et al. Subsyndromal depression in the United States: prevalence, course, and risk for incident psychiatric outcomes. Psychol Med 2013;43(7):1401–14.
11. Rodríguez MR, Nuevo R, Chatterji S, et al. Definitions and factors associated with subthreshold depressive conditions: a systematic review. BMC Psychiatry 2012; 12:181.
12. Bromberger JT, Kravitz HM. Mood and menopause: findings from the Study of Women's Health Across the Nation (SWAN) over 10 years. Obstet Gynecol Clin North Am 2011;38(3):609–25.

13. Bromberger JT, Schott L, Kravitz HM, et al. Risk factors for major depression during midlife among a community sample of women with and without prior major depression: are they the same or different? Psychol Med 2015;45:1653–64.

14. Freeman EW, Sammel MD, Lin H, et al. Associations of hormones and menopausal status with depressed mood in women with no history of depression. Arch Gen Psychiatry 2006;63:375–82.

15. Bromberger JT, Kravitz HM, Youk A, et al. Patterns of depressive disorders across 13 years and their determinants among midlife women: SWAN mental health study. J Affect Disord 2016;206:31–40.

16. Clayton AH, Pinkerton JV. Vulnerability to depression and cardiometabolic risk associated with early ovarian disruption. Menopause 2013;20(6):598–9.

17. Hickey M, Schoenaker DA, Joffe H, et al. Depressive symptoms across the menopause transition: findings from a large population-based cohort study. Menopause 2016;23(12):1287–93.

18. Bromberger JT, Kravitz HM, Chang Y, et al. Does risk for anxiety increase during the menopausal transition? Study of women's health across the nation. Menopause 2013;20(5):488–95.

19. Freeman EW, Sammel MD. Anxiety as a risk factor for menopausal hot flashes: evidence from the Penn Ovarian Aging cohort. Menopause 2016;23(9):942–9.

20. Kravitz HM, Zhao X, Bromberger JT, et al. Sleep disturbance during the menopausal transition in a multi-ethnic community sample of women. Sleep 2008; 31(7):979–90.

21. Joffe H, Soares CN, Thurston RC, et al. Depression is associated with worse objectively and subjectively measured sleep, but not more frequent awakenings, in women with vasomotor symptoms. Menopause 2009;16(4):671–9.

22. Joffe H, Massler A, Sharkey KM. Evaluation and management of sleep disturbance during the menopause transition. Semin Reprod Med 2010;28(5):404–21.

23. Joffe H, Crawford SL, Freeman MP, et al. Independent contributions of nocturnal hot flashes and sleep disturbance to depression in estrogen-deprived women. J Clin Endocrinol Metab 2016;101(10):3847–55.

24. Lampio L, Polo-Kantola P, Himanen SL, et al. Sleep during menopausal transition: a 6-year follow-up. Sleep 2017;40(7). https://doi.org/10.1093/sleep/zsx090.

25. McEwen BS, Alves SE. Estrogen actions in the central nervous system. Endocr Rev 1999;20(3):279–307.

26. Lokuge S, Frey BN, Foster JA, et al. Depression in women: windows of vulnerability and new insights into the link between estrogen and serotonin. J Clin Psychiatry 2011;72(11):e1563–9.

27. Yonkers KA, O'Brien PM, Eriksson E. Premenstrual syndrome. Lancet 2008; 371(9619):1200–10.

28. Deecher D, Andree TH, Sloan D, et al. From menarche to menopause: exploring the underlying biology of depression in women experiencing hormonal changes. Psychoneuroendocrinology 2008;33(1):3–17.

29. Genazzani AR, Bernardi F, Pluchino N, et al. Endocrinology of menopausal transition and its brain implications. CNS Spectr 2005;10(6):449–57.

30. Rubinow DR, Johnson SL, Schmidt PJ, et al. Efficacy of estradiol in perimenopausal depression: so much promise and so few answers. Depress Anxiety 2015;32(8):539–49.

31. Gundlah C, Lu NZ, Bethea CL. Ovarian steroid regulation of monoamine oxidase-A and -B mRNAs in the macaque dorsal raphe and hypothalamic nuclei. Psychopharmacology (Berl) 2002;160(3):271–82.

32. Bethea CL, Mirkes SJ, Su A, et al. Effects of oral estrogen, raloxifene and arzoxifene on gene expression in serotonin neurons of macaques. Psychoneuroendocrinology 2002;27(4):431–45.

33. Hiroi R, McDevitt RA, Neumaier JF. Estrogen selectively increases tryptophan hydroxylase-2 mRNA expression in distinct subregions of rat midbrain raphe nucleus: association between gene expression and anxiety behavior in the open field. Biol Psychiatry 2006;60(3):288–95.

34. Biegon A, Reches A, Snyder L, et al. Serotonergic and noradrenergic receptors in the rat brain: modulation by chronic exposure to ovarian hormones. Life Sci 1983; 32(17):2015–21.

35. Cyr M, Bosse R, Di Paolo T. Gonadal hormones modulate 5-hydroxytryptamine2A receptors: emphasis on the rat frontal cortex. Neuroscience 1998;83(3):829–36.

36. Moses-Kolko EL, Wisner KL, Price JC, et al. Serotonin 1A receptor reductions in postpartum depression: a positron emission tomography study. Fertil Steril 2008; 89(3):685–92.

37. Nelson HD. Menopause. Lancet 2008;371(9614):760–70.

38. Pau KY, Hess DL, Kohama S, et al. Oestrogen upregulates noradrenaline release in the mediobasal hypothalamus and tyrosine hydroxylase gene expression in the brainstem of ovariectomized rhesus macaques. J Neuroendocrinol 2000;12(9): 899–909.

39. Pérez-López FR, Pérez-Roncero G, Fernández-Iñarrea J, et al, MARIA (MenopAuse RIsk Assessment) Research Group. Resilience, depressed mood, and menopausal symptoms in postmenopausal women. Menopause 2014;21(2): 159–64.

40. Osterlund MK, Kuiper GG, Gustafsson JA, et al. Differential distribution and regulation of estrogen receptor-alpha and -beta mRNA within the female rat brain. Brain Res Mol Brain Res 1998;54(1):175–80.

41. Osterlund MK, Halldin C, Hurd YL. Effects of chronic 17beta-estradiol treatment on the serotonin 5-HT(1A) receptor mRNA and binding levels in the rat brain. Synapse 2000;35(1):39–44.

42. Srivastava DP, Woolfrey KM, Evans PD. Mechanisms underlying the interactions between rapid estrogenic and BDNF control of synaptic connectivity. Neuroscience 2013;239:17–33.

43. Rocca WA, Grossardt BR, Geda YE, et al. Long-term risk of depressive and anxiety symptoms after early bilateral oophorectomy. Menopause 2008;15(6): 1050–9.

44. Khoo SK, Coglan M, Battistutta D, et al. Hormonal treatment and psychological function during the menopausal transition: an evaluation of the effects of conjugated estrogens/cyclic medroxyprogesterone acetate. Climacteric 1998;1(1): 55–62.

45. Santoro N, Teal S, Gavito C, et al. Use of a levonorgestrel-containing intrauterine system with supplemental estrogen improves symptoms in perimenopausal women: a pilot study. Menopause 2015;22(12):1301–7.

46. Haines CJ, Yim SF, Chung TK, et al. A prospective, randomized, placebo-controlled study of the dose effect of oral oestradiol on menopausal symptoms, psychological well being, and quality of life in postmenopausal Chinese women. Maturitas 2003;44(3):207–14.

47. Girdler SS, O'Briant C, Steege J, et al. A comparison of the effect of estrogen with or without progesterone on mood and physical symptoms in postmenopausal women. J Womens Health Gend Based Med 1999;8(5):637–46.

48. Karsidag C, Karageyim Karsidag AY, Esim Buyukbayrak E, et al. Comparison of effects of two different hormone therapies on mood in symptomatic postmenopausal women. Archives of Neuropsychiatry 2012;49(1):39–43.

49. Almeida OP, Lautenschlager NT, Vasikaran S, et al. A 20-week randomized controlled trial of estradiol replacement therapy for women aged 70 years and older: effect on mood, cognition and quality of life. Neurobiol Aging 2006;27(1): 141–9.

50. Yalamanchili V, Gallagher JC. Treatment with hormone therapy and calcitriol did not affect depression in older postmenopausal women: no interaction with estrogen and vitamin D receptor genotype polymorphisms. Menopause 2012;19(6): 697–703.

51. Hlatky et al., 2002.

52. Resnick SM, Maki PM, Rapp SR, et al, Women's Health Initiative Study of Cognitive Aging Investigators. Effects of combination estrogen plus progestin hormone treatment on cognition and affect. J Clin Endocrinol Metab 2006;91(5):1802–10.

53. Resnick SM, Espeland MA, An Y, et al, Women's Health Initiative Study of Cognitive Aging Investigators. Effects of conjugated equine estrogens on cognition and affect in postmenopausal women with prior hysterectomy. J Clin Endocrinol Metab 2009;94(11):4152–61.

54. Welton AJ, Vickers MR, Kim J, et al, WISDOM team. Health related quality of life after combined hormone replacement therapy: randomised controlled trial. BMJ 2008;337:a1190.

55. Wittchen HU, Becker E, Lieb R, et al. Prevalence, incidence and stability of premenstrual dysphoric disorder in the community. Psychol Med 2002;32(1):119–32.

56. Gleason CE, Dowling NM, Wharton W, et al. Effects of hormone therapy on cognition and mood in recently postmenopausal women: findings from the randomized, controlled KEEPS-cognitive and affective study. PLoS Med 2015;12(6): e1001833.

57. Gordon JL, Rubinow DR, Eisenlohr-Moul TA, et al. Efficacy of transdermal estradiol and micronized progesterone in the prevention of depressive symptoms in the menopause transition: a randomized clinical trial. JAMA Psychiatry 2018; 75(2):149–57.

58. Cohen LS, Soares CN, Poitras JR, et al. Short-term use of estradiol for depression in perimenopausal and postmenopausal women: a preliminary report. Am J Psychiatry 2003;160(8):1519–22.

59. Rasgon NL, Altshuler LL, Fairbanks L. Estrogen-replacement therapy for depression. Am J Psychiatry 2001;158(10):1738.

60. Schmidt PJ, Nieman L, Danaceau MA, et al. Estrogen replacement in perimenopause-related depression: a preliminary report. Am J Obstet Gynecol 2000;183(2):414–20.

61. Soares CN, Almeida OP, Joffe H, et al. Efficacy of estradiol for the treatment of depressive disorders in perimenopausal women: a double-blind, randomized, placebo-controlled trial. Arch Gen Psychiatry 2001;58(6):529–34.

62. Amsterdam J, Garcia-Espana F, Fawcett J, et al. Fluoxetine efficacy in menopausal women with and without estrogen replacement. J Affect Disord 1999; 55(1):11–7.

63. Entsuah AR, Huang H, Thase ME. Response and remission rates in different subpopulations with major depressive disorder administered venlafaxine, selective serotonin reuptake inhibitors, or placebo. J Clin Psychiatry 2001;62(11):869–77.

64. Schneider LS, Small GW, Hamilton SH, et al. Estrogen replacement and response to fluoxetine in a multicenter geriatric depression trial. Fluoxetine Collaborative Study Group. Am J Geriatr Psychiatry 1997;5(2):97–106.

65. Schneider LS, Small GW, Clary CM. Estrogen replacement therapy and antidepressant response to sertraline in older depressed women. Am J Geriatr Psychiatry 2001;9(4):393–9.

66. Soares CN, Poitras JR, Prouty J, et al. Efficacy of citalopram as a monotherapy or as an adjunctive treatment to estrogen therapy for perimenopausal and postmenopausal women with depression and vasomotor symptoms. J Clin Psychiatry 2003;64(4):473–9.

67. Soares CN, Arsenio H, Joffe H, et al. Escitalopram versus ethinyl estradiol and norethindrone acetate for symptomatic peri- and postmenopausal women: impact on depression, vasomotor symptoms, sleep, and quality of life. Menopause 2006;13(5):780–6.

68. Soares CN. Menopausal transition and depression: who is at risk and how to treat it? Expert Rev Neurother 2007;7(10):1285–93.

69. Joffe H, Petrillo LF, Koukopoulos A, et al. Increased estradiol and improved sleep, but not hot flashes, predict enhanced mood during the menopausal transition. J Clin Endocrinol Metab 2011;96(7):E1044–54.

70. Schmidt PJ, Ben Dor R, Martinez PE, et al. Effects of estradiol withdrawal on mood in women with past perimenopausal depression: a randomized clinical trial. JAMA Psychiatry 2015;72(7):714–26.

71. Stahl S. Effects of estrogen on the central nervous system. J Clin Psychiatry 2001; 62(5):317–8.

72. Stahl SM. Vasomotor symptoms and depression in women, part I. Role of vasomotor symptoms in signaling the onset or relapse of a major depressive episode. J Clin Psychiatry 2009;70(1):11–2.

73. Morrison MF, Kallan MJ, Ten Have T, et al. Lack of efficacy of estradiol for depression in postmenopausal women: a randomized, controlled trial. Biol Psychiatry 2004;55(4):406–12.

74. Morrison JH, Brinton RD, Schmidt PJ, et al. Estrogen, menopause, and the aging brain: how basic neuroscience can inform hormone therapy in women. J Neurosci 2006;26(41):10332–48.

75. Rudolph I, Palombo-Kinne E, Kirsch B, et al. Influence of a continuous combined HRT (2 mg estradiol valerate and 2 mg dienogest) on postmenopausal depression. Climacteric 2004;7(3):301–11.

76. Santoro N. The menopausal transition. Am J Med 2005;118(Suppl 12B):8–13.

77. Maki PM, Freeman EW, Greendale GA, et al. Summary of the National Institute on Aging-sponsored conference on depressive symptoms and cognitive complaints in the menopausal transition. Menopause 2010;17(4):815–22.

78. Freeman MP, Cheng LJ, Moustafa D, et al. Vortioxetine for major depressive disorder, vasomotor, and cognitive symptoms associated with the menopausal transition. Ann Clin Psychiatry 2017;29(4):249–57.

79. Frey BN, Haber E, Mendes GC, et al. Effects of quetiapine extended release on sleep and quality of life in midlife women with major depressive disorder. Arch Womens Ment Health 2013;16(1):83–5.

80. Gambacciani M, Ciaponi M, Cappagli B, et al. Effects of low-dose, continuous combined estradiol and noretisterone acetate on menopausal quality of life in early postmenopausal women. Maturitas 2003;44(2):157–63.

81. Joffe H, Groninger H, Soares CN, et al. An open trial of mirtazapine in menopausal women with depression unresponsive to estrogen replacement therapy. J Womens Health Gend Based Med 2001;10(10):999–1004.
82. Joffe H, Soares CN, Petrillo LF, et al. Treatment of depression and menopause-related symptoms with the serotonin-norepinephrine reuptake inhibitor duloxetine. J Clin Psychiatry 2007;68(6):943–50.
83. Kornstein SG, Jiang Q, Reddy S, et al. Short-term efficacy and safety of desvenlafaxine in a randomized, placebo-controlled study of perimenopausal and postmenopausal women with major depressive disorder. J Clin Psychiatry 2010;71(8): 1088–96.
84. Soares CN, Kornstein SG, Thase ME, et al. Assessing the efficacy of desvenlafaxine for improving functioning and well-being outcome measures in patients with major depressive disorder: a pooled analysis of 9 double-blind, placebo-controlled, 8-week clinical trials. J Clin Psychiatry 2009;70(10):1365–71.
85. Soares CN, Thase ME, Clayton A, et al. Desvenlafaxine and escitalopram for the treatment of postmenopausal women with major depressive disorder. Menopause 2010;17(4):700–11.
86. Soares CN, Frey BN, Haber E, et al. A pilot, 8-week, placebo lead-in trial of quetiapine extended release for depression in midlife women: impact on mood and menopause-related symptoms. J Clin Psychopharmacol 2010;30(5):612–5.
87. Maki PM, Kornstein SG, Joffe H, et al, Board of Trustees for The North American Menopause Society (NAMS) and the Women and Mood Disorders Task Force of the National Network of Depression Centers. Guidelines for the evaluation and treatment of perimenopausal depression: summary and recommendations. Menopause 2018;25(10):1069–85.
88. Green SM, Key BL, McCabe RE. Cognitive-behavioral, behavioral, and mindfulness-based therapies for menopausal depression: a review. Maturitas 2015;80(1):37–47.

Management of Grief, Depression, and Suicidal Thoughts in Serious Illness

Kanako Y. McKee, MD[a,b,*], Anne Kelly, LCSW[c]

KEYWORDS

- Serious illness • Grief • Prolonged grief • Depression • Death contemplation
- Suicidal ideation • Antidepressants • Psychotherapy

KEY POINTS

- Psychological distress is a common cause of suffering in patients and families facing serious illness.
- Grief is an adaptive and individualized process that may occur in response to any form of loss.
- Prolonged grief and major depressive disorder (MDD) are discrete conditions that warrant individualized assessment and treatment.
- Differentiating between grief, prolonged grief, MDD, and other conditions marked by depressive symptoms is important to provide appropriate support and treatment.
- Although thoughts about death may be normative in patients nearing the end of life, they must be differentiated from active suicidal ideation in which a patient actively seeks to take one's own life.

INTRODUCTION

Serious illness causes a cascade of life changes for patients and their families. The varied physical, social, and psychological stressors that accompany advanced disease can be burdensome and cause intense emotional suffering, hindering the ability of patients to cope in day-to-day life and affecting their ability to endure or adhere to recommended treatments. Clinicians may find it challenging to distinguish normative symptoms of grief from other conditions that may have overlapping symptoms but require further clinical attention, such as prolonged grief and major depression.

This article originally appeared in *Medical Clinics*, Volume 104, Issue 3, May 2020.
[a] Division of Geriatrics, Department of Medicine, University of California San Francisco San Francisco, San Francisco, CA, USA; [b] San Francisco Veterans Affairs Health Care System, 4150 Clement Street, Box 181G, San Francisco, CA 94121, USA; [c] San Francisco Veterans Affairs Health Care System, 4150 Clement Street (NH 181), San Francisco, CA 94121, USA
* Corresponding author.
E-mail address: kanako.mckee@ucsf.edu

Clinics Collections 11 (2021) 233–254
https://doi.org/10.1016/j.ccol.2020.12.041
2352-7986/21/Published by Elsevier Inc.

Suicide assessments in this population are complicated by the reality that seriously ill patients and their caregivers may frequently contemplate or talk about death without having active suicidal thoughts. This article addresses key concepts for the assessment and management of commonly encountered types of psychological distress among patients and families living with serious illness.

GRIEF AND LOSS IN SERIOUS ILLNESS
Grief

Grief is a natural, albeit painful, response to a loss. Patients and families facing serious health conditions are likely to experience many types of loss over the course of illness, including physical functioning, cognitive functioning, meaningful social roles, and financial resources. They may also include loss of control, certainty, or hopes and expectations for the future. Bereavement is a term used to describe the event of losing of a loved one through death, which is considered to be among life's most stressful events and a time often marked by considerable grief.

Assessment and Diagnosis

Grief is a highly individualized process, although there are common traits that clinicians can identify or anticipate. Symptoms fluctuate and may manifest across multiple domains:

- Emotional—numbness, guilt, sadness, yearning, relief, anger
- Physical—decreased energy, tension in the body
- Cognitive—difficulty concentrating, thoughts focused on the loss
- Behavioral—changes in sleep and appetite, crying, social withdrawal
- Spiritual—questions of meaning, relationship to one's faith may be strengthened or challenged

Although grief is a dynamic process without prescribed stages, the difficulties experienced in grief dissipate with time. In the context of bereavement, surviving loved ones may initially feel an acute form of grief marked by strong waves of sadness, disbelief, and persistent yearning. Sleep disturbances and social withdrawal can occur, and some individuals report seeing, hearing, or feeling the presence of the deceased.[1,2] However, the intensity of grief subsides as the griever comes to grasp the reality of the loss and adapts to a changed life and future. As the loss is integrated into daily life, bereaved individuals regain the desire and ability to engage in pleasurable activity and meaningful relationships while maintaining a sense of connection to the deceased. Acute symptoms of grief commonly subside within 6 months to a year after the death has occurred.[3] However, important reminders of the loss, such as holidays, birthdays, and anniversaries may trigger strong feelings of grief to re-emerge.

Although grief is difficult and may cause temporary or intermittent changes in functioning, distress is largely attributed to the loss itself and does not preclude individuals from also experiencing pleasure, joy, and hope. A normative grief process is not characterized by problems with self-worth or sustained impairments in social or occupational functioning. The intensity, duration, and expression of grief is influenced by a variety of factors including the type of loss, how the loss occurred, gender, cultural and spiritual norms, age, health, and the griever's support system.[4]

Treatment

On its own, grief does not require formal medical or psychiatric intervention for distress levels to improve.[5] For many, the empathy and reassurance received from family, friends, or a spiritual community are enough to foster healthy coping. Clinicians can actively support grieving patients by offering empathic listening and normalizing their experience in the context of the loss. Educating patients and families about what to expect while grieving can help them navigate an unfamiliar and difficult process while also dispelling myths that grief adheres to prescribed traits or stages. In situations where an informal support system feels inadequate to the griever, a referral to a peer support group, chaplain, or mental health provider should be considered. For bereaved individuals seeking grief support, local hospice agencies may be an apt resource. Bereaved families of hospice may receive counseling services for up to a year after the death of a loved one and many hospices make their bereavement programs available to the wider public regardless of hospice enrollment.

The risk of developing distinct mood, anxiety, and substance use disorders is heightened during bereavement.[2,4] Because the symptoms that frequently characterize grief may also appear in other health conditions, a careful and culturally sensitive assessment is warranted to avoid either pathologizing a natural grief response or neglecting to identify and address a co-occurring illness. In circumstances where sleep disturbances are affecting daily functioning, it may be appropriate to consider targeted treatment of insomnia.

PROLONGED GRIEF

Prolonged grief is a severe and debilitating grief reaction that is estimated to occur in 10% of bereaved adults,[6] possibly affecting more than 1 million Americans annually.[7] Associated with reduced quality of life, poor health, and high-risk behaviors,[8,9] prolonged grief is a discrete mental health condition that can lead to substantial and long-lasting consequences.

The concept of prolonged grief in bereavement has been explored using different definitions and names, including complicated grief and traumatic grief. The World Health Organization included a new diagnosis of Prolonged Grief Disorder (PGD) in their release of the *International Classification of Diseases, 11th Revision*. The American Psychological Association's *Diagnostic and Statistical Manual, Fifth Edition (DSM-5)*[10] included a variant of this diagnosis, Persistent Complex Bereavement Disorder (PCBD), in section III, "Conditions for Further Study." The Yale Bereavement Study found no significant difference between the patient populations identified by PGD and PCBD.[11] For consistency, the term "prolonged grief" will be used throughout this article.

Assessment and Diagnosis

Prolonged grief is characterized not simply by the presence of grief symptoms over time but rather by the protracted duration of intense grief that causes impairments in daily functioning. In prolonged grief, acute cognitive, emotional, and behavioral grief symptoms remain unremitting for most of the time at least 6 months to a year after the death of a loved one and are inconsistent with cultural, spiritual, or social norms.[1,12–14]

Fundamental to this condition is the persistent yearning for or preoccupation with the deceased person. This is often accompanied by unrelenting feelings of anger, guilt, or shock. The griever may have difficulty accepting the reality of the death, feel they have lost a part of themselves, and/or actively avoid people, places, or things that trigger memories of the loss. Feelings of guilt may be centered around regrets related to the deceased or blaming themselves/others for their inability to prevent the death from happening. For the griever, the process may feel never-ending and worrisome or, alternatively, it may feel that grief is what maintains their connection to the deceased. Disturbed sleep and suicidal thinking can occur in prolonged grief independent of a comorbid mood or anxiety disorder.[8,15] Suicidal thoughts may particularly stem from the griever's longing to be with the deceased.

Prolonged grief is associated with other health problems including cardiac disease, hypertension, cancer, and substance use.[9] Bereaved people with a history of trauma, previous losses, mood and anxiety disorders, substance use disorders, inadequate social support, and women are among those more vulnerable to developing prolonged grief; losing a loved one in sudden or violent circumstances also raises the risk.[1,13,16]

Clinicians are cautioned not to screen for or diagnose PGD within the first 6 months of bereavement to avoid pathologizing a normative grief process, and guidelines proposed for PCBD do not allow a diagnosis to be made for at least 12 months into bereavement. If severe grief symptoms are persistent and causing impairments within important areas of functioning 6 months to a year after the death of a loved one, patients should be screened for prolonged grief. Because the presenting symptoms may initially appear similar to or exist alongside a mood or anxiety disorder (**Table 1**), clinicians should identify all presenting conditions to inform an appropriate treatment plan.

There are multiple assessment tools that have been shown to reliably distinguish normative grief from prolonged grief. Examples include:

- The Inventory of Complicated Grief: consists of 19 self-rated items; scores greater than 25 warrant further clinical assessment.[17]
- The Brief Grief Questionnaire: consists of 5 self-rated items; scores greater than 5 warrant further clinical assessment.[18,19]

Table 1
Differences between prolonged grief and major depression

Symptom	Prolonged Grief	Major Depression
Negative thoughts & emotions	Centered around the deceased and persistent longing	Generalized and pervasive, feelings of hopelessness
Feelings of pleasure	Able to experience positive emotions alongside preoccupation with the deceased	Inability to enjoy daily activities
Feelings of guilt	Centered around regrets in relation to the deceased	Global feelings of guilt, worthlessness, and being a burden on others
Avoidant behaviors	Avoidance of places, objects, and people that remind them of the reality of the loss	General avoidance and social withdrawal
Physical symptoms	Sleep disturbance	Sleep disturbance, changes in appetite/weight, psychomotor agitation/retardation, fatigue/loss of energy
Suicidal thoughts	Commonly associated with a wish to be with the deceased	Rooted in feelings of hopelessness and worthlessness, intolerable suffering, and feeling a burden to others

- Prolonged Grief Disorder-13: consists of 12 self-rated items; diagnostic criteria warranting further clinical assessment are specified.[14]

Treatment

When prolonged grief is suspected, patients should be referred to a mental health provider for specialized assessment and treatment. Psychotherapeutic interventions designed to treat prolonged grief seem to be more effective than standard interventions used in the treatment of depression.[7,20] Many targeted treatments have been studied with promising results.[21–24] One such intervention is Complicated Grief Treatment (CGT), which has demonstrated positive outcomes across 3 randomized control trials.[7,20,25] The treatment is a manualized, 16-session cognitive behavioral therapy which incorporates strategies used in interpersonal therapy and motivational interviewing.[26] The role of pharmacotherapy in treating prolonged grief remains unclear. Some studies have examined the concurrent use of antidepressants in patients receiving CGT, but the results are mixed and the evidence base remains limited.[27]

All clinicians caring for individuals with prolonged grief can offer added support through empathic listening and gentle reassurance around their attempts to resume daily activities. Educating the griever about prolonged grief may offer a framework for their distress and foster hope for improvement. They should be encouraged to use support available through their family, friends, and spiritual community. Clinicians should also remain vigilant to suicidal thinking or behaviors and assess a griever's risk for self-harm.

DEPRESSION IN SERIOUS ILLNESS

Depressive symptoms are common among patients with serious illness and take a major toll on quality of life. Depression can exacerbate the physical burdens of advanced disease including pain, fatigue, poor appetite, and sleep disturbance.[28] It has been associated with decreased treatment adherence,[29,30] increased disability,[31,32] increased health service costs,[33] increased caregiver burden,[34] poor prognosis,[35] and—in some diseases—higher mortality.[36–39] In addition, major depression is a well-established risk factor for suicide.[40] Although estimates of depression prevalence among the seriously ill vary widely due to differences in definitions used and populations studied, available studies consistently show that patients with serious illness experience depression at higher rates than the general population. Compared with a 4% 1-year pooled prevalence of major depressive disorder (MDD) in the general population,[41] a 2011 meta-analysis found prevalence ranges of 5% to 30% for depression among patients with cancer in palliative care settings, with a pooled prevalence of 15% for MDD and about 10% for minor depression.[42] Rates of depressive symptoms are also high at the very end of life: 1 study found that 43% of all home hospice patients experienced moderate-to-severe symptoms of depression, as rated by caregivers using the Edmonton Symptom Assessment Scale.[43] Unfortunately, clinical depression remains underdiagnosed and undertreated in palliative care.

Assessment and Diagnosis

The *DSM-5* defines a major depressive episode as greater than 2 weeks of pervasive and functionally debilitating depressed mood or anhedonia, accompanied by at least 4 of the following additional symptoms of depression:

1. Changes in weight or appetite
2. Insomnia or hypersomnia
3. Psychomotor agitation or retardation
4. Fatigue or loss of energy

5. Feelings of worthlessness or excessive guilt
6. Poor concentration or indecisiveness
7. Recurrent thoughts of death, suicidal ideation, or suicidal behavior[10]

Many screening instruments are used in clinical practice. The simplest of these is a 2-question screen, which is considered positive if a patient answers "Yes" to both of the following questions: "Are you depressed?" and "Have you experienced loss of interest in things or activities that you would normally enjoy?"[44] In a meta-analysis of 5 studies of patients with cancer and patients receiving palliative care, this 2-question screen had a pooled sensitivity of 91% and a specificity of 86%.[45] Other depression screening tools used in palliative care include the 4-question Brief Case Find for Depression,[46] Patient Health Questionnaire-9,[47] and the Hospital Anxiety and Depression Scale.[48]

In-Depth Assessment

For patients who screen positive for depression, clinicians should conduct a more detailed assessment starting with the history of present illness. The history is essential to establishing the presence of depressive symptoms and their chronology, their impact on functioning, any alleviating or aggravating factors, and comorbid medical and psychiatric conditions. Special attention should be paid to the patient's underlying serious illness—including disease and symptom burden, current and past treatment history, and medication review. Because the somatic symptoms of depression are often caused by the patient's underlying illness, assessments of depression in the seriously ill often give greater weight to psychological symptoms and require clinicians to carefully consider the time course of symptoms, changes from baseline, and proportionality or intensity of symptoms in relation to the situation.[49,50] Finally, clinicians should assess patients for suicidal ideation/risk, obtain a social history, and perform focused physical and mental status examinations.[51]

The differential diagnosis for MDD includes adjustment disorder with depressed mood, demoralization syndrome, and prolonged grief—all of which can present with symptoms of distress. Adjustment disorder with depressed mood occurs in response to an identifiable stressor, with patients experiencing distress out of proportion to the stressor itself; the distress resolves within 6 months of resolution of the identified stressor.[10] Demoralization syndrome, although not currently recognized as a distinct psychiatric syndrome, is marked by existential despair, hopelessness, and a profound sense of helplessness and incompetence. The distress arising from demoralization can be profound—even leading to a desire for hastened death—and studies suggest that it is clinically significant in 13% to 18% of patients with progressive disease or cancer.[52] Prolonged grief has been discussed in detail above. For cases in which making a diagnosis is particularly challenging, consultation with a specialist is recommended.

Treatment

Whenever possible, management of major depression in patients with serious illness should combine patient and family education/support, supportive psychotherapy, and antidepressant pharmacotherapy.

Nonpharmacologic Therapy

All health care providers can take an active role in providing psychosocial support for patients and families. Evidence from randomized controlled trials (RCTs) in patients with cancer shows that:

- Interactions that convey empathy and active listening promotes psychological adjustment

- Providing anticipatory guidance about what to expect in the future promotes psychological well-being
- Opportunities to discuss feelings with a health professional reduce psychological distress[53]

Offering compassion, listening deeply, clarifying and validating patient concerns, encouraging adaptive coping mechanisms, engaging existing social supports, reframing cognitive distortions, and helping patients with meaning-making are all interventions that can decrease psychological suffering.[49,54,55]

For more formal psychotherapy, patients should be referred to a mental health provider. Multiple RCTs have demonstrated that psychotherapy is an efficacious treatment of unipolar major depression in healthy adults, comparable with treatment with antidepressants.[56,57] A meta-analysis of psychotherapy for depression treatment in patients with advanced cancer found a statistically significant decrease in depression scores indicating a moderate clinical effect.[58] Cognitive behavioral therapy,[57,58] supportive-expressive therapy,[59] dignity therapy,[55,60] and meaning-centered psychotherapy[61] are examples of psychotherapies used in treatment of depression for patients with serious illness.

Pharmacotherapy

Antidepressants are prescribed at lower rates for depressed patients with concurrent physical illness compared with their physically healthy counterparts,[62] perhaps due to clinicians' uncertainty about the appropriateness and efficacy of pharmacotherapy.[62,63] A 2010 Cochrane systematic review and meta-analysis found antidepressants to be effective and appropriate for the treatment of depression in patients with physical illness,[64] and a follow-up study in 2011 reached a similar conclusion for depressed patients with life-threatening illness.[65] Specifically, the latter found antidepressants to be superior to placebo at every time point starting at 4 to 5 weeks after initiation, with effect size increasing over time up to 9 to 18 weeks. Interestingly, this meta-analysis also suggested that, in the palliative care population, antidepressants may be effective in reducing depressive symptoms not only in MDD, but also in milder mood disorders, such as adjustment disorder with depressed mood and dysthymia (now classified under persistent depressive disorder in the *DSM-5*).[65] As noted by a 2018 Cochrane review and meta-analysis of antidepressant use in patients with cancer, however, the evidence base remains limited and better trials are needed.[66]

Numerous studies on standard antidepressant pharmacotherapy in physically healthy patients demonstrate similar efficacy across and within antidepressant classes.[56] The choice of antidepressant in palliative care thus depends on factors such as the patient's symptoms, preferences, and prognosis; the medication's side effect profile and other distinguishing features; and drug-drug interactions (DDIs). **Table 2** summarizes commonly used antidepressants, recommended dosing ranges, and notable characteristics. Selective serotonin reuptake inhibitors (SSRIs), widely used as first-line therapy for depression, have a positive safety profile for patients with serious illness and have fewer autonomic and anticholinergic side effects than tricyclic antidepressants (TCAs).[56,65] Common side effects of SSRIs include transient nausea, gastrointestinal upset, headache, and sexual dysfunction; some (especially citalopram) can cause dose-dependent QTc prolongation.[56] Serotonin/norepinephrine reuptake inhibitors (SNRIs) have a similar antidepressant efficacy and side effect profile as SSRIs. In addition, SNRIs may be more effective than SSRIs in treating concomitant anxiety and are effective for the treatment of neuropathic pain—very useful in palliative care.[67] Two other first-line antidepressants with atypical mechanisms of

Table 2
Antidepressants commonly used in palliative care

Medication	Typical Starting Dosage	Typical Dosage Range	Notes on Titration & Available Formulations	Clinical Considerations
SSRIs				• Positive safety profile in patients with serious illness; generally well tolerated • Common side effects: transient nausea, gastrointestinal upset, headache, sexual dysfunction
Citalopram (Celexa)	10–20 mg/d	20–40 mg/d	• Start at 20 mg/d; may increase dose after >1 wk • Available as tabs, liquid	• Well tolerated • Few DDIs • Max dose 20 mg/d older patients • Significant risk of QTc prolongation at doses >40 mg/d
Escitalopram (Lexapro)	5–10 mg/d	10–20 mg/d	• Start at 5–10 mg/d; may increase dose after >1 wk • Available as tabs, liquid	• Well tolerated • Few DDIs • Max dose 10 mg/d in older patients • Dose-dependent QTc prolongation • Taper to DC when possible • Some evidence suggests that escitalopram and sertraline provide best combination of efficacy and acceptability among SSRIs
Fluoxetine (Prozac)	10–20 mg/d	20–60 mg/d	• Start at 10–20 mg/d; may increase dose after >1 wk • Available as tabs, capsules, liquid	• Many DDIs (potent CYP2D6 inhibition) • Associated with weight loss (most other SSRIs associated with weight gain) • May be activating in some patients • Wide dose range: up to 80 mg/d • Very long $t^{1/2}$ → tapering to DC less important

Paroxetine (Paxil)	10–20 mg/d	20–40 mg/d	• Start at 10–20 mg/d; may increase dose after >1 wk
			• Available as tabs, liquid
				• Many DDIs (potent CYP2D6 inhibition)
				• Very short $t^{1/2}$
				  ○ Taper to DC to avoid significant discontinuation syndrome
				  ○ Caution if oral route unreliable

Sertraline (Zoloft)	25–50 mg/d	50–200 mg/d	• Start at 25–50 mg/d; may increase dose by 50 mg weekly up to 200 mg/d • Available as tabs, liquid	• Well tolerated • Few DDIs • Taper to DC when possible • Some evidence suggests that escitalopram and sertraline provide best combination of efficacy and acceptability among SSRIs
SNRIs				• Similar antidepressant efficacy and side effect profile as SSRIs • May be more effective than SSRIs for concomitant anxiety • Effective treatment of neuropathic pain

Venlafaxine (Effexor)	37.5–75 mg/d	75–225 mg/d	• Start at 37.5–75 mg/d; may increase by 75 mg every 4 d up to 225 mg/d
			• Available as tabs, capsules
			• Capsule granules are difficult to administer through feeding tubes
			• Extended-release formulation can be given qd. Otherwise, divide the total daily dose bid-tid
				• Effective treatment of neuropathic pain (higher doses)
				• Very short $t^{1/2}$
				  ○ Taper to DC to avoid significant discontinuation syndrome
				  ○ Caution if oral route unreliable
				• Common side effects: insomnia, headache, hypertension
				• Decrease dose by 25%–50% in renal impairment and by 50% in mild-mod hepatic impairment.

(continued on next page)

Table 2
(continued)

Medication	Typical Starting Dosage	Typical Dosage Range	Notes on Titration & Available Formulations	Clinical Considerations

Duloxetine (Cymbalta)	30–60 mg/d	60–120 mg/d	• Start at 30–60 mg/d; may increase by 30 mg weekly
			• Available as capsules
			• Capsule granules are difficult to administer through feeding tubes
				• Effective treatment of neuropathic pain (higher doses)
				• Doses >60 mg/d are rarely more effective for depression, although ok to increase up to 120 mg/d for neuropathic pain.
				• Short t¹/²
				  ○ Taper to DC to avoid significant discontinuation syndrome (although less severe than venlafaxine)
				  ○ Caution if oral route unreliable
				  ○ Contraindicated in renal impairment (CrCl < 30) and hepatic impairment/cirrhosis.

Atypical agents			• Buproprion, mirtazapine, and methylphenidate may be used as single agents or in combination with SSRIs/SNRIs • Esketamine is currently available on a restricted basis only for treatment-resistant depression; it must be given with an oral antidepressant	
Bupropion (Wellbutrin)	150 mg/d	300–450 mg/d	• Start at 150 mg/d; may increase to 300 mg/d after 3 d and then to 450 mg/d after 2 wk • Available as tabs • Multiple formulations (IR, SR, XL); XL allows for once daily dosing	• Weak norepinephrine and dopamine reuptake inhibitor • Useful in patients working on smoking cessation • Lowers seizure threshold → contraindicated in seizure disorder and eating disorder • Mild stimulant effect → useful in fatigue, but may worsen anxiety or insomnia • May improve concentration • Minimal sexual side effects

Mirtazapine (Remeron)	7.5–15 mg/d	15–45 mg/d	• Increase dose by 15 mg every 1–2 wk	• Exact mechanism of action unknown. Increases central serotonergic and noradrenergic activity
				• Side effects include sedation and appetite gain
				  ○ Useful in patients with insomnia, anorexia, weight loss
				  ○ Dose at bedtime
				• May help with nausea
				• Common side effect: orthostatic hypotension
				• Antidepressant effect may peak at 30 mg/d, then decrease at higher doses
				• A few studies suggest slightly faster onset of action compared with standard antidepressants

Methylphenidate (Ritalin)	2.5–5 mg/d	10–30 mg/d	• Start at 2.5 mg once daily or 2.5 mg bid. Increase by 5 mg/d (or 2.5 mg/dose) every 5 d, up to 15 mg bid	• Psychostimulant medication • Rapid antidepressant effect (within 1–3 d) ○ Consider choosing as first-line therapy for patients with short prognoses (days to <2 mo) • Well tolerated in most patients • Most have good response at lower dosages • Dose qam or bid. If dosing bid, administer 2nd dose no later than 2 PM to avoid insomnia • May also help with fatigue, opioid-induced sedation, and appetite • Side effects: anxiety, restlessness, insomnia • Caution/avoid in patients with history of tachyarrhythmias

(continued on next page)

Table 2
(continued)

Medication	Typical Starting Dosage	Typical Dosage Range	Notes on Titration & Available Formulations	Clinical Considerations
Ketamine Esketamine (Spravato)	? 56 mg intranasally on day 1	? 56–84 mg intranasally twice weekly during 4-wk induction phase, then 56–84 mg q 1–2 wk during maintenance phase		• N-methyl-D-aspartate antagonist traditionally used as an anesthetic • Various dosing regimens studied (iv/po), but studies are small • Rapid onset of antidepressant effect (within minutes to hours) observed in studies • Esketamine: intranasal formulation Food and Drug Administration approved for treatment-resistant depression in conjunction with an oral antidepressant • Restricted distribution (Risk Evaluation and Mitigation Strategy) in the US: must be administered under observation • Side effects: dissociation, dizziness, nausea, sedation
TCAs				• Not a first-line medication class in palliative care due to side effect profile (anticholinergic/autonomic side effects are common), DDIs, and narrow therapeutic window with potential for overdose • Helps with neuropathic pain as well as depression

| Nortriptyline (Pamelor) | 10–25 mg/d | 50–150 mg/d | • Start at 10–25 mg/d; may increase by 25–50 mg/d every 2–3 d (10–25 mg/d every 2–3 d in older adults).
 • Available as tabs | • Side effects: sedation, delirium, urinary retention, orthostatic hypotension
   ○ Administer at bedtime
   ○ Nortriptyline has fewer anticholinergic adverse effects than amitriptyline
 • Many DDIs
 • Narrow therapeutic window; cardiotoxicity, risk of fatal overdose
 • Effective for neuropathic pain, but generally not used as first-line (SNRIs preferred) |

Abbreviation: DC, discontinuation

action deserve mention for their distinguishing features. Bupropion causes less sexual dysfunction than SSRIs, is useful in patients who want treatment of comorbid tobacco dependence, and has mild stimulant properties—which may be helpful to patients with significant fatigue, or potentially bothersome to patients with anxiety.[56] Mirtazapine is an effective antidepressant, with a few studies suggesting a faster time to onset than other antidepressants.[56] Its side effects of sedation and increased appetite are helpful to patients suffering from insomnia, anorexia, and weight loss, and data support its use in nausea management.[68] Finally, other patient factors may influence the choice of antidepressant. For patients with a history of abruptly stopping medications or for those at risk of losing the oral route in the near future, clinicians may want to avoid medications with significant discontinuation syndromes such as paroxetine or SNRIs (venlafaxine more so than duloxetine). For patients with severe depression expressing suicidal ideation, clinicians should exercise caution in prescribing TCAs, which carry the potential for fatal overdose. In fact, although TCAs are effective for depression and neuropathic pain, they are not considered first-line agents due to their side effect profile, narrow therapeutic window, and frequent DDIs.[56,67]

One challenge to treatment of MDD in palliative care is the lengthy time course to effectiveness for all of the antidepressants discussed above. Although early responders may see symptom improvement as early as 1 to 2 weeks after drug initiation, a 4- to 8-week trial at the target dose is necessary to ascertain effectiveness.[56] Patients nearing the end of life may die before standard antidepressants have had time to work. For patients with very short prognoses, alternatives should be considered. Psychostimulants such as methylphenidate can reduce depressive symptoms in the short term (up to 4 weeks),[69] and a therapeutic trial can be completed in a matter of days by initiating treatment at a low dose and titrating up daily or every few days until the clinical target or unwanted side effects are reached. Another option is ketamine: an N-methyl-D-aspartate receptor antagonist traditionally used as an anesthetic that has garnered attention as a promising new treatment of refractory depression. A 2019 review article examined 11 studies of ketamine used as an antidepressant in the palliative care population; all reported positive results.[70] In these studies, significant improvement in depressive symptoms occurred as early as 40 minutes to a few hours after administration, with the effect of a single dose typically lasting 6 to 7 days and daily dosing regimens showing sustained alleviation of depression for many weeks. In March 2019, the Food and Drug Administration-approved Spravato (esketamine) nasal spray, in conjunction with an oral antidepressant, for the treatment of treatment-resistant depression.[71]

SUICIDAL THOUGHTS IN SERIOUS ILLNESS

Living with a chronic or serious illness often prompts patients and their families to think about death and the way in which they might one day die. Death contemplation is increasingly common as people approach the end of life and is likely to be accompanied by a variety of emotional responses, possibly including passive suicidal ideation (SI). Passive SI is characterized by thoughts of wanting life to end and must be distinguished from active SI, which is marked by the desire and/or intent to end one's own life. In patients with advanced illness, active SI may also be expressed through the desire for a hastened death.

It is estimated that 4% of American adults report SI annually[72] with even higher rates noted among older adults,[73] the bereaved,[4] and as many as 30% of nursing home residents in a given month.[74] The palliative care patient population is at an increased risk for SI given that a number of the risk factors for suicide are inherent for many people living with serious illness. For example, having one or more physical illnesses that cause functional limitations, pain, respiratory problems, or impaired vision are associated with an increased risk for suicide.[75,76] Feeling a lack of control, a lack of meaning or purpose in one's life, and feeling a burden to others also pose greater risk for suicide and are not uncommon among people living with advanced illness.[77,78] Although a co-occurring mental illness, such as depression, is frequently present in patients who report SI, it is not requisite for suicidal thoughts and behaviors to occur.

Proactively identifying and assessing SI in seriously ill patients is an essential yet complex task for health care providers. Many professionals find it challenging to respond to psychosocial suffering and worry that discussing difficult issues could provoke strong emotions or intensify patients' psychological distress.[53] Their discomfort may lead them to avoid the topic of SI or change the subject for fear of saying the wrong thing in response. The perpetuation of common myths regarding suicide assessment is another factor that may inhibit professionals from exploring the topic with patients. Two common myths claim that asking about suicide could cause SI to occur and that there is nothing a clinician can do if a patient is determined to die

Table 3
Risk factors, warning signs, and protective factors for suicide

Risk Factors: Suggest Risk Over a Longer Timeframe (1 Year ~ Lifetime)	Warning Signs: Specific to the Current State; Implies Imminent Risk	Protective Factors: Need to Be Both Available & Accessible
• Previous history of psychiatric diagnoses 　○ Comorbidity and recent onset of illness increase risk • Previous suicide attempts • Male gender • Same-sex sexual orientation • Age (y): >45, highest risk >64 • Veteran status • History of abuse • Family history of suicide • Significant loss (actual or perceived) • Physical illness, pain, insomnia • Impaired functional capacity • Isolation, limited social connectedness • Hopelessness • Perceived burdensomeness • Impulsivity or aggressive tendencies • Easy access to lethal means	• Talking about wanting to die or kill oneself • Looking for ways to kill oneself: seeking access to pills, weapons, or other means • Increasing or excessive alcohol/drug use • Hopelessness • Purposeless: no reasons for living • Talking about being a burden to others • Withdrawing from friends, family, society • Feeling trapped—like there is no way out • Being in unbearable pain • Rage, anger, seeking revenge • Acting reckless or engaging in risky activities (unthinkingly) • Anxiety, agitation, sleeping too little or too much • Displaying extreme mood swings	• Effective & active medical and mental health care • Social supports • Connectedness • Reasons for living • Meaning & purpose in life • Hopefulness • Adaptive problem-solving skills • Cultural & religious beliefs that discourage suicide • Restricted access to lethal means • Children present in the home • Fear of death or suicide

Data from Refs.[40,79,80]

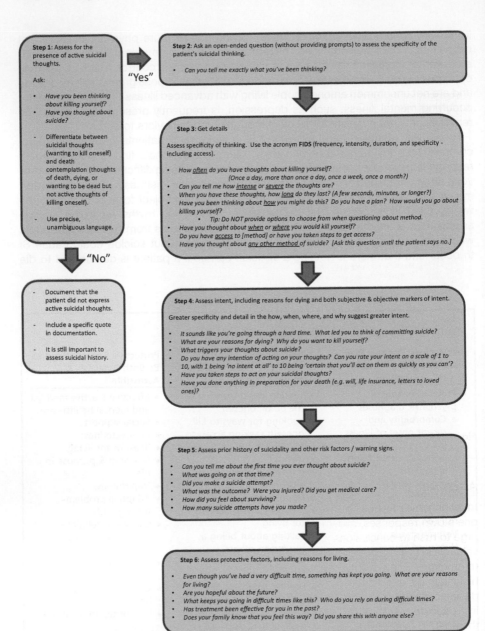

Fig. 1. Suggested framework for suicide assessment and risk stratification. (*Adapted from* Rudd MD. The assessment and management of suicidality. Journal of Contemporary Psychotherapy 2007;37(4):235; and Substance Abuse and Mental Health Services Administration (SAMHSA). SAFE-T: Suicide assessment five-step evaluation and triage. HHS Publication No. (SMA) 09-4432, CMHS-NSP-0193; Printed 2009; with permission.)

by suicide. However, evidence shows that asking about suicidal thoughts does not create SI in a patient's mind, and that accurate assessment for suicide risk gives clinicians the ability to intervene with a treatment plan to decrease suicidal behaviors, attempts, and ultimately death.

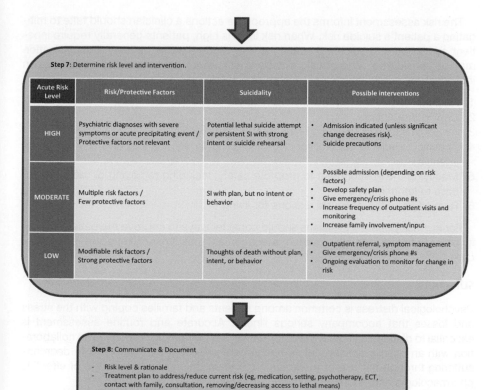

Step 7: Determine risk level and intervention.

Acute Risk Level	Risk/Protective Factors	Suicidality	Possible interventions
HIGH	Psychiatric diagnoses with severe symptoms or acute precipitating event / Protective factors not relevant	Potential lethal suicide attempt or persistent SI with strong intent or suicide rehearsal	• Admission indicated (unless significant change decreases risk). • Suicide precautions
MODERATE	Multiple risk factors / Few protective factors	SI with plan, but no intent or behavior	• Possible admission (depending on risk factors) • Develop safety plan • Give emergency/crisis phone #s • Increase frequency of outpatient visits and monitoring • Increase family involvement/input
LOW	Modifiable risk factors / Strong protective factors	Thoughts of death without plan, intent, or behavior	• Outpatient referral, symptom management • Give emergency/crisis phone #s • Ongoing evaluation to monitor for change in risk

Step 8: Communicate & Document

- Risk level & rationale
- Treatment plan to address/reduce current risk (eg, medication, setting, psychotherapy, ECT, contact with family, consultation, removing/decreasing access to lethal means)
- Follow-up plan

Fig. 1. (*continued*)

Assessment and Management

In responding to a patient expressing thoughts about death, it is important to be alert to one's own responses, allow for time to explore the patient's thoughts, and resist the urge to rush to conclusions. Serious illness communication techniques continue to be valuable in this setting. Active listening skills, the appropriate use of silence, responding to emotions with empathy, and acknowledging the patient's experience can all aid clinicians in the assessment, and can be done without actively supporting that person's desire to die. Using precise, unambiguous language is particularly important in performing a suicide assessment because it lays the foundation for honesty and bluntness in the therapeutic relationship, signals to a patient that the clinician will not shy away from painful details, and provides the details needed to make an accurate risk assessment. Precision and clarity in written documentation is likewise critical in this setting.[40]

Key components of an SI assessment include:

1. Differentiating between nonsuicidal death contemplation and SI/behavior
2. Assessing the patient's suicidal thoughts, intent, and planning behaviors
3. Assessing for risk factors, warning signs, and protective factors (**Table 3**)[40,79,80]

Based on these elements, a clinician makes a clinical judgment as to the patient's risk level for suicide. One framework for suicide assessment, adapted from "The Assessment and Management of Suicidality" by M. David Rudd,[40] is outlined in **Fig. 1**.

The risk assessment informs the appropriate actions a clinician should take to mitigating a patient's suicide risk. When risk level is high, patients generally require inpatient admission and suicide precautions. For moderate risk patients, hospitalization may be considered; alternatively, clinicians should work with patients to develop an individualized safety plan. Components of a safety plan include:

1. Helping the patient self-identify warning signs of a crisis
2. Coping strategies
3. Available supports, including safe people and places
4. Specific people to contact for help, including family, friends, and professionals/agencies
5. Modifying the environment to promote safety, including removing or reducing access to lethal means
6. Reminders of the patient's reasons for living

For low-risk patients, clinicians should consider ways to improve the patient's quality of life, whether through symptom management, psychosocial support, or spiritual care.[40,80]

SUMMARY

Psychological distress is common among patients and families coping with the stress and losses that accompany serious illness. Accurate and routine assessment is essential to distinguishing between normative and pathologic responses. In collaboration with an interdisciplinary team, health care providers can intervene to decrease suffering through the use of therapeutic communication and knowledge of effective pharmacologic and nonpharmacologic treatments.

REFERENCES

1. Shear MK. Clinical practice. Complicated grief. N Engl J Med 2015;372(2): 153–60.
2. Zisook S, Iglewicz A, Avanzino J, et al. Bereavement: course, consequences, and care. Curr Psychiatry Rep 2014;16(10):482.
3. Bonanno GA, Wortman CB, Lehman DR, et al. Resilience to loss and chronic grief: a prospective study from preloss to 18-months postloss. J Pers Soc Psychol 2002;83(5):1150–64.
4. Stroebe M, Schut H, Stroebe W. Health outcomes of bereavement. Lancet 2007; 370(9603):1960–73.
5. Jordan JR, Neimeyer RA. Does grief counseling work? Death Stud 2003;27(9): 765–86.
6. Lundorff M, Holmgren H, Zachariae R, et al. Prevalence of prolonged grief disorder in adult bereavement: a systematic review and meta-analysis. J Affect Disord 2017;212:138–49.
7. Shear K, Frank E, Houck PR, et al. Treatment of complicated grief: a randomized controlled trial. JAMA 2005;293(21):2601–8.
8. Latham AE, Prigerson HG. Suicidality and bereavement: complicated grief as psychiatric disorder presenting greatest risk for suicidality. Suicide Life Threat Behav 2004;34(4):350–62.
9. Prigerson HG, Bierhals AJ, Kasl SV, et al. Traumatic grief as a risk factor for mental and physical morbidity. Am J Psychiatry 1997;154(5):616–23.
10. Association AP. Diagnostic and statistical manual of mental disorders, fifth edition: DSM-5. 5th edition. Arlington (VA): American Psychiatric Association; 2013.

11. Maciejewski PK, Maercker A, Boelen PA, et al. "Prolonged grief disorder" and "persistent complex bereavement disorder", but not "complicated grief", are one and the same diagnostic entity: an analysis of data from the Yale Bereavement Study. World Psychiatry 2016;15(3):266–75.

12. Simon NM, Wall MM, Keshaviah A, et al. Informing the symptom profile of complicated grief. Depress Anxiety 2011;28(2):118–26.

13. Zisook S, Shear K. Grief and bereavement: what psychiatrists need to know. World Psychiatry 2009;8(2):67–74.

14. Prigerson HG, Horowitz MJ, Jacobs SC, et al. Prolonged grief disorder: psychometric validation of criteria proposed for DSM-V and ICD-11. PLoS Med 2009; 6(8):e1000121.

15. Hardison HG, Neimeyer RA, Lichstein KL. Insomnia and complicated grief symptoms in bereaved college students. Behav Sleep Med 2005;3(2):99–111.

16. Lobb EA, Kristjanson LJ, Aoun SM, et al. Predictors of complicated grief: a systematic review of empirical studies. Death Stud 2010;34(8):673–98.

17. Prigerson HG, Maciejewski PK, Reynolds CF 3rd, et al. Inventory of complicated grief: a scale to measure maladaptive symptoms of loss. Psychiatry Res 1995; 59(1–2):65–79.

18. Shear KM, Jackson CT, Essock SM, et al. Screening for complicated grief among Project Liberty service recipients 18 months after September 11, 2001. Psychiatr Serv 2006;57(9):1291–7.

19. Ito M, Nakajima S, Fujisawa D, et al. Brief measure for screening complicated grief: reliability and discriminant validity. PLoS One 2012;7(2):e31209.

20. Shear MK, Wang Y, Skritskaya N, et al. Treatment of complicated grief in elderly persons: a randomized clinical trial. JAMA Psychiatry 2014;71(11):1287–95.

21. Bryant RA, Kenny L, Joscelyne A, et al. Treating prolonged grief disorder: a randomized clinical trial. JAMA Psychiatry 2014;71(12):1332–9.

22. Kersting A, Dolemeyer R, Steinig J, et al. Brief Internet-based intervention reduces posttraumatic stress and prolonged grief in parents after the loss of a child during pregnancy: a randomized controlled trial. Psychother Psychosom 2013; 82(6):372–81.

23. Eisma MC, Boelen PA, van den Bout J, et al. Internet-based exposure and behavioral activation for complicated grief and rumination: a randomized controlled trial. Behav Ther 2015;46(6):729–48.

24. Rosner R, Pfoh G, Kotoucova M, et al. Efficacy of an outpatient treatment for prolonged grief disorder: a randomized controlled clinical trial. J Affect Disord 2014; 167:56–63.

25. Shear MK, Reynolds CF 3rd, Simon NM, et al. Optimizing treatment of complicated grief: a randomized clinical trial. JAMA Psychiatry 2016;73(7):685–94.

26. The Center for Complicated Grief CUSoSW. Complicated grief. 2017. Available at: www.complicatedgrief.columbia.edu. Accessed August 05, 2019.

27. Bui E, Nadal-Vicens M, Simon NM. Pharmacological approaches to the treatment of complicated grief: rationale and a brief review of the literature. Dialogues Clin Neurosci 2012;14(2):149–57.

28. Wilson KG, Chochinov HM, Skirko MG, et al. Depression and anxiety disorders in palliative cancer care. J Pain Symptom Manage 2007;33(2):118–29.

29. DiMatteo MR, Lepper HS, Croghan TW. Depression is a risk factor for noncompliance with medical treatment: meta-analysis of the effects of anxiety and depression on patient adherence. Arch Intern Med 2000;160(14):2101–7.

30. Mathes T, Pieper D, Antoine SL, et al. Adherence influencing factors in patients taking oral anticancer agents: a systematic review. Cancer Epidemiol 2014; 38(3):214–26.

31. Hays RD, Wells KB, Sherbourne CD, et al. Functioning and well-being outcomes of patients with depression compared with chronic general medical illnesses. Arch Gen Psychiatry 1995;52(1):11–9.

32. Wells KB, Stewart A, Hays RD, et al. The functioning and well-being of depressed patients. Results from the Medical Outcomes Study. JAMA 1989;262(7):914–9.

33. Unutzer J, Schoenbaum M, Katon WJ, et al. Healthcare costs associated with depression in medically ill fee-for-service medicare participants. J Am Geriatr Soc 2009;57(3):506–10.

34. Rhondali W, Chirac A, Laurent A, et al. Family caregivers' perceptions of depression in patients with advanced cancer: a qualitative study. Palliat Support Care 2015;13(3):443–50.

35. Hata M, Yagi Y, Sezai A, et al. Risk analysis for depression and patient prognosis after open heart surgery. Circ J 2006;70(4):389–92.

36. Frasure-Smith N, Lesperance F, Talajic M. Depression following myocardial infarction. Impact on 6-month survival. JAMA 1993;270(15):1819–25.

37. House A, Knapp P, Bamford J, et al. Mortality at 12 and 24 months after stroke may be associated with depressive symptoms at 1 month. Stroke 2001;32(3): 696–701.

38. Lloyd-Williams M, Shiels C, Taylor F, et al. Depression—an independent predictor of early death in patients with advanced cancer. J Affect Disord 2009;113(1–2): 127–32.

39. Pinquart M, Duberstein PR. Depression and cancer mortality: a meta-analysis. Psychol Med 2010;40(11):1797–810.

40. Rudd MD. The assessment and management of suicidality. Sarasota (FL): Professional Resource Press; 2006.

41. Waraich P, Goldner EM, Somers JM, et al. Prevalence and incidence studies of mood disorders: a systematic review of the literature. Can J Psychiatry 2004; 49(2):124–38.

42. Mitchell AJ, Chan M, Bhatti H, et al. Prevalence of depression, anxiety, and adjustment disorder in oncological, haematological, and palliative-care settings: a meta-analysis of 94 interview-based studies. Lancet Oncol 2011;12(2):160–74.

43. Kozlov E, Phongtankuel V, Prigerson H, et al. Prevalence, severity, and correlates of symptoms of anxiety and depression at the very end of life. J Pain Symptom Manage 2019;58(1):80–5.

44. Payne A, Barry S, Creedon B, et al. Sensitivity and specificity of a two-question screening tool for depression in a specialist palliative care unit. Palliat Med 2007;21(3):193–8.

45. Mitchell AJ. Are one or two simple questions sufficient to detect depression in cancer and palliative care? A Bayesian meta-analysis. Br J Cancer 2008; 98(12):1934–43.

46. Jefford M, Mileshkin L, Richards K, et al. Rapid screening for depression—validation of the Brief Case-Find for Depression (BCD) in medical oncology and palliative care patients. Br J Cancer 2004;91(5):900–6.

47. Kroenke K, Spitzer RL, Williams JB. The PHQ-9: validity of a brief depression severity measure. J Gen Intern Med 2001;16(9):606–13.

48. Zigmond AS, Snaith RP. The hospital anxiety and depression scale. Acta Psychiatr Scand 1983;67(6):361–70.

49. Block SD. Assessing and managing depression in the terminally ill patient. ACP-ASIM end-of-life care consensus panel. American College of Physicians—American Society of Internal Medicine. Ann Intern Med 2000;132(3):209–18.

50. Widera EW, Block SD. Managing grief and depression at the end of life. Am Fam Physician 2012;86(3):259–64.

51. Lyness JM. Unipolar depression in adults: assessment and diagnosis. Waltham, MA: UpToDate Inc; 2016. UpToDate Web site. Available at: https://www-uptodate-com.ucsf.idm.oclc.org. Accessed July 21, 2019.

52. Robinson S, Kissane DW, Brooker J, et al. A systematic review of the demoralization syndrome in individuals with progressive disease and cancer: a decade of research. J Pain Symptom Manage 2015;49(3):595–610.

53. Hudson PL, Schofield P, Kelly B, et al. Responding to desire to die statements from patients with advanced disease: recommendations for health professionals. Palliat Med 2006;20(7):703–10.

54. Onderdonk C, Thornberry K. Psychological aspects of care. In: Sumser B, Leimena ML, Altilio T, editors. Palliative care: a guide for health social workers. New York: Oxford University Press; 2019. p. 71–96.

55. Chochinov HM. Dying, dignity, and new horizons in palliative end-of-life care. CA Cancer J Clin 2006;56(2):84–103 [quiz: 104–5].

56. Simon G. Unipolar major depression in adults: choosing initial treatment. UpToDate; 2019. Available at: www.uptodate.com. Accessed July 22, 2019.

57. Hart SL, Hoyt MA, Diefenbach M, et al. Meta-analysis of efficacy of interventions for elevated depressive symptoms in adults diagnosed with cancer. J Natl Cancer Inst 2012;104(13):990–1004.

58. Okuyama T, Akechi T, Mackenzie L, et al. Psychotherapy for depression among advanced, incurable cancer patients: a systematic review and meta-analysis. Cancer Treat Rev 2017;56:16–27.

59. Kissane DW, Grabsch B, Clarke DM, et al. Supportive-expressive group therapy for women with metastatic breast cancer: survival and psychosocial outcome from a randomized controlled trial. Psychooncology 2007;16(4):277–86.

60. Chochinov HM, Kristjanson LJ, Breitbart W, et al. Effect of dignity therapy on distress and end-of-life experience in terminally ill patients: a randomised controlled trial. Lancet Oncol 2011;12(8):753–62.

61. Breitbart W, Poppito S, Rosenfeld B, et al. Pilot randomized controlled trial of individual meaning-centered psychotherapy for patients with advanced cancer. J Clin Oncol 2012;30(12):1304–9.

62. Kendrick T, Dowrick C, McBride A, et al. Management of depression in UK general practice in relation to scores on depression severity questionnaires: analysis of medical record data. BMJ 2009;338:b750.

63. Lloyd-Williams M, Friedman T, Rudd N. A survey of antidepressant prescribing in the terminally ill. Palliat Med 1999;13(3):243–8.

64. Rayner L, Price A, Evans A, et al. Antidepressants for depression in physically ill people. Cochrane Database Syst Rev 2010;(3):CD007503.

65. Rayner L, Price A, Evans A, et al. Antidepressants for the treatment of depression in palliative care: systematic review and meta-analysis. Palliat Med 2011;25(1):36–51.

66. Ostuzzi G, Matcham F, Dauchy S, et al. Antidepressants for the treatment of depression in people with cancer. Cochrane Database Syst Rev 2018;(4):CD011006.

67. Fairman N, Hirst JM, Irwin SA. Depression and anxiety: assessment and management in hospitalized patients with serious illness. In: Pantilat S, Anderson W,

Gonzales M, et al, editors. Hospital-based palliative medicine: a practical, evidence-based approach. Hoboken (NJ): John Wiley & Sons, Inc.; 2015. p. 71–91.

68. Theobald DE, Kirsh KL, Holtsclaw E, et al. An open-label, crossover trial of mirtazapine (15 and 30 mg) in cancer patients with pain and other distressing symptoms. J Pain Symptom Manage 2002;23(5):442–7.

69. Candy M, Jones L, Williams R, et al. Psychostimulants for depression. Cochrane Database Syst Rev 2008;(2):CD006722.

70. Goldman N, Frankenthaler M, Klepacz L. The efficacy of ketamine in the palliative care setting: a comprehensive review of the literature. J Palliat Med 2019;22(9):1154–61.

71. Administration UFD. FDA news release: FDA approves new nasal spray medication for treatment-resistant depression; available only at a certified doctor's office or clinic. 2019. Available at: https://www.fda.gov/news-events/press-announcements/fda-approves-new-nasal-spray-medication-treatment-resistant-depression-available-only-certified. Accessed July 20, 2019.

72. Substance Abuse and Mental Health Services Administration. 2017 National survey on drug use and health: detailed tables. Rockland (MD): Center for Behavioral Health Statistics and Quality; 2018.

73. Juurlink DN, Herrmann N, Szalai JP, et al. Medical illness and the risk of suicide in the elderly. Arch Intern Med 2004;164(11):1179–84.

74. Mezuk B, Rock A, Lohman MC, et al. Suicide risk in long-term care facilities: a systematic review. Int J Geriatr Psychiatry 2014;29(12):1198–211.

75. Harwood DM, Hawton K, Hope T, et al. Life problems and physical illness as risk factors for suicide in older people: a descriptive and case-control study. Psychol Med 2006;36(9):1265–74.

76. MacLean J, Kinley DJ, Jacobi F, et al. The relationship between physical conditions and suicidal behavior among those with mood disorders. J Affect Disord 2011;130(1–2):245–50.

77. Kanzler KE, Bryan CJ, McGeary DD, et al. Suicidal ideation and perceived burdensomeness in patients with chronic pain. Pain Pract 2012;12(8):602–9.

78. Rafanelli C, Guidi J, Gostoli S, et al. Subtyping demoralization in the medically ill by cluster analysis. Eur J Psychiatry 2013;27(1):7–17.

79. Rudd MD, Berman AL, Joiner TE, et al. Warning signs for suicide: theory, research, and clinical applications. Suicide Life Threat Behav 2006;36(3):255–62.

80. Substance Abuse and Mental Health Services Administration. SAFE-T: suicide assessment five-step evaluation and triage. In: .Rockland (MD) Substance Abuse and Mental Health Services Administration

Risk Versus Resiliency
Addressing Depression in Lesbian, Gay, Bisexual, and Transgender Youth

Brandon Johnson, MD[a],*, Scott Leibowitz, MD[b],
Alexis Chavez, MD[c], Sarah E. Herbert, MD, MSW[d,1]

KEYWORDS

- Lesbian • Gay • Bisexual • Transgender • Depression • Suicidality
- Gender dysphoria

KEY POINTS

- Lesbian, gay, bisexual, and transgender (LGBT) youth are at increased risk of depression due to stigma, discrimination, and victimization.
- Transgender youth often meet criteria for gender dysphoria, which may be associated with depression. This may additionally be alleviated by social and medical gender transition interventions (pubertal suppression and/or hormones).
- Targeting interventions to bolster supports in various environments (home, school, and community) is an important part of treating depression in LGBT youth in addition to other gold standard treatments.

INTRODUCTION

It has been widely established that youth who are minorities based on their sexual orientation and/or gender identity have a greater risk of negative mental health outcomes, including depression and suicidality.[1–6] Lesbian, gay, bisexual, and transgender (LGBT) youth have unique risk factors that predispose them to depression through the moderator of stigma. Experiences, such as family rejection, bullying,

This article originally appeared in *Child and Adolescent Psychiatric Clinics*, Volume 28, Issue 3, July 2019.
Disclosure Statement: S. Leibowitz—Royalties from Springer. No further disclosures.
[a] Mount Sinai St. Luke's Hospital, Icahn School of Medicine at Mount Sinai, 411 West 114th Street, 2nd Floor, New York, NY 10025, USA; [b] THRIVE Gender Development Program, Nationwide Children's Hospital, The Ohio State University College of Medicine, 555 South 18th Street, Columbus, OH 43205, USA; [c] Department of Psychiatry, University of Colorado, Anschutz, 13001 East 17th Place, Building 500, 2E, Aurora, CO 80045, USA; [d] Department of Psychiatry and Behavioral Sciences, Morehouse School of Medicine, Atlanta, GA, USA
[1] Present address: 160 Clairemont Avenue, Suite 445, Decatur, GA 30030.
* Corresponding author.
E-mail address: brandondjohnson@gmail.com

and lack of social acceptance, can contribute to negative health outcomes in this population. It can be difficult for clinicians to stay current with guidelines in a rapidly changing field, although the American Academy of Child and Adolescent Psychiatry Practice Parameter on Gay, Lesbian, or Bisexual Sexual Orientation, Gender Nonconformity, and Gender Discordance in Children and Adolescents can serve as a general guide.[7] This article discusses the current literature, describes the LGBT youth population, discusses the unique risk factors associated with this population, and identifies interventions to address both stigma and subsequent mental health outcomes.

TERMINOLOGY

Gender and sexuality are complex aspects of individuals' identities that include several components, including sex, gender identity, gender expression, and sexual orientation (**Fig. 1**). Although for many individuals, these identities align based on societal stereotypical grouping of categories (ie, male sex, male gender identity, masculine gender expression, and heterosexual orientation), for a significant subset of the population this is not the case. LGBT is an acronym that serves as an umbrella for several groups of individuals who have minority identities related to sexual orientation, gender expression, and/or gender identity. Although LGBT stands for lesbian, gay, bisexual, and transgender, there are many other identities that fall under the acronym.

Sex is a medical term determined by multiple factors, including internal anatomy (gonads), external anatomy (genitalia), genetics (chromosomes), hormones, and hormone receptors. Gender identity refers to a sense of self as male or female, having aspects of male and female genders, or neither. External genitalia typically are used at birth to assign a gender; this is known as the assigned sex at birth (ASAB). In Western culture, gender identity traditionally has been viewed as a binary system, including males and females. A more accurate depiction of gender identity reveals that gender lies on a spectrum, with many identities outside the binary. The term, *cisgender*, refers

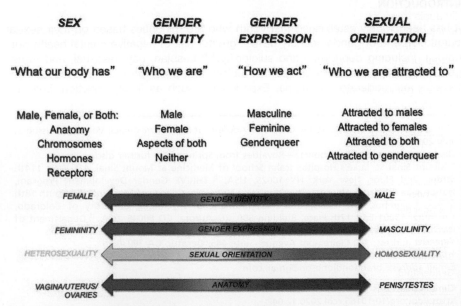

Fig. 1. Aspects of sexual orientation and gender identity.

to when gender identity is aligned with ASAB. *Transgender* refers to incongruence between gender identity and ASAB. **Table 1** depicts more colloquial terms that describe relationships between gender identity and ASAB.

Differences in gender identity are not pathologic; however, some individuals who identify as transgender meet criteria for the *Diagnostic and Statistical Manual of Mental Disorders* (Fifth Edition) (*DSM-5*) diagnosis, gender dysphoria (GD). This diagnosis refers to the distress related to the incongruence between gender identity and ASAB. Diagnostic criteria include distress related to socially expected gender expression based on ASAB and related to the anatomic incongruence. The *DSM-5* describes both childhood and adolescent/adult subtypes of GD, with differing criteria.[8]

Gender expression refers to outward expression of gender through dress, speech, mannerisms, and behavior. Expression of gender is culture-specific, with socially constructed ideals of what is masculine or feminine within each culture. Just as with gender identity, gender expression falls along a spectrum from typically feminine to typically masculine expression. Although gender expression and gender identity are related phenomena for a given person (ie, gender expression often aligns with gender identity), they are not inextricably linked. Gender expression that is different from expected societal norms does not necessarily mean that an individual identifies as LGBT, although many on the LGBT spectrum have diverse gender expressions within their culture.

Children and adolescents with diverse expressions of gender, who do not currently identify as another gender, have been described by various terms in the literature, including *gender nonconforming*, *gender variant*, *gender expansive*, *gender diverse*, and so forth. For the sake of uniformity, this population is referred in this article to as *gender diverse*.

Sexual orientation refers to the gender (or sex) of the people to whom one is sexually attracted or aroused by. With heterosexuality (attractions and arousal patterns to a different gender) as the majority status, other sexual orientations fall under the LGBT spectrum. Queer is a historically derogatory term reclaimed by some LGBT individuals that is often used to represent those who identify as nonheterosexual and/or noncisgender but without a specific label denoting gender identity and/or sexuality. **Table 2** depicts more colloquial terms used to describe various sexual orientations. Sexual orientation and gender identity are distinct aspects of identity. For instance, transgender individuals can identify as any sexual orientation (in relation to their affirmed gender identity), making it important to recognize that some youth identify as both transgender and gay, lesbian, or bisexual.

Table 1	
Terms related to gender identity	
Term	**Gender Identity**
Cisgender	ASAB matches gender
Transgender	ASAB is the opposite of gender
Intersex	Any identity but with ambiguous sexual anatomy
Agender	Does not identify with gender
Bigender	Aspects of both male and female genders
Genderfluid	Different genders at different times
Genderqueer	Outside of gender norms—defies categorization of gender
Nonbinary	Neither male nor female but elsewhere on the spectrum

Table 2 Terms related to sexual orientation		
Term	Individual's Gender	Gender Attracted to
Lesbian	Female	Female
Gay	Male	Male
Bisexual	Any	Male and female
Pansexual	Any	Any
Asexual	Any	None
Queer	Any	Nonheterosexual

METHODS

The authors highlight relevant literature and clinical guidelines related to LGBT youth and mental health outcomes, with a focus on depression and suicidal ideation as well as moderators of these outcomes in LGBT youth. The most widely known and relevant articles were used to compile data for this article. There is less research on transgender and gender diverse youth than on lesbian, gay, and bisexual (LGB) youth. In particular, the intersection of LGB and transgender or gender diverse identities has not been well studied. Where indicated, authors make a distinction between research that focuses specifically on LGB versus research on gender diverse identities.

EPIDEMIOLOGY

The number of people identifying as LGBT has been steadily increasing over the years.[9] Although many surveys have attempted to quantify the number of LGBT persons in the United States, differences in nomenclature and methodology have provided a range of estimates. These estimates of the adult LGB or LGBT population have ranged from 2.2% to 4%, or 5.2 million to 9.5 million adults.[10]

LGBT youth represent a significant percentage of young people, making the health disparities experienced by this population a serious and concerning problem. In the most recent Youth Risk Behavior Survey (YRBS) conducted by the Centers for Disease Control and Prevention,[1] 10.4% of high school students surveyed identified as LGB, which represents a larger percentage of teens than adults identifying as LGB.

UNIQUE RISK FACTORS FOR LESBIAN, GAY, BISEXUAL, AND TRANSGENDER YOUTH
Discrimination and Stigma

LGBT youth are at higher risk for depression, anxiety, suicide, and many other adverse mental and physical health outcomes.[1] When examining health disparities in minority populations, such as LGBT populations, it is important to consider the role that stress and stigma play to fully appreciate how these disparities are created, exacerbated, and perpetuated.

LGBT individuals can experience explicit legal discrimination (lack of same rights and protections as non-LGBT individuals) or noncodified discrimination through attitudes and behaviors used by the majority (bullying and exclusion) that restrict minority groups in the same manner.[11] Discrimination may prevent LGBT individuals from accessing important medical care either through refusal of care by the provider or through apprehension by the patient based on previous negative experiences.[12]

Chronic Stress and Internalizing Stigma

According to the minority stress model, discriminatory events lead to further expectation for future discriminatory events.[13] Persistent stigma creates a chronically elevated stress state in the individual, resulting in many negative mental and physical health conditions. When chronic stigma becomes internalized over time, this causes individuals to believe the discriminatory attitudes about them and leads to negative valuation of the self,[14] elevating the risk for depression. Internalized discriminatory attitudes can be directed toward one's own sexual orientation (internalized homophobia) or gender identity (internalized transphobia). Examples of internalized phobia are included in **Table 3**.

Family Rejection or Support

For all LGBT youth, a family's level of supportiveness is a major factor in a youth's self-esteem, health disparities, and overall well-being.[15] Unfortunately, gender diverse children are more likely to experience childhood physical, sexual, and psychological abuse by their parents.[16] Furthermore, LGBT youth from racial and ethnic minority groups experience parental rejection at a rate higher than racial majority groups.[17] Family rejection also may involve families sending a child to conversion therapy with the goal of changing the child's identity to cisgender and/or heterosexual. Efforts to change adolescents' identities through either parental efforts or conversion therapy have been associated with deleterious mental health and socioeconomic outcomes during young adulthood.[18]

Homelessness

In a 2012 study from the Williams Institute, 68% of LGBT homeless youth surveyed reported that family rejection was a major factor in their homelessness (by either running away or being forced out), making it by far the most commonly cited factor.[19] As many as 40% of transgender youth may experience homelessness at some point in their lives.[20] Lack of state funding, lack of local funding, and lack of federal funding were determined the top 3 barriers to preventing LGBT youth homelessness.[19]

Homelessness subsequently puts transgender youth at higher risk for many other negative outcomes. Homeless shelters or other types of emergency housing may deny transgender youth services outright due to religious beliefs or lack of comfort

Table 3
Examples of internalized phobia

Internalized Homophobia	Internalized Transphobia
"Men don't want to date other guys who are too 'faggy'."	"I'm not a 'real' man/woman."
"Women don't want to date other women who are too 'butch'."	"I don't want to transition if I can't pass because then I'll be a freak."
"I don't want my friends/family to meet my same-sex partner."	"I don't want to hang out with other transgender people if they don't pass."
"Gay relationships don't last as long as 'normal' relationships."	"If my friends or family don't use my name or pronouns it's okay as long as they don't kick me out of their lives."
"I refuse to hang out in LGBT spaces."	"Being transgender puts a burden on everyone around me and they are doing me a favor by accepting me."

in dealing with transgender populations.[20,21] When such emergency housing is available, they are more likely to experience victimization, including 50% or more of LGBT youth physically assaulted at larger shelters.[22]

School Environment

Targeting of LGBT youth can cause a hostile environment even in school. Data from the National School Climate Survey in 2011 found that large percentages of students felt unsafe due to their sexual orientation (63.5%) and gender expression (43.9%).[2] These unsafe feelings stemmed from high levels of verbal and electronic harassment and physical harassment or assault. The students who experienced higher levels of victimization due to their sexual orientation or gender expression had higher levels of depression than those with less victimization. Furthermore, the effects of LGBT-related school victimization persist and are strongly linked to negative young adult mental and physical health outcomes.[23]

Depression in Lesbian, Gay, Bisexual, and Transgender Youth

In summary, depression in LGBT youth is not a unique phenomenon that is unlike depression in any other youth. Whether there is a familial disposition, a break-up with a significant other, school pressure, or a loss of a family member, LGBT youth can suffer from depression for all of the same reasons as non-LGBT youth. Knowledge of the unique factors that may contribute to depression in LGBT youth is imperative, however, to understanding depression as a whole picture in this group.

DEPRESSION CHARACTERISTICS IN LESBIAN, GAY, AND BISEXUAL YOUTH

The mental health of LGB youth has been the subject of investigation for at least the past 30 years. Earlier research in the area of depression and suicidality in LGB individuals was done using convenience samples or selected population-based samples from 1 city or state. These older and less representative data found that LGB youth compared with non-LGB peers were more than 3 times as likely to have made a suicide attempt in the past 12 months.[3,4]

The 2017 YRBS showed some of the first data from a nationwide population-based sample of high school youth showing the prevalence of health-risk behaviors in LGB compared with non-LGB youth. The prevalence of most health-risk behaviors varied by the sexual identity and sex of a youth's sexual contacts.[1] Findings showed a striking difference on mental health measures between LGB and heterosexual youth. The YRBS asked about depression and suicidality to assess mental health risk with a question regarding feeling sad and/or hopeless with loss of pleasure for 2 weeks or more. This question was endorsed by 63% of LGB youth compared with 27.5% of heterosexual youth. Additionally, there were striking differences between the groups on measures related to suicidality (**Table 4**).

Whether there is a higher rate of actual suicide among LGB individuals is controversial because there are only a few psychological autopsy studies in the literature. Although there are not sufficient data to confirm a higher rate of completed suicide, there is evidence to suggest this could be the case.[24] More broadly, previous suicide attempts predict a greater likelihood of completed suicide, so it makes sense that LGB youth risk of completed suicide also is greater than that of their heterosexual counterparts.

Exploration of these nationwide data to understand the health risks faced by sexual minority youth still needs to take place. LGB youth also had higher rates of health risks related to driving, tobacco, alcohol, illegal drugs, exercise, and weight on the YRBS,

Table 4
Suicide-related outcomes reported by lesbian, gay, and bisexual youth in past 12 months on the Youth Risk Behavior Survey

Suicide-related Outcome	Rate Reported in Lesbian, Gay, and Bisexual Youth Versus Heterosexual Youth (%)
Seriously considered suicide	47.7 vs 13.3
Made a suicide plan	38 vs 10.4
Attempted suicide in the past 12 mo	23 vs 5.4
Suicide attempt requiring medical attention	7.5 vs 1.7

Data from Kann L, Olsen EO, McManus T, et al. Sexual identity, sex of sexual contacts, and health-related behaviors among students in grades 9-12—United States and selected sites, 2017. MMWR Surveill Summ 2018;67(No. SS-8):1–114.

but the differences were not as large as those related to depression, suicidality, and violence or victimization.[1] Understanding how these risk behaviors interact with the depression, suicidality, bullying, or violence experienced by sexual minority youth is important.

Protective Factors

There are many LGB youth who function well and are not depressed nor suicidal. Social relationships, self-concept, and coping style are known to be key factors in determining youth vulnerability to depressive symptoms.[25] So much of the focus on sexual minority youth has been on depression, suicide, victimization, and violence that clinicians do not always consider protective factors and resilience. For instance, family acceptance of LGB youth during adolescence has been shown to protect against depression, substance abuse, and suicidal ideation and behaviors.[15,26] Family connectedness seems to confer the most consistent protection against suicidal ideation and attempts among all youth regardless of sexual orientation. Stone and colleagues[27] found that although connectedness to adults outside the family was protective against suicidality for heterosexual youth, it was not protective for LGB youth. Furthermore, family connectedness was not more important for LGB youth, but it was the only type of adult connectedness associated with decreased suicide attempts in this population.

Additionally, sexual minority students living in states and cities with more protective school climates were found to have lower risk for suicidal thoughts, plans, and attempts. Protective school climates were defined as follows: having gay-straight alliances and safe spaces for LGBT youth, providing curricula on health matters relevant to LGBT youth, prohibiting harassment based on sexual orientation and gender identity, encouraging staff to attend trainings on creating supportive environments for LGBT youth, and facilitating access to off-site providers for health and other services targeted to LGBT youth. Sexual orientation disparities in suicidal thoughts were almost eliminated in states and cities that had the most protective school climates. Although the results were similar for suicidal plans and attempts, those measures did not reach statistical significance.[28]

Further evidence shows romantic involvement may be a protective factor for the psychological health of some sexual minority youth. One study of LGB youth found that romantic involvement was associated with lower psychological distress in lesbian and gay youth but with higher psychological distress in bisexual youth. The association between romantic involvement and psychological distress also differed by race/

ethnicity, with romantic relationships more protective for black and Latino youth than white youth.[29]

Assessment and Treatment Interventions for Lesbian, Gay, and Bisexual Youth

There are important ways in which issues specific to sexual orientation can be addressed in depressed LGB youth. It is imperative to ask about the sexual identity of all patients; clinicians should not avoid this subject or assume they know the answer. If an adolescent identifies as LGB, then clinicians need to be aware of all the aforementioned risk factors and protective factors.

Treatment involves creating an individualized treatment plan to bolster protective factors and reduce risk factors. This should include targeting interventions to the various environments where the youth interacts. It is important to learn what resources are available for LGB youth within these environments so that a clinician can recommend appropriate supportive interventions (**Table 5** lists examples).

Interventions with parents can increase their knowledge and acceptance of their child and are vitally important for youth still living at home or still dependent on family. Youth who have received even some support from family regarding their sexual orientation have a more positive outcome in young adulthood.[26] Attachment-based family therapy has been preliminarily studied as an intervention for addressing the needs of suicidal LGB adolescents with promising data.[30] Respect for youths' need for confidentiality regarding their sexual orientation is important, because they may need time to explore and understand their sexual orientation prior to disclosure to family members. If youths have disclosed bullying or discrimination (electronic or in person), it may be important to help them know how to advocate for themselves or to involve parents in advocating for their child.

DEPRESSION IN CHILDREN AND ADOLESCENTS WITH GENDER DYSPHORIA

Although a majority of individuals with GD identify as transgender, not all transgender youth meet criteria for GD. Because there are evidence-based treatments specific to youth with GD related to gender transition, these youth are referred to as meeting criteria for GD rather than using the identity term, transgender. Depression in children and adolescents presenting with GD is important to identify, classify, and treat considering this population of youth is a high-risk and vulnerable group. The presence of depression in a youth who may, or definitively does, meet criteria for GD evokes several considerations: (1) the relationship between depression and GD in terms of diagnostic clarity, (2) the clinician's ability to appreciate the relationship among various

Table 5 Resources in different environments to support lesbian, gay, and bisexual youth	
Environment	**Resource**
Home/family	Family Acceptance Project Parents and Friends of Lesbians and Gays support groups
School	Gay-straight alliance Supportive faculty/administration Protective policies
Community	LGBT community centers LGBT support groups LGBT-friendly shelters
Online	Hotlines, text lines, chat lines like The Trevor Project

etiologic factors (gender identity related and otherwise) that is leading to depression for the particular individual, and (3) developmental differences between children and adolescents in terms of treatment.

Depression Characteristics in Gender-Dysphoric Youth

Youth with GD experience depression and co-occurring psychiatric disorders at disproportionate rates from cisgender peers. Spack and colleagues[5] described that in their sample of 97 referred adolescents, 44.3% had a prior history of psychiatric diagnoses, 37.1% were taking psychotropic medications, and 21.6% had a history of self-injurious behavior. Another study describing the baseline characteristics of 101 adolescents with GD seeking medical intervention found clinically relevant depression scores, as measured by the Beck Depression Inventory,[31] in 35% of the sample (24% in the mild–moderate range and 11% in the severe range).[6] Additionally concerning data showed that half of the 55 transgender adolescents recruited from a community center had reported suicidal ideations and 25% had reported at least 1 suicide attempt.[32]

Assessment and Treatment Principles That Apply to All Youth with Gender Dysphoria

The 2017 Endocrine Society guidelines recommend a comprehensive mental health evaluation using a biopsychosocial model prior to the use of gender-affirming irreversible interventions in minors.[33] Diagnostic clarity for GD can be complicated by depression in the following way: a youth may be depressed for another reason and sees gender transition as a pathway toward reducing depression. Alternatively, the depression may, at least in part, stem from GD and the internal and external factors associated with the diagnosis (ie, the lack of intrinsic comfort with anatomy, potential stigma, potential lack of family acceptance or hostile school climates, and so forth). Diagnostic clarity is important because, regardless of the presence of GD, there are gender-affirming medical treatments to consider with increasing degrees of irreversibility based on the World Professional Association for Transgender Health (WPATH) Standards of Care, 7th edition.[34] Withholding medical interventions that are at least partially irreversible (such as hormones) in hopes that other interventions (such as psychopharmacology) might improve a youth's depression is not a neutral act, particularly when the source of the depression is related to the lack of secondary sex characteristics of a youth's affirmed gender. Conversely, moving forward with irreversible gender-affirming interventions (hormones and surgery) with the intention of alleviating depression is not without risk. This is of particular concern when a youth's depression might impair a clinician's ability to accurately confirm the definitive presence of GD (eg, the youth is acutely suicidal). Importantly, the WPATH *Standards of Care for the Health of Transsexual, Transgender, and Gender Nonconforming People*, 7th edition, describes that psychological interventions (social gender transition) alone also may help alleviate GD as a first step.

Where the presence of GD is clear, clinicians should avoid premature closure via the assumption that depression is the direct singular result of a lack of social and/or medical gender transition. Assessing etiologic factors in a depressed youth with GD guides clinicians in prioritizing the timing and sequence of interventions, which include both those that are gender-affirming and treatment modalities used for all youth. It is prudent to understand the contributions of multiple etiologies, including the gender-sex incongruence itself, internalized transphobia, stigma, biological predisposition, and stressor-dependent and psychological or interpersonal factors.

Prepubertal Children with Gender Dysphoria

Assessment of prepubertal children to determine whether or not they meet *DSM-5* criteria for GD requires a child to have "a strong desire to be of the other gender or an insistence that one is the other gender (or some alternative gender different from one's assigned gender)."[8] Without meeting this criterion, children cannot be diagnosed with GD of childhood, no matter how many additional indicators are met. This has increased the specificity of the diagnosis to more accurately distinguish children who are truly dysphoric from those who are potentially only gender diverse in their expression but not identity.

There is no official consensus regarding whether or not social gender transition is the universal best course of action for prepubertal children with GD. The details surrounding the controversial nature of prepubertal social gender transition are best summarized elsewhere; however, clinicians must consider the etiology of depression when considering how to best proceed.[35] In some situations, social transition in this age group can lead children to feel as though they must keep their transition a secret, which over time may inadvertently lead to shame around their gender-sex incongruence. Conversely, children who have not transitioned may develop depressive symptoms as a result of not being able to live and be perceived as their authentic gender. Data on prepubertal children who have transitioned to their affirmed gender demonstrate comparable (low) rates of depression and anxiety compared with siblings and community cisgender control groups.[36] It is important, however, to interpret these data cautiously because there were no control groups of transgender-identified children with supportive parents who did not transition nor are the data longitudinal. Therefore, social gender transition in children remains complex. Collaboratively navigating the pros and cons of transitioning (including the pace at which a child transitions) with the families and children remains a commonly described individualized approach. This approach considers the lack of predictability for how a child will identify later in life[37] and addresses the importance of how a social transition will potentially alleviate depression symptoms in a particular child.[35]

Adolescents with Gender Dysphoria

Adolescence marks a time when youth may seek physical interventions as part of a gender transition process. This may present in the context of worsening GD as physical pubertal changes occur. Interventions are tailored to the emotional and cognitive capacity of the adolescent in terms of medical decision making. More irreversible measures are deferred until the adolescents can conceptualize more fully how a particular intervention will affect their physical bodies and emotional wel-lbeing. In the United States, adolescents rely on parental consent for hormonal treatment in most multidisciplinary treatment centers, which adds a layer of family dynamics inherent in the assessment and treatment of these youth.

Puberty suppression is indicated for younger adolescents who have begun to experience pubertal changes (at least Tanner stage 2) through the use of a GnRH agonist, which ultimately delays the production of sex hormones by the gonads.[33] This allows time for a GD adolescent to explore gender identity further without the pressure of the development of irreversible secondary sex characteristics that would likely worsen GD. The most recent hallmark prospective study suggesting positive mental health outcomes after medical interventions was done by de Vries and colleagues[38] in 2014. The Amsterdam team studied youth who received puberty suppression, then gender-affirming hormones, and subsequently gender-confirming surgery. Their cohort was found to have comparable psychological adjustment to cisgender controls groups in young adulthood.

The Endocrine Society recommends, as adolescents mature, the potential use of gender-affirming sex hormones for individuals continuing to meet criteria for GD in adolescents and adults.[33] Transgender female youth (assigned males at birth) receive estrogen to create feminizing effects whereas transgender male youth (assigned female at birth) receive testosterone to create masculinizing effects. The complexity of these interventions often is discussed in a mental health setting prior to initiation.

For depressed adolescents with GD, the timing of the initiation of any physical intervention often depends on an assessment of the acuity of the depression and the family's readiness to consent. Some adolescents seeking hormonal treatment have depression that is multifactorial in nature. As such, advising families that depression may not fully remit once hormonal interventions begin can help reduce future concerns in the event that depressive symptoms persist. Understanding that adolescents with GD become depressed for all the same reasons other adolescents do, in addition to the external and internal challenges of inherently being transgender, helps guide a provider to fully understand and treat the patient.

SUMMARY

LGBT youth have disproportionate health disparities, including higher rates of depression, than their non-LGBT peers. Available evidence repeatedly shows that these higher rates of depression occur in the context of stigma, discrimination, and victimization. Assessment of depression in LGBT youth must take into account these additional risk factors as they have an impact on a particular youth. Treatment includes addressing these factors in addition to using other gold standard treatments for depression. Emerging evidence shows that LGBT youth who are in more supportive environments have better mental health outcomes, making the role of the mental health provider as an advocate even more important in this population.

Further research is needed to better understand various aspects of working with depressed LGBT youth. This is perhaps most notable in the area of youth with GD, where complex medical decision making is currently based on limited outcome data. What seems most clear is that there is no 1-size-fits-all approach for working with LGBT youth. Forming collaborative relationships with both youth and their families allows clinicians to create an individualized treatment plan to address their unique needs.

REFERENCES

1. Kann L, Olsen EO, Mcmanus T, et al. Sexual identity, sex of sexual contacts, and health-related behaviors among students in grades 9-12—United States and selected sites, 2017. MMWR Surveill Summ 2018;67(No. SS-8):1–114.
2. Kosciw JG, Greytak EA, Bartkiewicz MJ, et al. The 2011 National School Climate Survey: the experiences of lesbian, gay, bisexual and transgender youth in our nation's schools. New York: GLSEN; 2012.
3. Garofalo R, Wolf RC, Wissow LS, et al. Sexual orientation and risk of suicide attempts among a representative sample of youth. Arch Pediatr Adolesc Med 1999;153:487–93.
4. Stone DM, Luo F, Ouyang L, et al. Sexual orientation and suicide ideation, plans, attempts, and medically serious attempts: evidence from local youth risk behavior surveys, 2001-2009. Am J Public Health 2014;104:262–71.
5. Spack NP, Edwards-Leeper L, Feldman HA, et al. Children and adolescents with gender identity disorder referred to a pediatric medical center. Pediatrics 2012;129:418–25.

6. Olson J, Schrager SM, Belzer M, et al. Baseline physiologic and psychosocial characteristics of transgender youth seeking care for gender dysphoria. J Adolesc Health 2015;57:374–80.

7. Adelson SL. Practice parameter on gay, lesbian, or bisexual sexual orientation, gender nonconformity, and gender discordance in children and adolescents. J Am Acad Child Adolesc Psychiatry 2012;51:957–74.

8. American Psychiatric Association. Diagnostic and statistical manual of mental disorders. 5th edition. Arlington (VA): American Psychiatric Association; 2013.

9. Gates GJ. In U.S., more adults identifying as LGBT. In: Gallup, social and policy issues. 2017. Available at: https://news.gallup.com/poll/201731/lgbt-identification-rises.aspx. Accessed December 1, 2018.

10. Gates GJ. LGB/T Demographics: comparisons among population-based surveys. Williams Institute, UCLA School of Law; 2014.

11. Chavez A, Janssen A. Structural stigma in LGBTQ youth. JAACAP Connect, in press.

12. One Colorado Education Fund. Transparent: the state of transgender health in Colorado 2014. Available at: https://one-colorado.org/wp-content/uploads/2017/06/OC_Transparent_Download2mb.pdf. Accessed December 1, 2018.

13. Meyer IH, Link BG, Schwartz S, et al. Minority stress and mental health in gay men. J Health Soc Behav 1995;36:38–56.

14. Meyer IH. Prejudice, social stress, and mental health in lesbian, gay, and bisexual populations: conceptual issues and research evidence. Psychol Bull 2003; 129(5):674–97.

15. Ryan C, Russell ST, Huebner D, et al. Family acceptance in adolescence and the health of LGBT young adults. J Child Adolesc Psychiatr Nurs 2010;23(4):205–13.

16. Roberts AL, Rosario M, Corliss HL, et al. Childhood gender nonconformity: a risk indicator for childhood abuse and posttraumatic stress in youth. Pediatrics 2012; 129(3):410–7.

17. Richter BEJ, Lindahl KM, Malik NM. Examining ethnic differences in parental rejection of LGB youth sexual identity. J Fam Psychol 2017;31(2):244–9.

18. Ryan C, Toomey RB, Diaz RM, et al. Parent-initiated sexual orientation change efforts with LGBT adolescents: implications for young adult mental health and adjustment. J Homosex 2018;7:1–15.

19. Durso LE, Gates GJ. Serving our youth: Findings from a national survey of service providers working with lesbian, gay, bisexual, and transgender youth who are homeless or at risk of becoming homeless. Los Angeles (CA): The Williams Institute with True Colors Fund and The Palette Fund; 2012.

20. Ventimiglia N. LGBT selective victimization: unprotected youth on the streets. J Law Soc 2012;13(2):439–53.

21. Quintana NS, Rosenthal J, Krehley J. On the streets. Center for American Progress; 2010. Available at: https://www.americanprogress.org/wp-content/uploads/issues/2010/06/pdf/lgbtyouthhomelessness.pdf. Accessed on December 1, 2018.

22. Hunter E. What's good for the gays is good for the gander: making homeless youth housing safer for lesbian, gay, bisexual, and transgender youth. Fam Court Rev 2008;46(3):543–57.

23. Russell ST, Ryan C, Toomey RB, et al. Lesbian, gay, bisexual, and transgender adolescent school victimization: implications for young adult health and adjustment. J Sch Health 2011;81:223–30.

24. Plöderl M, Wagenmakers ER, Tremblay P, et al. Suicide risk and sexual orientation: a critical review. Arch Sex Behav 2013;42:715–27.

25. Martin-Storey A, Crosnoe R. Sexual minority status, peer harassment, and adolescent depression. J Adolesc 2012;35(4):1001–11.
26. Ryan C, Huebner D, Diaz RM, et al. Family rejection as a predictor of negative health outcomes in white and Latino lesbian, gay, and bisexual young adults. Pediatrics 2009;123(1):346–52.
27. Stone DM, Luo F, Lippy C, et al. The role of social connectedness and sexual orientation in the prevention of youth suicide ideation and attempts among sexually active adolescents. Suicide Life Threat Behav 2015;45(4):415–30.
28. Hatzenbuehler ML, Birkett M, Van Wagenen A, et al. Protective school climates and reduced risk for suicide ideation in sexual minority youths. Am J Public Health 2014;104(2):279–86.
29. Whitton SW, Dyar C, Newcomb ME, et al. Romantic involvement: a protective factor for psychological health in racially-diverse young sexual minorities. J Abnorm Psychol 2018;127(3):265–75.
30. Diamond GM, Diamond GS, Levy S, et al. Attachment-based family therapy for suicidal lesbian, gay, and bisexual adolescents: a treatment development study and open trial with preliminary findings. Psychotherapy 2012;49(1):62–71.
31. Beck AT, Steer RA, Brown GK. Manual for the Beck depression inventory-II. San Antonio (TX): Psychological Corporation; 1996.
32. Grossman AH, D'Augelli AR. Transgender youth and life-threatening behaviors. Suicide Life Threat Behav 2007;37:527–37.
33. Hembree WC, Cohen-Kettenis PT, Gooren L, et al. Endocrine treatment of gender-dysphoric/gender-incongruent persons: an Endocrine Society* clinical practice guideline. J Clin Endocrinol Metab 2017;102(11):3869–903.
34. Coleman E, Bockting W, Botzer M, et al. Standards of care for the health of transsexual, transgender, and gender-nonconforming people, version 7. Int J Transgend 2012;13(4):165–232.
35. Leibowitz S. Social gender transition and the psychological interventions. In: Janssen A, Leibowitz S, editors. Affirmative mental health care for transgender and gender diverse youth. Cham (Switzerland): Springer International; 2018. p. 31–48.
36. Olson KR, Durwood L, DeMeules M, et al. Mental health of transgender children who are supported in their identities. Pediatrics 2016;137(3):e20153223.
37. Steensma TD, McGuire JK, Kreukels BPC, et al. Factors associated with desistence and persistence of childhood gender dysphoria: a quantitative follow-up study. J Am Acad Child Adolesc Psychiatry 2013;52:582–90.
38. de Vries AL, McGuire JK, Steensma TD, et al. Young adult psychological outcome after puberty suppression and gender reassignment. Pediatrics 2014;134(4):696–704.

Depression in African American and Black Caribbean Youth and the Intersection of Spirituality and Religion
Clinical Opportunities and Considerations

Lisa M. Cullins, MD[a],*, Martine M. Solages, MD[b],
Shalice McKnight, DO[c]

KEYWORDS

- Depression • Children and adolescents • African American • Black Caribbean
- Spirituality • Religion • Culture

KEY POINTS

- Major risk factors for depression in African American and black Caribbean youth are lower socioeconomic status, substance use, family history, and exposure to violence, as well as overt racism, perceived racial discrimination, microaggressions/macroaggressions, and implicit bias.
- Community connectedness, spirituality/religion, and family cohesion are protective factors for depression in African American and black Caribbean youth and their families.
- Forging a healthy provider-patient alliance with a culturally sensitive lens is essential in effective service delivery models for the treatment of depression in African American and black Caribbean youth and their families.

Similar to any other illness, depression can seize any individual, child, or family and does not discriminate against age, socioeconomic class, race, or ethnicity. However, the risk factors, presentation, and diagnostic and treatment variables may differ in ethnic minorities. Just like their Latino peers, African American and black Caribbean children and adolescents continue to experience disparities in access to and quality of mental health services compared with non-Latino white peers. Exploring how

This article originally appeared in *Child and Adolescent Psychiatric Clinics*, Volume 28, Issue 3, July 2019.
Disclosures: None.
[a] George Washington University School of Medicine, Washington, DC, USA; [b] 10903 New Hampshire Avenue, Silver Spring, MD 20904, USA; [c] Fort Belvoir Community Hospital, 9300 DeWitt Loop, Fort Belvoir, VA 22060, USA
* Corresponding author. 4000 Blackburn Lane, Suite 260, Burtonsville, MD 20866.
E-mail address: lisacullins@yahoo.com

depression affects African American and black Caribbean youth and their families and current barriers to treatment may assist in closing this mental health disparity and gap, which is imperative. This article examines risk and protective factors, unique clinical presentation, and the poignant interface of spirituality and religion affecting depression in this population of youth.

Mental health within the African American community has reached a point of crisis, with increased chronicity and severity.[1] Depression rates, although lower than in other ethnic and racial counterparts, have resulted in greater lifetime functional impairment and association with serious sequelae, such as suicide.[1] However, African American youth have been unable to escape this daunting reality, as shown by an increased suicide rate among children 5 to 11 years old from 1993 to 1997 compared with 2008 to 2012.[1] This increase is concerning because, during the same time frame, there was a decreased rate among white children of the same ages. This age-related racial disparity highlights the need to explore hidden factors that are contributing to suicide and depression in African American youth, not readily captured through the standard assessment tools, measures, and processes.

Within the African American community, depression is often viewed as a great masquerader, leading to poor identification and misdiagnosis. Classic signs and symptoms are not always evident and may manifest through unconventional means, such as aggression, violence, irritability, frustration, and trauma. Although traditional risk factors, not limited to lower socioeconomic status, substance use, family history, and exposure to violence, do predispose African Americans to depression, there are additional systemic stressors and biases that increase vulnerability within this population. As times continue to evolve, it is important to understand how factors such as overt racism, perceived racial discrimination, implicit bias, social injustice, police brutality, and microaggressions/macroaggressions affect African American youth. In the absence of early interventions, the constant exposure to the aforementioned factors could result in insults to identity, self-esteem, confidence, and happiness. It is therefore important to identify depression early on and engage youth and families in order to mitigate adverse outcomes.

The basic signs and symptoms of depression are consistent in all children and adolescents. Along with irritability and/or depressed mood, there may be changes in sleep, appetite, energy level, interests, attention, concentration, and motivation. However, when integrating and fully acknowledging culture, race, and ethnicity in African American youth, differences do emerge in belief systems and perception of illness, adaptability, risk factors, protective factors, help-seeking behaviors, and the perceptions of the medical community that must be considered.

There are key risk and protective factors for depression to consider in African American youth. Risk factors may include poverty (ie, food, housing, and financial insecurities/instabilities), community trauma (ie, witnessing violence both at home and in the community), polyvictimization, neighborhood social disorganization, repeated experiences of discrimination, and chronic exposure to racism.[2] Many of these identifiable risk factors disproportionately affect minority children and their families. Parental conflict and/or lower levels of family cohesion and adaptability are associated with higher rates of suicide attempts in African American adolescents.[3] Albeit multifaceted, bullying could be understood as a traumatic event, given its impact on children and adolescents' wellbeing, and is an important risk factor to consider. Sexual minority youth in particular are exposed to heightened levels of bullying.[4] They also are more likely to have been victims of both physical and sexual abuse and may feel less social connectedness to their communities, their churches, and even family, despite these all serving as protective factors in the traditional African American culture. Thus, ethnic minority gay, lesbian, bisexual, and transgender youth have higher risk levels for depression.[4]

Protective factors may include community connectedness. Ethnic enclaves may provide mental health benefits by enhancing resident collective identity and reducing exposure to discrimination. These benefits may attenuate some of the socioeconomic disadvantages that typically characterize racially segregated communities and facilitate psychosocial adjustment.[5] Links to the church, close interpersonal relationships, and family cohesion have been found to be protective factors for African American youth. Research has suggested that religion has a positive impact as a protective factor to suicide. In particular, involvement in the church can encourage social connection, improve self-esteem, and may provide a sense of meaning to the person's life.[3] Individual factors such as active coping or dynamic and adaptive response to stress can be features in African American culture that may serve as protective factors.[6] Similar to the known benefits of social and community supports, positive early teacher interactions have been found to enhance resilience, adaptability, and self-esteem, ameliorating mental health risks and other psychosocial stressors.[7]

There are numerous elements that influence help-seeking behaviors, perceptions of illness, and adaptive coping strategies. In African American families, early identification and intervention for depression in youth relies on the family's perception and understanding of illness. The association of changes in mood, sleep, appetite, interests, and energy level may not be understood as symptoms of depression. Instead, these changes could be viewed as a typical and normative response to psychosocial stressors, which African American families disproportionately experience, with greater intensity, frequency, and chronicity in their communities. There are many instances in which opportunities for early identification and intervention are missed, simply because the youth and the caregiver do not assign their feelings, thoughts, and behaviors to symptoms of depression. Previous research supports this notion by indicating that African American youth do not recognize depression as a medical disease but view it as a concern that can be controlled through strong will and religious faith.[8]

It has also been shown that not only are these opportunities to intervene missed by youth and caregivers, they may also be missed by medical professionals. African American children are less likely to be referred for mental health services by their primary care provider compared with white children.[9,10]

Even after both the child and caregiver embrace the possibility of depression and the primary care provider has referred them for mental health services, factors such as stigma, structural barriers, faith-based cultural attributions, and mistrust of the medical community may emerge as impediments to pursuing and accessing care, especially quality care. With regard to stigma, African American families may fear that a diagnosis of mental illness might adversely label their child and disadvantage their child throughout life in educational, social, financial, and vocational realms.[9]

Systemic barriers to the pursuit and acquisition of quality mental health care for African American families are overwhelming. Population-level barriers include socioeconomic disparities, stigma, poor health education, and lack of activism/advocacy; provider factors include deficits in cross-cultural knowledge, skills, patient orientation, attitudinal sensitivity, and language, and a dearth of bicultural providers; systemic factors include services location, cost, convenience, wait times, depth and breadth of clinical training, and culturally competent care.[10,11]

In addition, the notion that African American families may delay recommended receipt of mental health care for their children because of their mistrust of the medical community is not farfetched. It has both historical and contemporary roots. In the Tuskegee Experiment, which lasted for more than 40 years, investigators failed to obtain informed consent from the participants and withheld readily available syphilis treatment from African American men.[12] African American and Hispanic/Latino youth are more likely to be diagnosed with psychotic disorders and behavioral problems, whereas white youth are more likely to be diagnosed with depressive disorders and bipolar disorder.[13] Such trends have been shown in both pediatric inpatient and outpatient settings. This diagnostic trend in ethnic minority children and adolescents was consistent with previous research that found that African American adult patients were diagnosed at higher rates with psychotic disorders and at lower rates of mood disorders; white adult patients were diagnosed with higher rates of mood disorders and lower rates of psychotic disorders across mental health settings.[13] This stark contrast may be caused by a possible delay in treatment, with African American families presenting to psychiatric emergency services once the child had significantly declined only after community and family supports were ineffective. These contrasts could have also been secondary to provider bias, cultural variations in clinical presentations, stress adaptation, clinical misperceptions, and stereotypes of mental disorder leading to diagnostic errors and misdiagnosis.[13] Further, these clinical diagnostic disparities have led African American youth to be more likely to receive treatment in more restrictive environments. Therefore, even now, mistrust of the medical community continues to be fueled by costly diagnostic errors, misdiagnosis, and greater restrictive dispositions for African American youth.

The term community connectedness is intended to describe strength-based properties of neighborhoods, including social cohesion, collective efficacy, social capital, and social support.[2] Community connectedness may increase an individual's motivation and ability to adaptively respond to adversity. Greater community connectedness may provide adolescents with coping resources outside their homes, including having additional adults to talk with, persons to provide aid in times of need, and feelings of protection. These protective factors may guard against depression and other problem behaviors.[13]

Once depression is diagnosed in an African American youth, effective treatments exist. The presence and engagement of a culturally sensitive and competent provider fosters a therapeutic alliance with both the child and the family.[14] If this therapeutic alliance is absent it is extremely difficult for any meaningful treatment to ensue even with medications, because this omission could lead to missed appointments and medication noncompliance. As a component of both the therapeutic alliance and treatment process, psychoeducation is essential to treatment adherence and success. There are numerous evidence-based treatments that are effective in this population of youth. Of note, African American families may be more likely to explore and use complimentary alternative medicine and approaches such as prayer, herbal remedies, and relaxation. These remedies may have been explored before seeking mental health care or concurrently. Providers should ask about this use and integrate this information into their clinical decision-making strategies and psychoeducation with the youth and their families.[14]

Research in this important area has outlined clear, attainable recommendations for prevention, early identification, and intervention for depression in African American children and adolescents. Social awareness and education of the signs and symptoms of depression in African American communities are paramount, especially in schools, faith-based institutions, and primary care clinics. Services need to be developed and implemented in natural settings that are in close proximity to the communities, with flexible hours that can accommodate caregivers who are employed in positions that do not provide flexible time off at varying hours. Pediatric medical homes and schools are excellent natural settings to house treatment services.

Services also need to be delivered by culturally aware, sensitive, and competent providers open to listening to their patients' stories, validating, partnering, and learning from them. Services must be consistent and stable with limited turnover and disruptions. It is important to expand the treatment team to include supportive teachers, appropriate academic supports, coaches, and faith-based and community mentors. Extracurricular activities, faith-based youth groups, academic enrichment, and opportunities for African American youth to develop their passions and cultivate their strengths are protective factors. The roadmap exists, but it takes a collective, diverse global body surrounding the youth to actualize, mobilize, and maintain it.

APPRECIATING THE DIVERSITY OF BLACK YOUTH: BLACK CARIBBEAN YOUTH AND DEPRESSION

Clinical studies frequently represent the black American population as a monolith, with few attempts to examine the potential significance of the diverse spectrum of black identities. Black Caribbean American youth are a growing population whose mental health needs are poorly understood. Although migration from the Caribbean to the United States has occurred since the 1800s, changes in immigration policies in 1965 led to a significant increase in the numbers of Caribbean migrants. There are now 4 million Caribbean immigrants in the United States, 50% of whom identify as black. Fifty percent of black immigrants in the United States have origins in the Caribbean.[15,16] Only limited data exist about how black Caribbean Americans and other subgroups of the black American population may be distinct in terms of their experiences with mental health issues.

Black immigrant communities have described themselves as underrepresented or invisible in broader dialogues about immigration, but nonetheless contend with the stressors of immigration.[17,18] Within the black Caribbean population in the United States, the limited available data suggest that risk of psychiatric illness may vary across generations, genders, and socioeconomic classes. Greater length of stay in the United States may be associated with a higher risk of mental health problems.[19] Black Caribbean immigrant and second-generation youth may struggle with acculturation, language barriers, family separation, and discrimination, all of which can affect their risk of mood, anxiety, and posttraumatic disorders and inform the pivotal childhood task of identity formation. Idioms of distress from a youth's country of origin may persist, transmute, or dissipate during the process of immigration and acculturation, complicating psychiatric diagnosis and formulation. Immigration can powerfully shape parent-child relationship dynamics; for example, by shifting children into translator roles or other positions of authority within the family.[20]

Although immigration and acculturation stress may have adverse psychological impacts, more research is needed about factors that protect or buffer against the development of mental health problems. For example, a family's socioeconomic status or educational attainment before migration, family and community connectedness, and a strong sense of ethnic identity may be protective against the development of psychological or social difficulties. However, it is likely that the relationship between these factors and an immigrant or second-generation youth's mental health is nonlinear. For example, family connectedness may bolster resilience but may also slow a youth's integration into the community outside of the home.[20] In one study, high levels of identification with an ethnic identity seemed to protect against negative outcomes such as depression in US-born immigrant-origin youth but not in foreign-born youth.[21]

In addition to facing stressors related to the immigration and second-generation experience, black Caribbean American youth must navigate entry into the black

American population as a whole. Notably, immigrants become exposed to race-based discrimination that they may not have encountered overtly in their countries of origin. Reports of discrimination seem to increase with the length of time in the United States, perhaps indicating that time in the United States increases both the likelihood of experiencing discrimination and recognition of discriminatory forces.[22] However, discrimination has been associated with depression in US born immigrant-origin youth, but not necessarily for foreign-born youth.[21] Further exploration into the complex process of racial group identification for black Caribbean youth is needed.

INTERSECTION OF SPIRITUALITY/RELIGION AND DEPRESSION IN AFRICAN AMERICAN YOUTH AND FAMILIES

The protective values and omnipresence of spirituality and religion has been a common theme deeply threaded in the black diaspora that warrants its own spotlight in the discourse pertaining to depression in African American children and adolescents. Failing to delve into and crystallize an understanding about its cultural underpinnings and influence would be a serious oversight and missed opportunity to further sharpen clinical acumen.

It is estimated that 84% of the world's population ascribes to a spiritual belief with guiding principles to govern their individual and communal practices.[23] These practices often help to shape these people's identities and worldviews. In some instances, this leads to revelation, enlightenment, or awakening, which in turn, has the ability to change a life for the better. In the United States, African Americans are reported to be markedly more religious on a variety of measures than the US population as a whole, with 79% versus 56% overall citing spirituality as a significant part of their lives.[24] Historically, African Americans have leaned on spiritual tenets to combat adverse experiences, believing that faith in God brings solace, hope, and healing, especially in times of peril and discord. Because spirituality has been a pillar of support within the African American community, it is important to explore ways in which to leverage this differentiating factor in the context of mental health assessment and treatment.

SPIRITUALITY: WHAT IS IT AND WHY SHOULD CLINICIANS CARE?

Spirituality has long been regarded as an integral part of people's composition: body, soul, and spirit. Here the spirit represents the intangible part of a person that connects with God/a higher power. It houses emotions and character, serves as the life-giving part of human beings, and through communion with God/higher power, allows self-reflection, conviction, and surrender. It is an internal force that is often overlooked or disregarded by the outside observer; however, many rely heavily on this spiritual sense to navigate the issues of life. According to the US Religious Landscape Survey, conducted by Pew Research in 2007, more than half of African Americans attended religious services regularly, at least once a week; 76% prayed at least daily; and nearly 90% were certain of God's existence.[20] Brown and Gary's[25] research found that religious involvement was inversely related to depressive symptoms among African American people. When it comes to religious practices and beliefs, studies have shown that there is a protective factor against the development and persistence of mental health conditions. This spiritual regard and subsequent benefit applies to the younger generations of this subpopulation.

SPIRITUALITY: ITS PROTECTIVE NATURE AND BENEFITS

Research posits that the protective nature of spirituality does extend to youth and often in a greater capacity compared with adults.[26] The search for meaning and purpose in life that typically occurs during adolescence drives many to seek religion for answers.[26] Ninety-five percent of youth 13 to 17 years of age currently believe in God, with 85% to 95% stating that spiritual/religious beliefs and practices play an important role in their lives.[27] Compared with other ethnic and racial groups, African American youth are more likely to identify with a religious affiliation and to rely on spiritual beliefs and practices to cope with life stressors.[28] Holder and colleagues[29] found that African American youth reporting greater importance of religion engaged less frequently in voluntary sexual activity. Additional research showed a decrease in substance use and abuse when adolescents had a personal experience with God and were socially integrated within a spiritual community. Furthermore, African American youth with serious or chronic medical conditions were more likely to use spiritual coping to address their concerns and find meaning. With approximately 70% of African Americans reporting an increased sense of spiritual peace and well-being with regular religious involvement, it is only natural to consider spirituality as an effective means to improve mental health within the African American community.[24,26,29]

SPIRITUALITY AND MENTAL HEALTH: AN UNCONVENTIONAL APPROACH TO TREATMENT

The interplay between spirituality and mental health presents a rich opportunity to reach African American youth and their families. Research has found that many African Americans rely on faith, family, and social communities for emotional support rather than turning to health care professionals. Spirituality within the African American community is deeply relational and community-oriented and naturally lends itself to community-based care as a viable service delivery model. For example, faith-based programs have been instrumental in identifying those at risk by raising health awareness through screenings and health-related activities, resulting in positive outcomes.[30] Although this has largely focused on diabetes, high blood pressure, cancer, weight loss, smoking cessation, and cardiovascular disease, there is reason to believe that such faith-based promotion and screening would be beneficial in the area of mental health. In 2015, Hankerson and colleagues[31] published the first study of depression screenings conducted among African American adults in predominately African American churches, finding that it is feasible to screen for mental health disorders while partnering with pastors and church stakeholders. More research is needed regarding how best to cultivate such partnerships to aid in the identification and engagement of African American youth.

Despite scant literature, the following should be considered when establishing collaborative community/faith-based initiatives to address depression in youth:

1. Forge a healthy provider-patient relationship: the success of a meaningful collaboration begins with the doctor-patient relationship. The relationship between provider and patient must be fortified and built on trust. It is imperative that providers are unbiased and possess a willingness to reach beyond levels of comfort to best support the patient, including being aware of their own beliefs, attitudes, and perceptions.
2. Assess the role of spirituality in the youth and family's life: understanding cultural dynamics and identity assists in accuracy of diagnosis and development of an appropriate treatment plan. Mathai and North[32] (2003) found that more than 50% of parents indicated that not only was spirituality important to them but they thought it should be addressed in the treatment of their children. The Diagnostic and Statistical Manual of Mental Disorders, Fifth Edition, Cultural Formulation is an invaluable tool that provides an adaptable framework to support cultural dialogue between providers and patients.

3. Identify and consult appropriate community/faith-based services: it is critical to work with agencies or key stakeholders that reflect the cultural, linguistic, racial, and ethnic differences of the population they serve. This approach assists in facilitating access to and use of appropriate resources. When appropriately matched, there is a mutual benefit between provider and clergy where mental health providers are able to learn from spiritual leaders regarding their practices/beliefs, with clergy receiving educational and professional strategies to assist in the delivery of care.

4. Implement effective service delivery models: although strategies and models may vary, there are key considerations to keep in mind when devising a program. Research has found that intervention has been most effective when targeted toward specific subgroups.[33] Pearce and colleagues[34] highlighted 2 factors, interpersonal religious experience and considering oneself spiritual, as being associated with lower levels of depression, with interpersonal religious experience having the stronger association. Youth need to be and to feel connected. This connection provides a level of support and buffers the youth from negative social and peer influences. Positive examples include church youth groups, mentorship programs, as well as general support from a congregation or spiritual friends.[35] However, there exists a slippery slope in the quality of social connectedness because negative interpersonal religious experiences can lead to increased depressive symptoms among youth. Age and gender differences within African American youth warrant additional exploration to further customize intervention.

Spirituality is an integral part of the lives of almost all African American youth. It is a logical entry point to address mental health issues with notable benefits. With more than 90% of youth currently reporting a belief in God, it is vital that providers inquire as to the role this belief plays in their lives. Community/faith-based partnerships hold promise in combating stigma and reducing institutional mistrust, thereby increasing accessibility and early identification. Such partnerships are an effective way to engage African American youth and families in order to bridge the gap between spirituality and mental health.

SUMMARY

African American and black Caribbean youth and their families have rich, bountiful cultural origins. These cultural complexities and intricacies deserve understanding and should not be contrived or stereotyped. Every patient encounter can be an opportunity for the clinician to be open and objective, hear the voices, and learn the unique stories of the children, adolescents, and families they have the privilege to serve. Depression pervades all socioeconomic levels, race, and ethnicities. If left unrecognized and untreated, depression can be devastating to the life trajectory of any child or adolescent. The tools to detect, comprehensively assess, and treat depression in children and adolescents exist. Research has led to advancements for these clinical tools to be refined and integrate linguistic and cultural factors when treating children and adolescents and their families. However, significant health care disparities continue to prevail in the access and quality of care for African American and black Caribbean youth. These children continue to experience inequities in the health care system. Progress has been made, but much more work needs to, and can, be done.

REFERENCES

1. Bridge JA, Horowitz LM, Fontanella CA, et al. Age-related racial disparity in suicide rates among U.S. youths between 2001 and 2015. JAMA Pediatr 2018;172(7):697–9.

2. Matlin S, Molock SD, Tebes JK. Suicidality and depression among African American adolescents: the role of family and peer support and community connectedness. Am J Orthopsychiatry 2011;81(1):108–17.
3. Balis T, Postolache T. Ethnic differences in adolescent suicide in the United States. Int J Child Health Hum Dev 2008;1(3):281–96.
4. Cook S, Valera P, Calebs B, et al. Adult attachment as a moderator of the association between childhood I traumatic experiences and depression symptoms among young black gay and bisexual men. Cultur Divers Ethnic Minor Psychol 2017;23(3):388–97.
5. Alegría M, Molina K, Chen C. Neighborhood characteristics and differential risk for depressive and anxiety disorders across racial/ethnic groups in the United States. Depress Anxiety 2014;31(1):27–37.
6. Breland-Noble A, Bell C, Burriss A. "Mama just won't accept this": adult perspectives on engaging depressed African American teens in clinical research and treatment. J Clin Psychol Med Settings 2011;18(3):225–34.
7. Scott S, Wallander J, Cameron L. Protective mechanisms for depression among racial/ethnic minority youth: empirical findings, issues, and recommendations. Clin Child Fam Psychol Rev 2015;18:346–69.
8. Breland-Noble A, Burriss A, Poole HK. Engaging depressed African American adolescents in treatment: lessons from the AAKOMA PROJECT. J Clin Psychol 2010;66(8):868–79.
9. Alegría M, Chatterji P, Wells K, et al. Disparity in depression treatment among racial and ethnic minority populations in the United States. Psychiatr Serv 2008;59(11):1264–72.
10. Nestor B, Cheek S, Liu R. Ethnic and racial differences in mental health service utilization for suicidal ideation and behavior in a nationally representative sample of adolescents. J Affect Disord 2016;202:197–202.
11. Alegria M, Vallas M, Pumariega A. Racial and ethnic disparities in pediatric mental health. Child Adolesc Psychiatr Clin N Am 2010;19(4):759–74.
12. Department of Health and Human Services. Centers for disease Control and Prevention. U.S. Public health service Syphillis study at Tuskegee. Available at: www.cdc.gov. Accessed December 14, 2015.
13. Muroff J, Edelsohn G, Joe S, et al. The role of race in diagnostic and disposition decision-making in a pediatric psychiatric emergency service (PES). Gen Hosp Psychiatry 2008;30(3):269–76.
14. Barner J, Bohman T, Brown C, et al. Use of complementary and alternative medicine (CAM) for treatment among African-Americans: a multivariate analysis. Res Social Adm Pharm 2010;6(3):196–208.
15. Thomas KJA. A demographic profile of Black Caribbean immigrants in the United States. Washington, DC: Migration Policy Institute; 2012.
16. Zong J, Batalova J. Caribbean immigrants in the United States. Washington, DC: Migration Policy Institute; 2016. Available at: https://www.migrationpolicy.org.
17. Guy TC. Black immigrants of the Caribbean: an invisible and forgotten community. Adult Learning 2001;13(1):18–21.
18. Easter M. For Black immigrants here illegally, a battle against both fear and historic discrimination. Los Angeles Times 2018. Available at: www.latimes.com.
19. Williams DR, Haile R, González HM, et al. The mental health of Black Caribbean immigrants: results from the national Survey of American life. Am J Public Health 2007;97:52–9.
20. Rothe EM, Pumariega AJ, Sabagh D. Identity and acculturation in immigrant and second generation adolescents. Adolesc Psychiatry 2011;1(1):72–81.

21. Tummala-Narra P, Claudius M. Perceived discrimination and depressive symptoms among immigrant-origin adolescents. Cultur Divers Ethnic Minor Psychol 2013;19(3):257–69.
22. Gee GC. Self-reported discrimination and mental health status among African descendants, Mexican Americans, and other latinos in the New Hampshire REACH 2010 initiative: the added dimension of immigration. Am J Public Health 2006; 96(10):1821–8.
23. Pew Research Center Religion and Public Life. The global religious Landscape. 2012. Available at: http://www.pewforum.org/2012/12/18/global-religious-landscape-exec/. Accessed December 18, 2012.
24. Pew Research Center Religion and Public Life. A religious Portrait of African-Americans. 2009. Available at: http://www.pewforum.org/2009/01/30/a-religious-portrait-of-african-americans/. Accessed January 30, 2009.
25. Brown DR, Gary LE. Religious involvement and health status among African-American males. J Natl Med Assoc 1994;86:825–31.
26. Miller L, Davies M, Greenwald S. Religiosity and substance abuse among adolescents in the national comorbidity Survey. J Am Acad Child Adolesc Psychiatry 2000;39:1190–7.
27. Gallup GJ, Bezilla R. The religious life of young Americans. Princeton (NJ): The George H. Gallup International Institute; 1992.
28. Pearce MJ, Little TD, Perez JE. Religiousness and depressive symptoms among adolescents. J Clin Child Adolesc Psychol 2003;32(2):267–76.
29. Holder DW, Durant RH, Harris TL, et al. The association between adolescent spirituality and voluntary sexual activity. J Adolesc Health 2000;26(4):295–302.
30. DeHaven MJ, Irby B, Hunter MD, et al. Health programs in faith-based organizations: are they effective. Am J Public Health 2004;94:61030.
31. Hankerson SH, Lee YA, Brawley DK, et al. Screening for depression in african-american churches. Am J Prev Med 2015;49:526–33.
32. Mathai J, North A. Spiritual history of parents of children attending a child and adolescent mental health service. Australas Psychiatry 2003;11:172–4.
33. Cotton S, Zebracki K, Rosenthal SL, et al. Religion/spirituality and adolescent health outcomes: a review. J Adolesc Health 2006;38(4):472–80.
34. Pearce MJ, Little TD, Perez JE. Religiousness and depressive symptoms among adolescents. J Clin Child Adolesc Psychol 2003;32(2):267–76.
35. Cotton S, Larkin E, Hoopes A, et al. The impact of adolescent spirituality on depressive symptoms and health risk behaviors. J Adolesc Health 2005; 36(6):529.

Depression in Latino and Immigrant Refugee Youth
Clinical Opportunities and Considerations

Milangel T. Concepcion Zayas, MD, MPH[a,1],
Lisa R. Fortuna, MD, MPH[b], Lisa M. Cullins, MD[c,]*

KEYWORDS

- Depression • Children and adolescents • Latino • Immigrant • Refugee • Culture

KEY POINTS

- Over the past decade there has been burgeoning research in the epidemiology, prevalence, and health disparities in the identification, clinical presentation, and treatment approaches in Latino and immigrant refugee children and adolescents.
- Policies that protect against parental deportation and promote family stability can assist in improving child mental health and development and reducing childhood depression in Latino and other immigrant refugee populations.
- Evidence-based research has increased regarding effective diagnostic and treatment approaches for Latino and immigrant refugee children and adolescents, but these recommendations have been sparsely and inadequately disseminated and implemented across the country, leading to ongoing and persistent suboptimal outcomes for this population of youth, which is unacceptable.
- Extensive and thoughtful efforts should be made to thread these pieces together to create a system of care that addresses the unmet mental health needs of all children and adolescents, especially for vulnerable populations such as Latino and immigrant refugee youth.

Depression carries one of the highest global disease burdens. Better understanding of signs, symptoms, and effective treatments for depression is of utmost importance.[1] Further, given that depression is one of the leading risk factors of suicide and that suicide is now the second foremost cause of death in adolescents and young adults,

This article originally appeared in *Child and Adolescent Psychiatric Clinics*, Volume 28, Issue 3, July 2019.
Disclosures: None.
[a] Dartmouth Geisel School of Medicine, Dartmouth-Hitchcock Medical Center, West Central Behavioral Health; [b] Boston Medical Center, Boston University School of Medicine, Doctors Office Building, 720 Harrison Avenue, Room 907, Boston, MA 02118, USA; [c] George Washington University School of Medicine, Washington, DC, USA
[1] Present address: 3 Placid Square, Lebanon, NH 03766.
* Corresponding author. 4000 Blackburn Lane, Suite 260, Burtonsville, MD 20866.
E-mail address: lisacullins@yahoo.com

Clinics Collections 11 (2021) 279–291
https://doi.org/10.1016/j.ccol.2020.12.044

comprehensively examining prevention, early identification, and intervention for depression in children and adolescents is critical.[2]

Latino children and youth are the fastest growing population in the United States.[3] Latino youth have the highest rates of depression among minority groups, but this population remains undertreated and has limited access to mental health services.[4] Child and adolescent mental health providers may not be equipped to provide the necessary mental health care unless the cultural and linguistic needs of this population are addressed. This article:

1. Describes risk and protective factors in the emergence of depressive symptoms in Latino and immigrant refugee children and adolescents
2. Elucidates the clinical presentation of depression, opportunities, barriers, and treatment considerations for Latino and immigrant refugee children and adolescents
3. Provides practical recommendations for clinicians assessing Latino and immigrant refugee youth

LATIN AMERICAN CHILDREN AND ADOLESCENTS

Latin American/Hispanic youth (herein referred to as Latino youth) are the fastest growing population segment, representing 25% of the total US pediatric population, with continued future growth projections.[5] Latino youth originate from more than 20 countries of Central America, South America, and the Caribbean arbitrarily grouped into a homogenous population. They are in fact a heterogeneous group with diverse nationalities, race, socioeconomic and educational levels, citizenship status, and geographic locations within the United States.[6]

Most Latino children and adolescents are US born, and some of their families have lived in the United States for several generations. However, some of these youth are foreign born and recently moved to the United States (first generation). More than half of Latino youth have a foreign-born parent (second generation), with different types of sociohistorical backgrounds depending on their country of origin and immigration experiences.[3] Regardless of the generation, the immigration process can be distressing, rendering Latino youth and their families vulnerable to adverse outcomes and mental health problems.[7]

Violence exposure and displacement, prominent factors in many migration experiences, can increase the risk for depression.[8,9] Frequently, migrants from countries such as Colombia, Venezuela, Honduras, and Guatemala have faced violence in the context of political and civil strife, including civil war, coup d'états, and genocides.[10] Displacement secondary to acts of violence continues to affect many countries in Latin America. In Mexico, Honduras, Nicaragua, and El Salvador this violence is often the catalyst behind the surge of unaccompanied minors that have entered the United States since 2014.[11] Natural disasters have also led to the displacement of entire families. Most recently, Hurricane Maria ravaged Puerto Rico and displaced countless families.[10]

DEPRESSION IN LATINO YOUTH

Depression, a chronic disease that can have an early onset and lead to substantial disability, often goes unrecognized in children and adolescents.[2] The Diagnostic and Statistical Manual, Fifth Edition (DSM 5), is the classification system for depression used in the United States. Although different DSM versions have been widely referenced, limitations exist in its integration of cultural attributions and cross-cultural validity in the criterion and disease process of depression in children and adolescents.[12]

Compared with non-Latino youth in the United States, Latino youth consistently reported higher levels of sadness and hopelessness,[13] both known as indicators for depression.[14] Studies have shown that Latino children and adolescents have higher rates of depression and suicide attempts compared with non-Latino white and African American youth.[15] Nativity also is an important factor: US-born Latino youth have higher rates of depression and are more likely to attempt suicide than their foreign-born Latino peers.[16] Latina (feminine version of Latino) women are reportedly twice as likely as Latino men to have suicidal ideation, have a suicide plan, and/or attempted suicide over a 12-month duration.[13]

Depression can have different manifestations based on ethnicity. Culturally related beliefs about the cause of depression, its clinical presentation, and its treatment can influence approaches to clinical interventions.[17] A recent study described variations in the manifestation of anxiety/depression in an adult Hispanic/Latino population from different ethnic groups.[18] Although these results could be extrapolated to apply to Latino children and adolescents, limited research has been done to corroborate these findings in a pediatric population. In a qualitative study of Mexican American youth that examined youth's attitudes about depression, participants were able to identify symptoms that are common to depression as per the DSM 5. Participants most often recognized social withdrawal as an early sign of depression. They thought that a nonsupportive family environment could be the cause of depression. Regarding treatment, most participants thought that they were exclusively responsible for their own recovery.[19]

A multimodal approach to treatment that includes psychoeducation, individual therapy, family interventions, and medications (when indicated) is the recommended treatment of depression in children and adolescents.[20] Cognitive behavior therapy and interpersonal psychotherapy are treatments with empirical support for depression in Latino youth.[21,22] Notably, both group and family interventions have shown positive benefits for Latino children and adolescents. It has been posited that group interventions may be as efficacious as individual therapy for Latino youth[23] and family interventions may decrease internalizing symptoms in high-risk Latino youth in particular.[24] In summary, devising a multimodal treatment approach that focuses on the individual child or adolescent and the family as a whole is essential. Family involvement and interactions have been extremely influential in the onset and prognosis of depression in this population of youth.

Latino children and adolescents with depression additionally experience inequities in health and health care access.[4] Studies have shown that Latino youth are less likely than non-Hispanic white youth to receive mental health services,[25] including being offered psychotherapy or receiving antidepressants.[26] Further, lack of insurance coverage disproportionately affects Latino youth and has been linked to their limited access to care.[27]

SOCIOCULTURAL VARIABLES AND DEPRESSION IN LATINO YOUTH

Understanding concepts such as acculturation, acculturative stress, and discrimination is essential when providing clinical care to Latino youth with depression. Several scholars have shown that variables such as poverty, the immigration experience, acculturation, discrimination, and acculturative stress may adversely affect children and adolescents' psychological well-being and lead to depression in Latino youth.[28–30]

Acculturation, the process whereby individuals from one cultural group learn and adopt elements of another cultural group and integrate them into their original culture,[31] is a known risk factor of depression for Latino youth. Acculturative stress, the level of psychosocial strain experienced by immigrants and their descendants and their response to immigration-related challenges that they encounter as they adapt to the new country, can affect many aspects of the family unit.[32] Language barriers are also a component of acculturative stress that should be considered. Latino youth often must assume the role of language brokers for their parents or other adult family members. When adolescents perceive this role as a burden, it can transform into a risk factor for family-based acculturation stress, which can lead to an increase in alcohol and marijuana use in these adolescents.[33] Further, alcohol and marijuana use are known risk factors for depression. Language brokering at home for items such as housing, banking, and insurance forms can at times negatively affect the parent-child relationship, frequently altering the power of authority in the home. This shift in power can result in youth having more autonomy and parents having less control over their children's behavior.[34] Being a primary language broker in the family can lead to discrimination, another risk factor for depression.[35] Perceived discrimination can be detrimental to mental health outcomes and strongly associated with depression. Combined legal status of the parents or having family members with undocumented status can also increase the risk for depression.[36] In contrast, strong family values can serve as protective factors to mitigate acculturative stress in Latino youth. Values such as respeto (respect) and familismo (strong family connections, active coping strategies, and social supports) can minimize the detrimental influences of acculturative stress.[37] The following clinical case of an adolescent Latino youth with depression provides examples of some of these sociocultural variables (**Box 1**).

SUMMARY

Latino youth, the largest fastest growing minority group, are disproportionately affected by depression. Context and culturally related characteristics of depression are important given the different idiosyncrasies among and within ethnic groups in a

---

Box 1
Clinical case

Mercedes is a 16-year-old US-born Mexican American adolescent girl in 10th grade who presents after ingesting a bottle of her mother's blood pressure medication, with the intent to kill herself. She describes feelings of sadness and hopelessness. Although she enjoys listening to music and doing karate, she has lost interest in interacting with her friends and family, and complains of feeling tired, experiencing both problems with sleep initiation and hypersomnia. This clinical presentation has transpired over the past year in the context of multiple school stressors, including bullying. Mercedes has always been a good student, but since entering high school she has had some difficulties with peers and her grades have worsened. She identifies herself as a millennial. She lives at home with her parents, 2 siblings, and some extended family members. Both of her parents are first-generation immigrants from Mexico (father) and El Salvador (mother), and have limited English proficiency. Mercedes shares that there are some financial hardships at home and both her parents have 2 jobs. There have also been recent discussions with some family members around recent governmental policy changes that have them concerned. Mercedes' paternal grandmother recently died and since then her father has been isolative and drinks more frequently, refusing any type of help. In their household, her mother always goes to church and prays to "la Virgencita" whenever emotionally burdened. Her father always says that "Boys do not cry." The father often mentions his childhood hardships in Mexico.

globalized world. Misunderstandings of these variations can lead to incorrect diagnosis and treatment. Thus, the need to better understand these cultural variations is compelling. Researchers have posited that the development of instruments such as the DSM 5 Cultural Formulation Interview Fidelity Instrument offers an opportunity to explore how cultural competence improves mental health outcomes.[38,39] As this pivotal work proceeds, mental health clinicians should provide safe spaces and cultivate a level of trust with the children and adolescents they treat to foster the youth's sense of self, build on their family's strengths, and champion their cultural heritage. This step in treating depression in Latino youth is critical. If the richness of Latino culture is not appreciated and values of the dominant culture are imposed at any stage of treatment, it is possible that this special population of youth may feel marginalized and not fully benefit from the care they are receiving.

DEPRESSION IN IMMIGRANT REFUGEE YOUTH

Depression in the general, multifaceted, multicultural pediatric Latino population was discussed earlier. However, it is important to specifically and more comprehensively discuss how depression may emerge in Latino immigrant refugee youth to better comprehend this unique population. The immigrant population is projected to almost double in size and account for 18% of the US population by 2060; the health and mental health needs of this growing population are important to understand.[40–42] Population growth estimates only account for foreign-born children and do not take into account second-generation immigrants, which consist of another 38 million individuals. US births are expected to be a major factor for future population growth.[43] Immigrants face high levels of premigration and postmigration stressors that are expected to be detrimental to their mental health, including discrimination and acculturative stress.[44,45] However, despite these challenges, most research since the 1980s has shown that foreign-born immigrants may be less likely to develop mental disorders and more likely to be physically healthy than their US-born counterparts.[46,47] This finding is sometimes referred to as the healthy-immigrant paradox because, despite experiencing more stressors, which in turn usually increase the risk of mental and physical disorders, the first generation of immigrants seems to have reduced risk. However, across generations, the health advantage of immigrant children fades.[48] For example, researchers have found that the percentage of youth who are overweight or obese, a key indicator of physical health, is lowest for foreign-born youth.[49,50] The prevalence of mental health and substance use disorders is also lower for foreign-born youth compared with US-born counterparts. However, the prevalence of these problems grows larger for each generation, increasing as youth transition into adulthood.[51–53] Female gender, younger age, living in the United States for a longer period of time, and exposure to political violence in the country of origin are associated with developing depression.[54]

Both preimmigration-related and resettlement-related factors are associated with depression. Stressful migration and acculturation experiences of first-generation Latino youth negatively affect their psychological well-being. Potochnick and Perreira[7] conducted a study using the Latino Adolescent Migration, Health, and Adaptation (LAMHA) study, which surveyed 281 first-generation Latino immigrant youth, aged 12 to 19 years. They evaluated how migration stressors (ie, traumatic events, choice of migration, discrimination, and documentation status) and postmigration supports (ie, family and teacher support, acculturation, and personal motivation) were associated with mental health and well-being. The investigators found that migration stressors, including acculturative stress, poverty, and displacement, increased the risk of both depression and anxiety.[7] This study and others have found that receiving support from family and teachers reduces the risk for both depressive symptoms and anxiety. Immigration status also significantly influences the risk for depression. Compared with documented adolescents, undocumented adolescents were found to be at greater risk of developing anxiety disorder, and children in mixed-status families were also at greater risk of anxiety and depression.[7]

Refugee youth and families migrate to the United States fleeing wars, mass disasters, and political unrest. Because of trauma exposure, the more common mental health diagnoses associated with refugee populations include posttraumatic stress disorder (PTSD), major depressive disorder (MDD), generalized anxiety disorder, panic disorder, adjustment disorder, and somatization disorders.[55] Different studies have shown rates of PTSD and MDD in settled refugees to range from 10% to 40% and 5% to 15%, respectively. Children and adolescents exposed to psychological trauma have been found to have higher levels of PTSD compared with adults with similar exposure. Studies have revealed rates of PTSD from 50% to 90% and MDD from 6% to 40% among youth exposed to severe traumatic experiences.[55] Risk factors for PTSD and depression include the number of traumatic exposures, delayed asylum application processes, detention and traumatic separations, and the loss of culture and support systems. Interpersonal conflict, especially family conflict regarding expectations for cultural norms and behaviors, are other potential risk factors for depression and suicidal ideation.[51] Perceived discrimination represents an obstacle to community integration, especially for second-generation immigrants, and perceived discrimination is directly associated with lower psychological well-being and depression.[56]

Similar to immigrant youth, traditionally the refugee experience is divided into 3 categories: preflight, flight, and resettlement. The preflight phase may include, for example, physical and emotional trauma to the individual or family, the witnessing of murder, and social upheaval. Adolescents may also have participated in violence, voluntarily or not, as child soldiers or militants. Flight involves an uncertain journey from the host country to the resettlement site and may involve arduous travel, refugee camps, and/or detention centers. Children and adolescents are often separated from their families and at the mercy of others for care and protection. The resettlement process includes challenges such as the loss of culture, community, and language as well as the need to adapt to a new and foreign environment.[57] Children often straddle the old and new cultures because they learn new languages and cultural norms more quickly than their elders. Adolescent well-being is significantly affected by caregiver mental health, including depression in this refugee context.[57,58] However, opportunities to integrate child behavioral health programming with prevention and treatment of caregivers' mental health symptoms are limited.

There are many challenges in the detection and effective treatment of depression in immigrant and refugee youth. Often language and cultural barriers, and biases, whether of the refugee or the provider, can hinder identification of problems and the development of a therapeutic relationship.[59] Furthermore, there is little evidence for the efficacy of any particular treatment strategy. Much work remains to be done to develop culturally competent means of screening immigrant and refugee youth for depression and then implementing evidence-based interventions. Interventions designed to address prevention, treatment, and recovery from depression among Latino, immigrant, and refugee youth in the United States need to consider the importance of supportive communities and relationships; improving access to mental health care through expanded services, like behavioral health care integration in primary care, and overcoming cultural and systematic barriers to care are essential for addressing depression among youth in all of these groups.

While these challenges in the assessment process and lack of evidence-based interventions for Latino and immigrant refugee youth are being elucidated, individual clinicians have a unique opportunity to advocate for and to provide a space of healing for these children and adolescents and their families within their systems. Some practical clinical recommendations when assessing Latino and immigrant refugee youth are provided here.

PRACTICAL RECOMMENDATIONS

Recognizing the cultural diversity within Latino and immigrant refugee youth and their context is an essential first step when assessing these youth and their families. As with any child or adolescent psychiatric evaluation, Latino youth assessment should occur within the frame of reference of the ecosystem (family, school, community, culture) and the presenting concerns should be appraised within a developmental context with a biopsychosocial approach.

- Explore English language proficiency in the family. Parents of Latino youth and some first-generation Latino youth themselves may have limited English proficiency.
  - Before the appointment, arrange for the use of medical interpreters when needed.[60] Refrain from using the youth or any other family member as interpreters.
  - At the appointment, assess whether the youth is used as a language broker.
  - Integrate linguistic sensitivity when eliciting symptoms and in the evaluation, diagnostic formulation, and intervention recommendations in order to develop comprehensive and effective treatment plans.
  - Consider an extended appointment time when using interpreters.
- Build trust with the youth and the family member. The family is a significant part of the Latino youth culture.[61,62]
  - Before the appointment, prepare the office for multiple persons.
  - Offer to bring all the family members to the office for a formal introduction and openly explore the youth and the family preference for visits.
  - Explore family values, belief systems, and level of connectedness.
  - Family interventions that improve communication among the parent-child dyad are encouraged.
- Clinicians should learn about the immigration status of the family and listen to their unique story and strive to understand how their life experiences have affected their mental health and well-being. Most importantly, clinicians must be open to their patients and families educating them about their cultural similarities and differences.
  - Inquire about the country of origin and cultural identification.
  - Respect and validate the family's possible political and historical experiences.
  - Explore exposure to violence that the family (or individual members of the family) may have experienced.
  - Explore intergenerational trauma.
  - Explore possible fears of deportation.
- Clinicians should develop an understanding of how acculturative stress threatens the emotional well-being of the child.
  - Explore gender roles and perceptions in the family. This point is particularly important for adolescent girls in the context of safety planning for suicide attempts.
  - Inquire about number of generations in the United States and explore challenges related to intergenerational conflicts, social supports, and available resources for the family.

- ○ Explore and screen for polyvictimization. This information becomes critically important for sexual minority Latino youth because the risks of depression and suicide are even higher. These populations of youth are more likely to have been physically or sexually abused and/or bullied and may have more limited social supports and community connectedness.[63]
- Explore beliefs around mental illness, reasons for seeking treatment, and expectations of the doctor-patient relationship.
  - ○ Explore the idioms of distress, such as decaimiento, agitamiento, locura, and ataque de nervios (nerve attack).[61,64] In female Latino youth, researchers have contrasted the suicide attempt phenomenon in female Latino youth to ataque de nervios and hypothesize whether the attempts are a developmental or cultural variant of el ataque de nervios.[65]
  - ○ Inquire about idioms of distress when inquiring about the family history of psychiatric illness.
  - ○ Explore how stigma might play a role in their approach to mental health treatment and services.
  - ○ Explore the use of other family members, religion/spirituality, and/or the use of healers as alternative mental health supports in the family.
- Actively collaborate with primary care providers. Studies of Latino populations have found that they show more somatic complaints and will discuss them with their primary care providers.
- Engage Latino youth and their families in activities that promote resilience.
  - ○ Activities that promote social support at home and school can improve the effects of acculturation.
  - ○ Encourage the use of all forms of media to increase awareness, educate, and promote mental health and well-being, and also engage Latino youth and their families in psychiatric care, when indicated. For example, a recent study used entertainment-education to increase depression literacy, decrease stigma, and increase help-seeking knowledge and behavior in Latino youth. The intervention showed improvements in depression knowledge, self-efficacy to identify the need for treatment, and decreased stigma.[66]

SUMMARY

Over the past decade there has been burgeoning research in the epidemiology, prevalence, and health disparities in the identification, clinical presentation, and treatment approaches in Latino and immigrant refugee children and adolescents. This research has enlightened clinicians about opportunities, challenges, and substantive service deliveries and effective treatment modality recommendations for this population of youth that intricately integrate sociocultural factors.

At the policy level, the evidence has identified opportunities as well. One recent study found that mothers' Deferred Action for Child Arrivals eligibility significantly decreased adjustment and anxiety disorder diagnosis among their children.[67] Policies that protect against parental deportation and promote family stability can assist in improving child mental health and development. Advocacy for immigration policies that protect child and family well-being are important to consider in reducing childhood depression in Latino and other immigrant refugee populations.

Evidence-based research has increased regarding effective diagnostic and treatment approaches for Latino and immigrant refugee children and adolescents, but these recommendations have been sparsely and inadequately disseminated and implemented across the country, leading to ongoing and persistent suboptimal outcomes for this population of youth, which is unacceptable. Extensive and thoughtful efforts should be made to thread these pieces together to create a system of care that addresses the unmet mental health needs of all children and adolescents, especially for vulnerable populations such as Latino and immigrant refugee youth. Child and adolescent psychiatrists and mental health clinicians have an opportunity and responsibility to enhance service delivery with advocacy and clinical excellence for this population of youth.

REFERENCES

1. Kessler RC. The costs of depression. Psychiatr Clin North Am 2012;35(1):1–14.
2. Thapar A, Collishaw S, Pine DS, et al. Depression in adolescence. Lancet 2012; 379(9820):1056–67.
3. Bureau UC. Hispanic heritage month 2018. Available at: https://www.census.gov/newsroom/facts-for-features/2018/hispanic-heritage-month.html. Accessed September 7, 2018.
4. Alegria M, Vallas M, Pumariega A. Racial and ethnic disparities in pediatric mental health. Child Adolesc Psychiatr Clin N Am 2010. https://doi.org/10.1016/j.chc.2010.07.001.
5. Interagency Forum on Child F, Statistics F. America's children: key national indicators of well-being, 2017 2017. Available at: https://www.childstats.gov/pdf/ac2017/ac_17.pdf. Accessed September 18, 2018.
6. Foxen P, Mather M, Foxen P, et al. Towards a more equitable future the trends and challenges facing America's Latino children population. Washington D.C., National Council of La Raza 9-2016. Washington, DC. 2016. Available at: www.nclr.org. Accessed March 7, 2018.
7. Potochnick SR, Perreira KM. Depression and anxiety among first-generation immigrant Latino youth: key correlates and implications for future research NIH public access. J Nerv Ment Dis 2010;198(7):470–7.
8. Lê F, Tracy M, Norris FH, et al. Displacement, county social cohesion and depression after a large-scale traumatic event. Soc Psychiatry Psychiatr Epidemiol 2013. https://doi.org/10.1007/s00127-013-0698-7.
9. Fazel M, Reed RV, Panter-Brick C, et al. Mental health of displaced and refugee children resettled in high-income countries: risk and protective factors. Lancet 2012;379(9812):266–82.
10. Rodríguez J, De La Torre A, Miranda CT. Mental health in situations of armed conflict. Biomedica 2002;22(Suppl 2):337–46 [in Spanish]. Available at: http://www.ncbi.nlm.nih.gov/pubmed/12596454. Accessed August 16, 2018.
11. Boehner N, Goldberg P, Schmidt S, et al. Children on the run: unaccompanied children leaving Central America and Mexico and the need for international protection. Washington, DC: The United Nations High Commissioner For Refugees Regional Office For The United States and Caribbean; 2014.
12. Canino G, Alegría M. Psychiatric diagnosis - is it universal or relative to culture? J Child Psychol Psychiatry 2008;49(3):237–50.
13. Kann L, McManus T, Harris WA, et al. Youth risk behavior surveillance — United States, 2017. MMWR Surveill Summ 2018;67(8):1–114.
14. Horwitz AG, Berona J, Czyz EK, et al. Positive and negative expectations of hopelessness as longitudinal predictors of depression, suicidal ideation, and suicidal behavior in high-risk adolescents. Suicide Life Threat Behav 2017;47(2):168–76.
15. Guzmán Á, Koons A, Postolache T. Suicidal behavior in latinos: focus on the youth. Int J Adolesc Med Health 2009;21(4):431–40.

16. Fortuna LR, Perez DJ, Canino G, et al. Prevalence and Correlates of Lifetime suicidal ideation and attempts among Latino Subgroups in the United States NIH Public access. J Clin Psychiatry 2005;68:572–81. Available at: https://www.ncbi.nlm.nih.gov/pmc/articles/PMC2774123/pdf/nihms154115.pdf.   Accessed February 8, 2019.

17. Jimenez DE, Bartels SJ, Cardenas V, et al. Cultural beliefs and mental health treatment preferences of ethnically diverse older adult consumers in primary care. Am J Geriatr Psychiatry 2012. https://doi.org/10.1097/JGP.0b013e318227f876.

18. Camacho Á, Gonzalez P, Buelna C, et al. Anxious-depression among hispanic/latinos from different backgrounds: results from the hispanic community health study/study of latinos (HCHS/SOL). Soc Psychiatry Psychiatr Epidemiol 2015. https://doi.org/10.1007/s00127-015-1120-4.

19. Fornos LB, Seguin Mika V, Bayles B, et al. A qualitative study of Mexican American adolescents and depression. J Sch Health 2005;75(5):162–70.

20. Birmaher B, Brent D, AACAP Work Group on Quality Issues, Bernet W, et al. Practice parameter for the assessment and treatment of children and adolescents with depressive disorders. J Am Acad Child Adolesc Psychiatry 2007;46(11):1503–26.

21. Huey SJ Jr, Polo AJ. Evidence-based psychosocial treatments for ethnic minority youth. J Clin Child Adolesc Psychol 2008;37(1):262–301. Available at: https://www.ncbi.nlm.nih.gov/pmc/articles/PMC2413000/pdf/nihms51473.pdf.   Accessed February 8, 2019.

22. Rosselló J, Bernal G, Rivera-Medina C. Individual and group CBT and IPT for Puerto Rican adolescents with depressive symptoms. Cultur Divers Ethnic Minor Psychol 2008;14(3):234–45.

23. Cumba-Avilés E. Cognitive-behavioral group therapy for Latino youth with type 1 diabetes and depression: a case study. Clin Case Stud 2017;16(1):58–75.

24. Perrino T, Brincks A, Howe G, et al. Reducing internalizing symptoms among high-risk, hispanic adolescents: mediators of a preventive family intervention HHS public access author manuscript. Prev Sci 2016;17(5):595–605.

25. Marrast L, Himmelstein DU, Woolhandler S. Racial and ethnic disparities in mental health care for children and young adults. Int J Health Serv 2016;46(4):810–24.

26. Olfson M, He J-P, Merikangas KR. Psychotropic medication treatment of adolescents: results from the national comorbidity survey-adolescent supplement. J Am Acad Child Adolesc Psychiatry 2013;52(4):378–88.

27. Kirby JB, Hudson J, Miller GE. Explaining racial and ethnic differences in antidepressant use among adolescents. Med Care Res Rev 2010;67(3):342–63.

28. Goodman E, Slap GB, Huang B. The public health impact of socioeconomic status on adolescent depression and obesity. Am J Public Health 2003;93(11):1844–50. Available at: http://www.ncbi.nlm.nih.gov/pubmed/14600051. Accessed February 8, 2019.

29. Denavas-Walt C, Proctor BD. Income and poverty in the United States: 2014 current population reports. 2015. Available at: https://www.census.gov/content/dam/Census/library/publications/2015/demo/p60-252.pdf. Accessed September 8, 2018.

30. Ornelas IJ, Perreira KM. The role of migration in the development of depressive symptoms among Latino immigrant parents in the USA. Soc Sci Med 2011;73(8):1169–77.

31. Schwartz SJ, Unger JB, Zamboanga BL, et al. Rethinking the concept of acculturation: implications for theory and research. Am Psychol 2010;65(4):237–51.
32. Revollo H-W, Qureshi A, Collazos F, et al. Acculturative stress as a risk factor of depression and anxiety in the Latin American immigrant population. Int Rev Psychiatry 2011;23(1):84–92.
33. Kam JA, Lazarevic V. The stressful (and not so stressful) nature of language brokering: identifying when brokering functions as a cultural stressor for Latino immigrant children in early adolescence. J Youth Adolesc 2014;43(12): 1994–2011.
34. Roche KM, Lambert SF, Ghazarian SR, et al. Adolescent language brokering in diverse contexts: associations with parenting and parent-youth relationships in a new immigrant destination area. J Youth Adolesc 2015;44(1):77–89.
35. Benner AD, Graham S. Latino adolescents' experiences of discrimination across the first 2 years of high school: correlates and influences on educational outcomes. Child Dev 2011;82(2):508–19.
36. Arbona C, Olvera N, Rodriguez N, et al. Acculturative stress among documented and undocumented Latino immigrants in the United States. Hisp J Behav Sci 2010;32(3):362–84.
37. Lorenzo-Blanco EI, Unger JB, Baezconde-Garbanati L, et al. Acculturation, enculturation, and symptoms of depression in Hispanic youth: the roles of gender, Hispanic cultural values, and family functioning. J Youth Adolesc 2012;41(10): 1350–65.
38. Aggarwal NK, Glass A, Tirado A, et al. The development of the DSM-5 cultural formulation interview-fidelity instrument (CFI-FI): a pilot study. J Health Care Poor Underserved 2014;25(3):1397–417.
39. Lewis-Fernández R, Aggarwal NK, Bäärnhielm S, et al. Culture and psychiatric evaluation: operationalizing cultural formulation for DSM-5. Psychiatry 2014; 77(2):130–54.
40. Howe Hasanali S, De Jong GF, Roempke Graefe D. Hispanic-asian immigrant inequality in perceived medical need and access to regular physician care. J Immigr Minor Health 2016;18(1):219–27.
41. Colby SL, Ortman JM. Population estimates and Projections Current population Reports. 2015. Available at: www.census.gov. Accessed September 8, 2018.
42. Faq E, Costa D, Cooper D, et al. Economic policy institute answers to frequently asked questions the immigrant population 1. How many immigrants reside in the United States?. 2014. Available at: http://www.fiscalpolicy.org/FPI_NewAmericansOnLongIsland_20120119.pdf. Accessed September 8, 2018.
43. Pew Research Center. Modern immigration Wave brings 59 million to U.S., driving population growth and change through 2065: View of Immigration's impact on U.S. Society Mixed. 2015. Available at: www.pewresearch.org. Accessed September 8, 2018.
44. Pumariega AJ, Rothe E, Pumariega JB. Mental health of immigrants and refugees. Community Ment Health J 2005;41(5):581–97.
45. George U, Thomson MS, Chaze F, et al. Immigrant mental health, a public health issue: looking back and moving forward. Int J Environ Res Public Health 2015; 12(10):13624–48.
46. Burnam MA, Hough RL, Karno M, et al. Acculturation and lifetime prevalence of psychiatric disorders among Mexican Americans in Los Angeles. J Health Soc Behav 1987;28(1):89–102. Available at: http://www.ncbi.nlm.nih.gov/pubmed/3571910. Accessed February 8, 2019.

47. Vega WA, Kolody B, Aguilar-Gaxiola S, et al. Lifetime prevalence of DSM-III-R psychiatric disorders among urban and rural Mexican Americans in California. Arch Gen Psychiatry 1998;55(9):771–8. Available at: http://www.ncbi.nlm.nih.gov/pubmed/9736002. Accessed February 8, 2019.
48. Marks AK, Ejesi K, García Coll C. Understanding the U.S. Immigrant paradox in childhood and adolescence. Child Dev Perspect 2014;8(2):59–64.
49. Crosnoe R, Ramos-Wada A, Bonazzo C. Paradoxes in physical health. Fac Publ - Dep World Lang Sociol Cult Stud. 2015. Available at: https://digitalcommons.georgefox.edu/lang_fac/23. Accessed February 8, 2019.
50. McCullough MB, Marks AK. The immigrant paradox and adolescent obesity: examining health behaviors as potential mediators. J Dev Behav Pediatr 2014;35(2):138–43.
51. Fortuna LR, Álvarez K, Ramos Ortiz Z, et al. Mental health, migration stressors and suicidal ideation among Latino immigrants in Spain and the United States. Eur Psychiatry 2016;36:15–22.
52. Porche MV, Fortuna LR, Lin J, et al. Childhood trauma and psychiatric disorders as correlates of school dropout in a national sample of young adults. Child Dev 2011;82(3):982–98.
53. Alegría M, Canino G, Shrout PE, et al. Prevalence of mental illness in immigrant and non-immigrant U.S. Latino groups. Am J Psychiatry 2008;165(3):359–69.
54. Wong EC, Miles JNV. Prevalence and correlates of depression among new U.S. Immigrants. J Immigr Minor Health 2014;16(3):422–8.
55. Silove D, Ventevogel P, Rees S. The contemporary refugee crisis: an overview of mental health challenges. World Psychiatry 2017;16(2):130–9.
56. Giuliani C, Tagliabue S, Regalia C. Psychological well-being, multiple identities, and discrimination among first and second generation immigrant muslims. Eur J Psychol 2018;14(1):66–87.
57. Betancourt TS, Abdi S, Ito BS, et al. We left one war and came to another: resource loss, acculturative stress, and caregiver-child relationships in Somali refugee families. Cultur Divers Ethnic Minor Psychol 2015;21(1):114–25.
58. Meyer SR, Steinhaus M, Bangirana C, et al. The influence of caregiver depression on adolescent mental health outcomes: findings from refugee settlements in Uganda. BMC Psychiatry 2017;17(1):405.
59. Lincoln AK, Lazarevic V, White MT, et al. The impact of acculturation style and acculturative hassles on the mental health of Somali adolescent refugees. J Immigr Minor Health 2016;18(4):771–8.
60. Leng JCF, Changrani J, Tseng C-H, et al. Detection of depression with different interpreting methods among Chinese and Latino primary care patients: a randomized controlled trial. J Immigr Minor Health 2010;12(2):234–41.
61. Zayas LH, Pilat AM. Suicidal behavior in Latinas: explanatory cultural factors and implications for intervention. Suicide Life Threat Behav 2008;38(3):334–42.
62. Shetgiri R, Kataoka SH, Ryan GW, et al. Risk and resilience in Latinos. Am J Prev Med 2009;37(6):S217–24.
63. Cook SH, Valera P, Calebs BJ, et al. Adult attachment as a moderator of the association between childhood traumatic experiences and depression symptoms among young Black gay and bisexual men. Cultur Divers Ethnic Minor Psychol 2017;23(3):388–97.
64. Lewis-Fernández R, Gorritz M, Raggio GA, et al. Association of trauma-related disorders and dissociation with four idioms of distress among Latino psychiatric outpatients. Cult Med Psychiatry 2010;34(2):219–43.

65. Zayas LH, Gulbas LE. Are suicide attempts by young Latinas a cultural idiom of distress? Transcult Psychiatry 2012;49(5):718–34.
66. Hernandez MY, Organista KC. Entertainment-education? A fotonovela? A new strategy to improve depression literacy and help-seeking behaviors in at-risk immigrant Latinas. Am J Community Psychol 2013;52(3–4):224–35.
67. Hainmueller J, Lawrence D, Martén L, et al. Protecting unauthorized immigrant mothers improves their children's mental health. Science 2017;357(6355): 1041–4.

Depression and Cardiovascular Disorders in the Elderly

Wei Jiang, MD[a,b,*]

KEYWORDS

- Elderly • Depression • Cardiovascular disease • Prevalence • Mechanisms
- Intervention

KEY POINTS

- Both depression and cardiovascular diseases are highly prevalent in elder individuals.
- Depression and cardiovascular diseases have a synergetic impact on prognosis of elder patients and they share similar pathologic mechanisms.
- Prompt recognition of depression in patients with cardiovascular disease is necessary.
- Applying evidence-based intervention that targets depression in elderly patients, especially those with cardiovascular diseases, will improve the outcomes of these patients.

The world's older population continues to grow at an unprecedented rate. Currently, 8.5% of people worldwide (617 million) are 65 years and older and this percentage is projected to jump to nearly 17% of the world's population by 2050 (1.6 billion).[1] Cardiovascular disease (CVD) and depression are among the most common diseases experienced by this older population. According to the statistics of *Aging in the United States* (2016),[2] the present population of 46 million Americans aged 65 years and older is projected to more than double to more than 98 million by 2050, and this group's share of the total population will increase to nearly 24% from 15%. This trend amplifies the necessity of improving care for older patients with chronic health problems. Of those with chronic health problems, those with CVD and depression are particularly challenging due to the multifaceted nature of these conditions. This review focuses on the significance of this aging trend and ways to better care for this particular population.

This article originally appeared in *Clinics in Geriatric Medicine*, Volume 36, Issue 2, May 2020.
This article originally appeared in Psychiatric Clinics, Volume 41, Issue 1, March 2018.
Disclosure Statement: The author does not have any financial relationship with any companies.
[a] Department of Psychiatry and Behavioral Sciences, Duke University Health System, Durham, NC 27710, USA; [b] Department of Medicine, Duke University Health System, Durham, NC 27710, USA
* 1108 Grogans Mill Drive, Cary, NC 27519.
E-mail address: jiang001@mc.duke.edu

Clinics Collections 11 (2021) 293–301
https://doi.org/10.1016/j.ccol.2020.12.045
2352-7986/21/© 2020 Elsevier Inc. All rights reserved.

THE SIGNIFICANCE OF DEPRESSION AND CARDIOVASCULAR DISEASE IN THE ELDERLY

The growing population of elderly is a sign of success reflecting several merits in societal enhancement. However, although people are living longer, they are increasingly battling chronic diseases of the heart, respiratory system, and the brain. With the growth of the younger population slowing, meeting the demand of the health care needs of the elderly has emerged as a significant public health burden for prevention and treatment. Of these chronic diseases, CVD has been the largest global disease burden in people aged 60 years and older, occupying about one-third of the total global disease burden.[3] An estimated 85.6 million of American adults (>1 in 3) have 1 or more types of CVD. Of these, more than a half (43.7 million) of are estimated to be 60 years of age or older. The prevalence of CVD is positively related to age. For instance, in the age group from 60 to 79 years old, 69.1% of men and 67.9% of women experience CVD; in the 80 years and older group, 84.7% of men and 85.9% of women have CVD. The leading causes of death in men and women 65 years of age or older are diseases of the heart.[4] Elderly patients with CVD account for more than 65% of the total spending of US CVD patients on personal health care and public health.[5]

Mental health concerns are also age-related issues. It is estimated that 20% of people aged 55 years or older experience some type of mental health concern,[6] with the most common conditions being anxiety, severe cognitive impairment, and depression. Depression affects approximately 20 million Americans every year, regardless of age, race, or gender. Depression in the elderly is generally considered to be 2 types: late-onset that develops when an individual reaches 60 years or older, and younger onset that persists into late life.[7] Recognizing certain features of these 2 kinds of depression can be helpful when developing appropriate care plans (**Table 1**). Although depression is not a normal part of the aging process, there is a strong likelihood of it occurring when other physical health conditions are present. For example, nearly one-fourth of the 600,000 people who experienced a stroke in a given year experienced clinical depression.[8] Differing rates of depression in the elderly have been reported due to variations in study designs, including the population studied, study size, tools of assessments, and so forth.

Table 1
Features differ between and early-onset and late-onset of depression

Features of Depression	Early-Onset	Late-Onset
Genetic	Higher with more family history of mental illnesses	Low
Risk factors	Higher rate of personality disorders	Higher rate of CVD risk factors
Brain abnormality	Functional	Structural
Cognitive or neurologic	Fewer issues	More issues
Depression manifestation	Expressive depressive symptoms	Somatic and cognitive
Obtain psychiatric care	More likely to need formal mental health care	Generally not recognized until late
Comorbidities	Greater substance abuse and dependence	Greater physical comorbidities
Suicide	At risk for suicide	Highest risk of suicide
Response to depression intervention	More responsive	More resistant

Studies investigating whether the prevalence of depression is more or less common in the elderly compared with younger individuals have generally shown younger adults to have a higher frequency of depression. The prevalence of past-year mood, anxiety, and substance use disorders, as well as lifetime personality disorders, in a nationally representative sample of 12,312 US adults, aged 55 years and older, were collected from wave 2 of the National Epidemiologic Survey on Alcohol and Related Conditions.[9] The investigators found the youngest group, aged 55 to 64 years, had the highest prevalence (8.75%) of major depressive disorder (MDD) plus dysthymia. The prevalence of the depressive disorders declined as age increased (5.25% for ages 65–74 years, 4.41% for ages 75–84 years, and 5.0% for ages ≥85 years).[10] The investigators explained that the age difference of depression prevalence; that is, the leveling off in prevalence rates among adults aged 85 years and older, may be explained by the overall pattern of decreased prevalence of psychiatric disorders with increased age as in (1) the socioemotional selectivity theory[11] or (2) the strength and vulnerability integration theory.[12] The elderly who were reported having the lower prevalence of depression were generally without significant medical comorbidities. In reality, approximately 92% of older adults have at least 1 chronic disease and 77% have at least 2. Four chronic diseases (heart disease, cancer, stroke, and diabetes) cause almost two-thirds of all deaths each year. There are recognized causes leading to early-onset and late-onset depression (see **Table 1**). Clinically, however, many elderly depressed patients who had had remitted depression at younger ages and became depressed later in life. Care for these patients can be more challenging because these patients' biopsychosocial profiles tend to differ significantly from patients who have only late-onset depression. Therefore, knowing whether an elder person's depression may be a mixed type is important.

According the 2017 report from the Centers for Disease Control and Prevention, depression in older people living in the community ranges from less than 1% to about 5% but increases to 13.5% in those who require home health care and to 11.5% in older hospital patients.[13] Rates of depression may vary among different medical conditions. MDD and mild and subclinical depression have been found to be highly prevalent in patients with CVD. Abundant evidence suggests that approximately 15% to 20% of patients with ischemia heart disease and/or chronic heart failure experience MDD and another 15% to 20% of these patients may have subthreshold depressive symptoms.[14,15] Most cardiac subjects studied were older than 55 years.

Like a double-edged sword, comorbid depression and CVD hurt elder individuals bidirectionally in many aspects in their lives, with a synergetic impact. It is well known that individuals with depression have a higher incidence of CVD and individuals with CVD have a higher incidence of depression.[15,17] The impact of depression on the incidence of CVD events has been found to range from a relative risk of 2.3 to 5.4 in many studies. Greater prevalence of depression occurs in CVD patients and these patients experience greater mortality and medical morbidity compared with CVD patients without depression.[15,18] Depression also negatively affects quality of life, resulting in more social isolation, fragility, poor adherence to effective intervention and lifestyle modifications, the need for assistance with daily living, and so forth. Consequently, the health care expenditure for elderly individuals with CVD and depression grows into a major burden on the patients, their families, and society. For example, US expenditures on personal health care and public health in 2013 totaled $2.1 trillion, from which 14.39% was for CVD ($231.1 billion) and depressive disorders ($71.1 billion).[5] Older patients with depression have roughly 50% higher health care costs than nondepressed seniors.[5] Furthermore, depression is a significant predictor of suicide in elderly Americans. Comprising only 13% of the US population, individuals aged

65 years and older account for 20% of all suicide deaths, with white men being particularly vulnerable. Suicide among white men aged 85 years and older (65.3 deaths per 100,000 persons) is nearly 6 times the suicide rate (10.8 per 100,000) in the United States.[19]

DIAGNOSING DEPRESSION IN ELDERLY PATIENTS WITH CARDIOVASCULAR DISEASE

Depression is neither a normal response to life stress, nor a normal consequence of aging. It is a serious brain disease that can be effectively treated at any age if the treatment is appropriate. Symptomatology of depression can be easily assessed by the Patient Health Questionnaire, version 9, which can be easily self-administered by patients who are not cognitively compromised.[20] Unfortunately, symptoms of depression are often overlooked and untreated, especially when they coexist with other medical illnesses or life events that commonly occur as people age (eg, loss of loved ones). The following elements learned from the 1999 Mental Health America survey on attitudes and beliefs about clinical depression[19] may help in understanding this phenomenon:

- Approximately 68% of adults aged 65 years and older know little or almost nothing about depression.
- Only 38% of adults aged 65 years and older believe that depression is a health problem.
- If suffering from depression, older adults are more likely than any other group to handle it themselves. Only 42% would seek help from a health professional.
- Signs of depression are mentioned more frequently by people younger than age 64 years than by people aged 65 years and older. These include a change in eating habits (29% vs 15%), a change in sleeping habits (33% vs 16%), and sadness (28% vs 15%).
- About 58% of people aged 65 years and older believe that it is normal for people to get depressed as they grow older.

Several features must be kept in mind when making a diagnosis of depressive disorders in elderly individuals. Depression may present more subtly in the elderly, with patients frequently not endorsing low or depressed mood as the primary complaint, even if asked directly. Somatic complaints tend to overshadow the emotional struggles of elderly. Therefore, predominant somatic complaints, particularly when symptoms are diffuse, nonspecific, or chronic, that are not explained by revealing organic causes are often manifestations of underlying depression. Feeling overwhelmed, stressed out, and fatigued, and/or being burdened, is also highly suggestive of depression. Increased irritability, social withdrawal, or isolation may be signs of patients feeling they are unable to engage in tasks as they typically would, which is also a common sign of depression in the elderly. The early stages of depression are often not recognized in older patients; therefore, they may not be diagnosed until they reach more advanced stage; for example, when they have stopped eating, which may or may not be an expression of suicidal intent. Psychotic features, such as nihilistic and negativistic delusions, including themes of poverty and poor health, are common in older depressed patients. Prolonged or intensive grief from losses (of relationships, independence, health, comforts, activities; although grief can be a normal experience with advancing age), especially when accompanied by reduction of social interaction, food intake, and/or physical activities, deserves the attention of a mental care provider. Because active and passive suicidal ideation is common among elderly patients and difficult to detect, it is important for mental health professionals to be highly sensitive to signs of suicidal risk, especially for recently bereaved, isolated men who are in physical pain and drinking. Anxiety symptoms that may impede the appropriate diagnosis and management of depression tend to occur in elderly depressed patients.[21] Cognitive decline and dementia can mask the presentation of depression in the elderly who, at times, may have symptoms of pseudodementia as well. Obtaining collateral information from patients' family members or close friends is generally necessary when caring for depression in elderly patients.

Promptly diagnosing depression in patients with significant CVD can be more challenging because these patients rarely present to typical psychiatric care services and their physical symptoms are often hard to differentiate from depression. Financial constraints are also a significant factor preventing patients from receiving appropriate mental health care.

PATHOMECHANISMS UNDERLYING DEPRESSION AND CARDIOVASCULAR DISEASE IN THE ELDERLY

Several biological systems have been recognized to be dysfunctional and overlapping in CVD and in depression (**Fig. 1**). Aging is also associated with almost all of these identified dysfunctional features.[22] What may explain that approximately 50% of older adults have no CVD and depression? Investigations aimed at understanding the features and mechanisms of mental stress–induced myocardial ischemia or left ventricular dysfunction (MSILVD) have provided some helpful insight.

Mental stress tasks in a laboratory setting, such as a mental serial subtraction of 7 or giving a 3-minute speech about things that had been upsetting recently, trigger occurrence of MSILVD in approximately 50% of subjects who have clinically stable coronary heart disease (CHD).[22] Being a woman or living alone as a man increases the risk of having MSILVD. Alterations of C-reactive protein and cortisol in plasma induced by the mental stress tasks are associated with MSILVD. Also, mental stress task–induced platelet hyperaggregation occurred in subjects with MSILVD.[23] Those

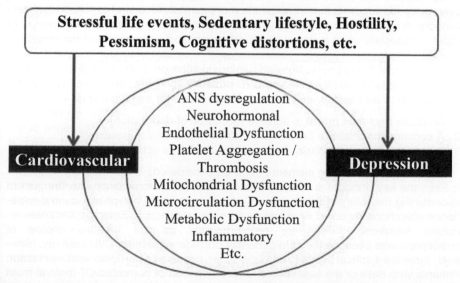

Fig. 1. Underlying pathomechanisms shared by depression and CVD in elderly. ANS, autonomic nerve system.

clinically stable CHD subjects who responded normally to the challenge of mental tasks had no such alterations. Metabolomics research hinted that mental stress induced changes of metabolites reflecting mitochondrial dysregulation.[24] Resting measurements of these biomarkers, however, did not differ between subjects who had normal responses and patients who developed MSILVD to mental tasks (unpublished data). Multiple investigations demonstrate symptoms of depression are associated with development of MSILVD.[22] MSILVD has been found consistently to be a significant and independent predictor for adverse CVD outcomes in clinically stable CHD patients.[25]

MSILVD investigations have revealed a critical interwoven mechanism underlying the adversity of CVD with comorbid depression. Such investigations, in addition, are reminders that certain patients' cardiovascular systems will respond to commonly encountered mental stressors more adversely than others. Mental stress–induced dynamic changes indicate that application of mental stress testing may be an effective measure to identify individuals who are more susceptible to emotional stressful experiences.

IMPROVING THE CARE FOR ELDERLY PATIENTS WITH CARDIOVASCULAR DISEASE AND DEPRESSION

Depression in the elderly seems to respond to common pharmacologic and psychosocial-behavioral interventions as effectively as that in younger individuals.[27] Bartels and colleagues[26] provide a thorough overview of empirically validated treatments and conclude that antidepressants are generally effective for treating geriatric depression, with most studies showing that more than half of older adults treated with antidepressants experience at least a 50% reduction in depressive symptoms. Furthermore, these investigators report that cognitive-behavioral therapy has the greatest empirical support for effectiveness in the treatment of geriatric depression among several forms of psychosocial interventions, such as problem-solving therapy, interpersonal therapy, brief psychodynamic therapy, and reminiscence therapy. Moreover, evidence suggests that a combination of pharmacologic and psychosocial interventions is more effective than either intervention alone in preventing recurrence of MDD,[27] especially when a clearly identified psychosocial stressor is at the root of its cause.

Promptly identifying depression and beginning appropriate interventions are essential components for the care of elderly CVD patients. There are usually 3 phases for the intervention to successfully achieve the effective care for these patients:

1. An acute treatment phase to achieve remission of depression
2. A continuation phase to prevent recurrence of depression (relapse)
3. A maintenance (prophylaxis) phase to prevent future episodes (recurrence).[28]

In addition, the following elements must be considered.

First, the key principle is to appropriately select antidepressants with the goal of ascertaining the safety of these patients who tend to be on polypharmacy and experience alterations in normal drug metabolism and elimination. Selective serotonin reuptake inhibitors (SSRIs) are recommended as the first-line choice of antidepressants because they are generally considered safe for CVD patients. However, there are 4 critical points to consider when choosing a particular antidepressant. Patients who have or are susceptible for prolongation of corrected QT interval must avoid citalopram and escitalopram.[16] Adverse drug-drug interaction can be common in elderly patients and usually requires a thorough review of medications, including health supplements and close monitoring of unanticipated symptoms. The Flockhart Table, or P450 Drug Interaction Table, consists of detailed cytochrome P (CYP) 450 enzyme-related drug interactions (available at http://medicine.iupui.edu/clinpharm/ddis/clinical-table). Fluoxetine has a long half-life and, therefore, should be avoided if frequent medication change is an issue for a patient. Although most adverse effects caused by SSRIs are short-lasting, the sexual dysfunction of SSRIs needs to be clearly discussed with these elderly patients without assuming that they do not care about their sexuality. Initiating a lower dose of the recommended drug for nonmedically ill patients tends to minimize adverse effects. Other antidepressants, such as venlafaxine, duloxetine, bupropion, and mirtazapine, may be considered as single agents, or as augmentation for the treatment of depression in CVD patients. However, close monitoring of blood pressure and heart rate with those medications may be required, especially when the doses are altered. Tricyclic antidepressants should be avoided owing to the known cardiac conduction system[16] adverse effects of these medications.

Second, depression in elderly CVD patients tends to be chronic with fluctuation from milder to severe. Therefore, preparing patients and their loved ones for committing to long-term intervention and aiming at functional improvement rather than simple symptom reduction may enhance the compliance and effectiveness of the intervention.

Third, despite the previously mentioned interventions, patients' depression may regress. Therefore, the clinician must be sensitive to certain symptoms, such as notable reduction of interaction with family, eating little or nothing, reduced verbal communication (even muteness), or being delusional, which may warrant medical and/or mental hospitalization and/or receiving electroconvulsive interventions.

There is evidence indicating that SSRIs may have cardiovascular protective effects, though several clinical trials have not been able to show that SSRIs improve CVD outcomes.[29] It was demonstrated that 6 weeks of escitalopram resulted in about 2.5 times reduction of MSILVD compared with the matched placebo in clinically stable CHD subjects.[29] Kamarck and colleagues[30] reported 2-month citalopram favorably changed metabolic risk factors, such as waist circumference ($P = .003$), glucose ($P = .02$), high-density lipoprotein cholesterol ($P = .04$), triglycerides ($P = .03$), insulin sensitivity ($P = .045$), and diastolic blood pressure by automated assessment ($P = .0021$) compared with placebo in 159 healthy adults with elevated hostility scores.

Regardless of the pharmacologic therapy chosen, it is important to consider the psychological, social, and environmental context of each patient. Various psychosocial behavioral interventions, such as life review, exercise,[31] music therapy, stress management,[31] and many others,[18] benefit the elderly. Tailoring interventions to the needs and acceptance of particular individuals can be challenging but necessary, especially in consideration of the accessibility and resources of each patient. Establishing tangible plans with the patients and their loved ones can be invaluable.

Integrated collaborative care with a systematic approach and targeting effective primary and secondary preventions has been considered most cost-effective in caring for medically ill patients with comorbid depression and other mental health conditions[32] but implementation of such caring mechanisms may take time to be effective.

In summary, comorbid CVD and depression constitutes a huge challenge for these patients, their loved ones, health providers, and the entire society globally. Greater attention, effort, and resources with integrated collaboration are needed to overcome this upcoming disastrous matter.

REFERENCES

1. Wan He, Daniel Goodkind, and Paul Kowal (2016). An Aging World: 2015 International Population Reports (Issued March 2016 P95/16–1). Available at: https://www.census.gov/content/dam/Census/library/publications/2016/demo/p95-16-1.pdf. Accessed November 24, 2017.
2. Fact sheet: aging in the United States (2016). Available at: http://www.prb.org/Publications/Media-Guides/2016/aging-unitedstates-fact-sheet.aspx. Accessed June 10, 2017.
3. Prince MJ, Wu F, Guo Y, et al. The burden of disease in older people and implications for health policy and practice. Lancet 2015;385(9967):549–62.
4. Mozaffarian D, Benjamin EJ, Go AS, et al, on behalf of the American Heart Association Statistics Committee and Stroke Statistics Subcommittee. Heart disease and stroke statistics—2016 update: a report from the American Heart Association. Circulation 2016;133:e38–360.
5. Dieleman JL, Baral R, Birger M, et al. US spending on personal health care and public health, 1996-2013. JAMA 2016;316(24):2627–46.
6. American Association of Geriatric Psychiatry (2008). Geriatrics and mental health—the facts. Available at: http://www.aagponline.org/prof/facts_mh.asp. Accessed June 23, 2008.
7. Bukh JD, Bock C, Vinberg M, et al. Differences between early and late onset adult depression. Clin Pract Epidemiol Ment Health 2011;7:140–7.
8. Blazer DG. Depression in late life: review and commentary. J Gerontol A Biol Sci Med Sci 2003;58:249–65.
9. Hasin DS, Grant BF. The national epidemiologic survey on alcohol and related conditions (NESARC) waves 1 and 2: review and summary of findings. Soc Psychiatry Psychiatr Epidemiol 2015;50:1609–40.
10. Reynolds K, Pietrzak RH, El-Gabalawy R, et al. Prevalence of psychiatric disorders in U.S. older adults: findings from a nationally representative survey. World Psychiatry 2015;14:74–81.
11. Carstensen LL, Isaacowitz DM, Charles ST. Taking time seriously: a theory of socioemotional electivity. Am Psychol 1999;54:165–81.
12. Charles ST. Strength and vulnerability integration: a model of emotional well-being across adulthood. Psychol Bull 2010;136:1068–91.
13. CDC 2017. Available at: https://www.cdc.gov/aging/mentalhealth/depression.htm. Accessed May 15, 2017.
14. Jiang W, Alexander J, Christopher E, et al. Relationship of depression to increased risk of mortality and rehospitalization in patients with congestive heart failure. Arch Intern Med 2001;161:1849–56.
15. Jiang W, Krishnan RR, O'Connor CM. Depression and heart disease: evidence of a link, and its therapeutic implications. CNS Drugs 2002;16:111–27.
16. Khawaja IS, Westermeyer JJ, Gajwani P, et al. Depression and coronary artery disease: the association, mechanisms, and therapeutic implications. Psychiatry (Edgmont) 2009;6:38–51.
17. Rozanski A. Behavioral cardiology: current advances and future directions. J Am Coll Cardiol 2014;64:100–10.
18. National Institute of Mental Health: older adults: depression and suicide fact sheet. Accessed August 1999. Netscape: Available at: http://www.nimh.nih.gov/publicat/elderlydepsuicide.cfm. Accessed on June 10, 2017.

19. Haddad M, Walters P, Phillips R, et al. Detecting depression in patients with coronary heart disease: a diagnostic evaluation of the PHQ-9 and HADS-D in primary care, findings from the UPBEAT-UK study. PLoS One 2013;8(10):e78493.
20. King-Kallimanis B, Gum A, Kohn R. Comorbidity of depressive and anxiety disorders for older Americans in the national comorbidity survey-replication. Am J Geriatr Psychiatry 2009;17:782–92.
21. Paneni F, Diaz Cañestro C, Libby P, et al. The aging cardiovascular system: understanding it at the cellular and clinical levels. J Am Coll Cardiol 2017;69: 1952–67.
22. Jiang W. Emotional triggering of cardiac dysfunction: the present and future. Curr Cardiol Rep 2015;17:635.
23. Jiang W, Samad Z, Boyle S, et al. Prevalence and clinical characteristics of mental stress-induced myocardial ischemia in patients with coronary heart disease. J Am Coll Cardiol 2013;61:714–22.
24. Boyle SH, Matson WR, Eric J, on behalf of the REMIT Investigators. Metabolomics analysis reveals insights into biochemical mechanisms of mental stress-induced left ventricular dysfunction. Metabolomics 2015;11(3):571–82.
25. Sun JL, Boyle SH, Samad Z, et al. Mental stress-induced left ventricular dysfunction and adverse outcome in ischemic heart disease patients. Eur J Prev Cardiol 2017;24:591–9.
26. Bartels SJ, Dums AR, Oxman TE, et al. Evidence-based practices in geriatric mental health care: an overview of systematic reviews and meta-analyses. Psychiatr Clin North Am 2003;26(4):971–90, x–xi.
27. Alexopoulos GS, Katz IR, Bruce ML, et al. Remission in depressed geriatric primary care patients: a report from the PROSPECT study. Am J Psychiatry 2005; 162(4):718–24.
28. Echols MR, Jiang W. Clinical trial evidence for treatment of depression in heart failure. Heart Fail Clin 2011;7:81–8.
29. Jiang W, Velazquez EJ, Kuchibhatla M, et al. Responses of mental stress-induced myocardial ischemia to escitalopram treatment: results from the REMIT trial. JAMA 2013;309:2139–49.
30. Kamarck TW, Muldoon MF, Manuck SB, et al. Citalopram improves metabolic risk factors among high hostile adults: results of a placebo-controlled intervention. Psychoneuroendocrinology 2011;36:1070–9.
31. Blumenthal JA, Sherwood A, Babyak MA, et al. Effects of exercise and stress management training on markers of cardiovascular risk in patients with ischemic heart disease: a randomized controlled trial. JAMA 2005;293(13):1626–34.
32. Katon WJ, Lin EH, Von Korff M, et al. Collaborative care for patients with depression and chronic illnesses. N Engl J Med 2010;363:2611–20.

Sadness and Worry in Older Adults
Differentiating Psychiatric Illness from Normative Distress

Julie Lutz, PhD, Kimberly A. Van Orden, PhD*

KEYWORDS

- Depression • Anxiety • Suicide • Grief • Bereavement • Social connectedness
- Social isolation • Geriatrics

KEY POINTS

- Later life is generally associated with greater emotional well-being.
- However, in certain contexts older adults may be more at risk for bereavement and grief, social isolation and loneliness, and suicide.
- Self-reported symptoms of depression and anxiety may differ for older adults, necessitating developmentally appropriate assessment of symptoms.
- It is critical to consider the balance of risk and resilience factors for depression and anxiety in late life, as well as developmental trajectories, rather than assessing each factor in isolation.

INTRODUCTION, BACKGROUND, AND DEFINITIONS

Although later life is broadly associated with greater emotional well-being,[1] older adults face a number of developmental changes that have the potential to negatively impact their mood and emotional well-being. This dichotomy between emotional well-being and emotional vulnerability in late life may be demonstrated by the relatively low rates of depression in this age group[2] compared with the fact that older men compose the demographic group with the highest risk of suicide in the United States[3] and around the world.[4] Further, older adults may present with a different array of risk factors and symptoms of depression or anxiety than younger adults.[2,5] Additionally, older adults may be at greater risk for changes that may frequently be comorbid with, but do not automatically confer a diagnosis of, depression or anxiety, such as grief, social isolation

This article originally appeared in *Medical Clinics*, Volume 104, Issue 5, September 2020.
Department of Psychiatry, University of Rochester Medical Center, Center for the Study and Prevention of Suicide, 300 Crittenden Boulevard, Box PSYCH, Rochester, NY 14642, USA
* Corresponding author.
E-mail address: Kimberly_Vanorden@URMC.Rochester.edu
Twitter: @kimvanorden (K.A.V.O.)

Clinics Collections 11 (2021) 303–314
https://doi.org/10.1016/j.ccol.2020.12.046

and/or loneliness, and thoughts of death. The aim of this review is to distinguish these phenomena from each other and from a major depressive disorder or anxiety disorder in late life, to clarify normative and non-normative changes in emotional well-being among older adults, and to provide recommendations for assessment and intervention.

There is a common misconception of aging that depression or poor emotional well-being is common, or even normal, in late life.[6,7] This notion likely stems from a societal ageist bias, and beliefs that it is normal for late life to be characterized by poor health and poor functioning and, therefore, poor mental health.[7,8] It additionally stems from a lack of understanding of normative developmental changes throughout adulthood and late life. Emotional experiences can be understood in a developmental context, such that certain experiences are normative at certain times in life, whereas others are not normative in certain contexts. Without an understanding of these contexts, a developmentally normal experience may be mistaken to be pathologic, whereas an experience of suffering may be overlooked owing to an incorrect assumption that it is typical of a certain age. With greater knowledge of the developmental trajectory of emotional well-being in late life, a clinician may more accurately assess whether a patient's experience represents a divergence from a healthy trajectory, and what interventions may support that patient in getting back "on track."

For the purpose of this review, "normative" refers to phenomena appearing in research to be developmentally appropriate, or to occur among a large portion of the population without diagnosable mental illness. "Non-normative" refers to phenomena that are associated with maladaptive coping or adjustment, and possibly (but not necessarily) mental illness, that may be the target of intervention/treatment. The terms "depression" and "anxiety" refer to diagnosable disorders per the *Diagnostic and Statistical Manual of Mental Disorders* (DSM) 5th edition[9] and/or *International Classification of Diseases*, 10th edition,[10] such as major depressive disorder, generalized anxiety disorder, and so on. There will also be some discussion of subthreshold syndromes, in which an older adult may not meet criteria for a disorder, but experiences some symptoms with a significant effect on his or her quality of life.

NORMATIVE EMOTIONAL DEVELOPMENT IN LATE LIFE

Research to date on lifespan development has shown that, generally, later life is associated with greater emotional well-being, including less frequent negative affect and more frequent positive affect, and decreased lability in emotions.[1,11] One prominent theory posited to explain this phenomenon is the socioemotional selectivity theory.[12] The socioemotional selectivity theory posits that, as the end of life is perceived to draw nearer, people shift their goals from the acquisition of knowledge or exploration of new experiences, to the regulation of emotion and enhancement of positive emotional and relational experiences. In other words, as people perceive their time becoming more limited, they focus more on maximizing positive emotional states and minimizing negative emotional states in the present, often via seeking out stable and positive social contexts.

Taking a more expanded view by considering the age-related physiologic factors in emotional experience in addition to the psychological factors, the strength and vulnerability integration theory posits that later life is associated with both psychological enhancements in adaptive emotion regulation strategies (as described in the socioemotional selectivity theory) as well as physiologic vulnerabilities to situations involving higher, more prolonged negative emotional arousal.[13] With age, people build and hone effective psychological strategies for regulating average, common emotional experiences, therefore leading to a decrease in exposure to negative emotional experiences, improved ability to rebound after minor negative experiences, and a general increase in emotional well-being. However, aging is also associated with decreased physiologic flexibility and resilience, leaving older adults more vulnerable to distress when they experience high levels of physical arousal associated with an unavoidable, prolonged state of stress or negative emotional arousal.

In behavioral and imaging studies of the brain as people age, patterns of resilience to negative emotional experience and reactivity to positive emotional experience are borne out, despite the general reality of physiologic and cognitive decline in later life.[14] Older adults exhibit less reactivity to negative stimuli, and greater memory for positive information. However, older adults who have damage to areas of the prefrontal cortex related to emotion regulation are more likely to experience negative outcomes such as depression.[14]

These results indicate that, contrary to a common misconception that growing older is associated with a decline in emotional well-being,[6] the majority of older adults will experience a general improvement in emotional well-being in late life. However, older adults who are exposed to significant, unavoidable, prolonged stressors may be especially vulnerable to negative outcomes, such as mood or anxiety disorders, or even suicidal thoughts or behaviors.

MOOD AND ANXIETY DISORDERS IN LATE LIFE

Numerous studies have documented that older adults have a lower prevalence of mood and anxiety disorders than younger adults,[15–17] which may be accounted for, in part, by increased levels of emotional well-being in later life. However, many believe that these estimates can be misleading, owing to issues of accurately detecting depression and anxiety in this population.[18] Under-recognition may occur due to underreporting of symptoms by older adults owing to stigma, or internalized ageism whereby older adults—and providers—expect depressed mood to accompany aging and thus do not think it warrants treatment. Physicians and other clinicians are less likely to ask older adults about psychological symptoms, including suicide ideation, than for younger adults.[18,19]

Older adults' presentation of mood or anxiety disorders often differ from younger adults, meaning that the symptoms older adults experience and describe differ from those of younger patients. Older adults are less likely to report sad or depressed mood, but more likely to report anhedonia (lack of pleasure),[5] apathy, and irritability.[20] In addition, older adults are more likely to describe somatic symptoms as their primary concern, such as those related to sleep, fatigue, and psychomotor slowing, as well as cognitive symptoms such as deficits in memory, concentration, processing speed, and executive functioning.[2] Depression in late life commonly co-occurs with gastrointestinal and other somatic symptoms.[20] Older adults may also be more likely to present with a subthreshold depression, meaning that clinically significant depression symptoms are present, but not enough symptoms to meet the criteria for a major depressive episode. The clinical importance of subthreshold syndromes should not be minimized, because this syndrome is associated with a greater odds of lifetime psychiatric disorders and of developing major depressive disorder or an anxiety disorder in the subsequent years.[21] Finally, because older adults are more likely to experience multiple health problems, differentiating a depressive disorder from an underlying medical condition is essential and can be complex. Nonspecific physical symptoms, such as fatigue, loss of appetite, weakness, diffuse physical pain, and sleep problems, can be signs of a depressive illness or symptoms of an underlying medical condition. Depressive disorders and medical illnesses also frequently co-occur (and share symptoms) and can increase risk in both directions—a depressive disorder is associated with poor health and many medical illnesses are associated with increased risk for a depressive disorder.[2]

Older adults' presentations of anxiety disorders may differ somewhat from those of younger adults, including the topics of worry (eg, more concerns about health and fewer about work or school),[5,22] but there are fewer differences than regarding depression. Older and younger adults report comparable symptoms of anxiety disorders, but they may describe their symptoms differently, using terms such as "stressed" or "tense" rather than "anxious," "worried," or "nervous."[5] Given these differences in the presentation of anxiety in late life, recommendations for future diagnostic classifications have included attention to the heterogeneity of anxiety symptoms and experiences in older adults, the use of language appropriate to the older adult in the assessment of anxiety, consideration of comorbidities (eg, comorbid depression, medical illness, and cognitive impairment), and attention to variants of anxiety that are mostly exclusive to late life (eg, fear of falling).[23]

As clinicians assess for the presence of mood or anxiety disorders among older adults, they should be alert to these possible differences in presentation and use appropriate assessment strategies and instruments. The use of assessment instruments developed and validated specifically for use in older adults (eg, Geriatric Depression Scale,[24] Geriatric Anxiety Inventory[25]) is recommended, because such instruments take into account differences in symptom presentations and measurement in older adults and are designed to be easy to administer, with yes/no response choices. Additionally, best judgment should be used regarding the presence of distressing subthreshold mood symptoms that may merit an intervention, although they may not meet diagnostic criteria.

BEREAVEMENT AND GRIEF

Losses become a normative part of life in older adulthood, including bereavement (death of a loved one) and loss of prior levels of health and physical functioning. However, although loss is a common experience in later life, that does not mean that all grief reactions will resolve on their own or do not warrant intervention. For example, individuals who have experienced bereavement are at greater risk for declines in health and functioning, potentially increased risk of mortality, decline in socioemotional well-being, and increase in loneliness and social isolation.[26] Prolonged grief around decline in health or physical functioning may be associated with greater use of health care services (eg, emergency room visits, hospitalizations).[27] Further, up to 25% of older adults who have experienced a major bereavement may go on to experience complicated grief, which refers specifically to an atypical, maladaptive, and prolonged grief reaction.[28–30] The boundary between what is normal after a loss and what constitutes a disorder is a topic of debate, including regarding the recent change in the fifth version of the DSM released in 2013.[9] In this version, a controversial change was made to remove an exclusion for a major depressive episode for bereavement, which in previous DSM versions had ruled out a diagnosis of major depressive disorder for individuals within 2 months after bereavement except in severe cases.[31] Although there are several arguments both in support and opposition of this change,[31] the implication for clinicians is the critical need to use best judgment in distinguishing a normative grief reaction from complicated grief or a depressive syndrome. Some of the research to date on differences between normal or uncomplicated grief, complicated grief, and depression or anxiety may be useful in making diagnostic decisions.

Common predictors for a greater risk of complicated grief across studies are female gender, older age, lower education, and poorer cognitive functioning.[28,29,32] Anticipation or expectancy around the loss (ie, whether an older widow expected the death of her spouse to occur) has not been shown to be predictive of differences in grief.[33] Among those with complicated grief, up to 10% may experience comorbid depression and 17% comorbid anxiety.[29] Of note, the emotional responses to bereavement may mitigate across time; for example, in 1 study, differences in depressive symptoms and psychopathology between widowed older adults and nonwidowed older adults that had been evident 2 months after a loss faded to nonsignificance within 12 months, although differences in grief-specific symptoms remained to some extent even up to 2.5 years after the loss.[34] Given that the DSM's bereavement exception extended only to 2 months after a loss, these results highlight the more protracted trajectory that recovery from grief and its emotional associates may take.

Research indicates that there is not a consistent, clear definition and boundary between complicated grief and uncomplicated or normal grief and, throughout the literature, symptoms of complicated grief and depression or anxiety significantly overlap.[30] Also, a comprehensive framework of bereavement and grief must take into account preloss factors (eg, preexisting depression), interpersonal and intrapersonal factors (eg, social support, physical health and functioning), and cognitive coping (eg, cognitive appraisal, emotion regulation), all of which influence grief outcomes and resilience.[30] Finally, cultural sensitivity to grief and mourning-related norms and practices is critical, although little is currently known about cultural differences in this area.[30]

Grief may present in many heterogeneous ways among older adults who have experienced bereavement and has the potential to impact risk for depression and anxiety. Clinicians should use their best judgment to distinguish normative grief responses, complicated grief, and depression or anxiety syndromes. Preloss functioning, as well as current functioning and the individual's trajectory of change in grief symptoms over time, may help to distinguish these phenomena.

SOCIAL ISOLATION AND LONELINESS

Aging is associated with changes in the size and composition of social networks, such that, as we age, the size of our social networks tends to decrease, with decreases primarily seen regarding friends and other nonfamily connections.[1] This finding was originally attributed to the many losses that occur in later life, including retirement (and loss of work relationships), declining health, and deaths of friends and family. However, gerontologists have documented that the decreased size of social networks associated with aging is actually due, in large part, to an active process by older adults to "prune" their networks and discard the less meaningful and valued ties to devote more energy and time to the most meaningful relationships.[1] Thus, although social networks tend to be smaller in later life, older adults report greater satisfaction with their social networks. Further, although loneliness and social isolation are often described as a problem of old age in the popular media, loneliness and social isolation are not the norm in later life. In fact, a recent study with a large sample representative of the US population found that the prevalence of loneliness decreases with age.[35] In contrast, up to one-third of community-dwelling older adults report that they expect to become lonely as they grow older or that they agree with the statement, "old age is a time of loneliness."[36] In turn, those who agree with these stereotypes of aging are then more likely to actually experience loneliness in the future, consistent with a "self-fulfilling prophecy."[36] Addressing expectations about aging to be more positive and realistic can be a useful intervention for individuals at all ages, patients, caregivers, and clinicians.

This is not to say that social isolation and loneliness are not relevant issues for older adults. Although social isolation and loneliness are not the norm in later life, when they do occur, they may have even more deleterious effects on health and well-being than at younger ages owing to the body's decreased capacity for managing stress (cf., the strength and vulnerability integration theory discussed in the Introduction). Further, social isolation and loneliness may be key targets of intervention to promote health and well-being in later life because these aspects of our social health remain malleable throughout our lives, whereas some factors, such as sensory impairment or loss of mobility may be less amenable to intervention. Thus, promoting social connectedness and social well-being is a promising intervention strategy in later life. However, the research literature on *how* to promote social connectedness and decrease loneliness is in its infancy for individuals at any age.[37] What is known, however, suggests that, to effectively help an older patient with isolation and/or loneliness, it is useful to understand the context in which these experiences are occurring and what the older adult believes is the primary cause. Research with older adults has confirmed that loneliness is due in part to objective circumstances—increasing disability and frailty, environmental barriers to socialization, and bereavement, whereas other research emphasizes the role of subjective perceptions, such as thinking of oneself as useless, in causing and perpetuating loneliness.[38,39] Each of these potential contributors to loneliness and isolation can be addressed through various interventions, such as care management to address transportation barriers, hearing aids to promote communication, psychotherapy to promote motivation to engage, and access to meaningful social activities, such as volunteering or educational opportunities.

For older adults with moderate to advanced dementia, or other illnesses that impact the ability to understand and communicate one's needs, a lack of social stimulation and loneliness can be one contributor to agitation or aggressive behavior that is distressing to both the patient and caregivers. These types of behaviors that are considered abnormal and problematic can sometimes occur when an older person is not able to communicate a very normal and healthy need, such as social connections and comfort. All humans have an innate need to belong to social relationships and groups.[40] When this need is not met, loneliness and distress emerges at all ages. When working with older adults who may be demonstrating abnormal behaviors, it is useful to consider whether a normal and healthy unmet need is contributing to the behavior.

SUICIDAL IDEATION AND BEHAVIOR

Older adults, specifically older men, have the highest rates of suicide in the United States[3] and around the world,[4] with risk increasing with age through late life. In the United States, white men aged 85 and older have the highest rates of suicide deaths, almost four times the rate in the general population (ie, 47.17 per 100,000 vs 14.21 per 100,000).[3] Among older Americans who reported suicidal ideation in the past year, 12.7% reported at least 1 suicide attempt in the past year.[41] Older adults who attempt suicide are known to be at exponentially greater risk for death, although exact statistics are difficult to find; some estimates state that whereas there are 25 attempts for every suicide death nationally within the United States, among older adults there are only 4 attempts to every suicide death,[42] therefore making nonlethal suicide attempts less common. Therefore, it is critically important to identify suicidal ideation and risk early in this age group, before it escalates into an attempt. Risk factors for suicide among older adults include the "5 Ds": depression and other psychiatric illnesses, disease (physical illness), disability (pain and functional impairment), social disconnectedness, and access to deadly means (such as firearms).[43,44]

Given the importance of identifying suicidal ideation early, understanding the difference between normative thoughts or attitudes about death in late life and maladaptive thoughts that could contribute to risk for suicide is critical. Older adults do demonstrate differences in their attitudes and reactions toward death compared with younger and middle-aged adults, such that they report overall less fear of death and greater acceptance of death,[45] and exhibit less attentional avoidance to death-related information.[46,47] Acceptance of death can be a neutral view of death as natural and inevitable, or even a positive view of death as a gateway to a positive afterlife. However, a lesser fear of death and greater acceptance of death with a particular focus on escaping negative situations or experiences in life are associated with a wish to die.[48] Passive suicidal ideation—going beyond just acceptance of death—refers to thoughts of being better off dead, or a desire to die, without specific thoughts of ending one's own life. (Active) suicidal ideation—refers to thoughts of ending one's own life. One study estimated that 10% to 13% of all adults age 50 and older experience passive suicidal ideation.[49] Despite misconceptions that passive suicidal ideation is less concerning than active suicidal ideation, or even normal among older adults, studies have shown that even passive suicidal ideation is associated with an increased risk for suicidal behavior and should not be considered normative.[50,51] Further, some research has shown that individuals may transition between passive and active suicidal ideation in a given episode.[52] The studies reviewed here suggest that, although older adults may exhibit less avoidance of death-related topics and greater overall acceptance of death, it is problematic when older adults express a desire for their life to end, even without active thoughts of ending one's own life.

Assessment of suicide risk by health care providers is essential, because many older adults who die by suicide have had recent contact with a health care provider, but may not have contact with any mental health provider. More than three-quarters (77%) of adults age 55 and older who die by suicide have had contact with a primary care physician within the past year, with 58% having contact within the past month, compared with 8.5% in the past year and 11.0% in the past month having contact with mental health care.[53] Almost one-third (29%) of adults age 50 and older who die by suicide have contact with a primary health care provider within 1 week of their death.[54] However, general medical providers may be less likely to screen for suicidal ideation and risk and implement important interventions. Among Veterans Affairs patients who attempted suicide, older adults' charts were less likely to show documentation by general medical providers of assessment for certain risk factors for suicide (eg, access to firearms) or interventions to reduce suicide risk (eg, safety planning, mental health care referrals) compared with younger adults.[19]

Although assessment for suicidality should occur for all patients with depression, suicidal ideation can also occur among those without depression, and therefore it is important to use best judgment in screening for suicide risk in a primary care or other medical population.[55,56] Although a clinician may use an assessment instrument to screen for suicidal ideation, such as the Patient Health Questionnaire-9, it is important to follow-up with specific questions about types of suicidal thoughts, plans, access to means, intent, and so on.[55,56] The P4 Screener may be a useful tool, because it was designed as a brief follow-up to the Patient Health Questionnaire-9.[57] Also, relying on assessments of depression may miss older adults who have suicidal ideation but are not reporting symptoms of depression.[55] It is important to have mental health care, implemented within an effective referral and transfer of care system, available for

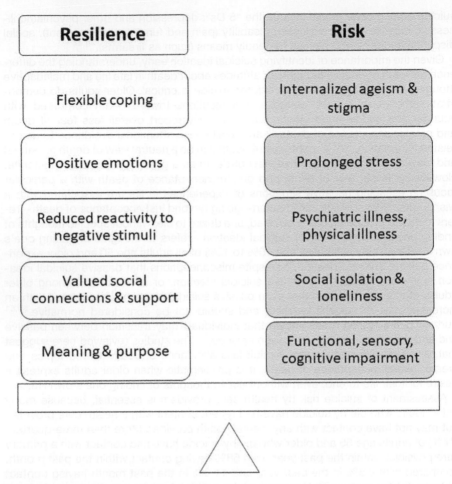

Resilience	Risk
Flexible coping	Internalized ageism & stigma
Positive emotions	Prolonged stress
Reduced reactivity to negative stimuli	Psychiatric illness, physical illness
Valued social connections & support	Social isolation & loneliness
Meaning & purpose	Functional, sensory, cognitive impairment

Fig. 1. Late life is associated with a number of both risk and resilience factors for depression and anxiety. Although older adulthood is generally a time of positive affective well-being owing to resilience factors pictured, the presence of the outlined risk factors may contribute to negative affective outcomes.

those who do exhibit an increased risk for suicide.[55,56] In addition to referrals to more intensive mental health care, brief interventions such as safety planning[58] may be implemented within medical clinics and emergency departments.

DISCUSSION AND SUMMARY

A common misconception, likely rooted in ageist societal biases, is that emotional turmoil or negative affective experiences are the norm in later life[6–8]; lifespan theory and research demonstrates that this is not true, and can negatively impact diagnosis and treatment by providers as well as expectations and physical and mental health outcomes in patients themselves.[7,8] However, in certain contexts older adults may be vulnerable to experiencing grief, social isolation, and/or loneliness and have a heightened risk of suicide. Although older adults experience greater psychological resilience to negative affect, they also experience age-related physiologic vulnerabilities.[14] **Fig. 1** illustrates the risk and resilience factors for affective well-being commonly experienced in late life, as discussed throughout this review, as weights on a balance scale. Although the majority of older adults benefit in late life from greater positive affect via flexible coping and decreased reactivity to negative affect, as well as more meaningful and valued social connections, those who experience prolonged stressors, physiologic risk factors such as illness or impairment and decreased physiologic resilience to stress, as well as social isolation or loneliness, along with internalized ageist views of late life may be at elevated risk for depression, anxiety, or other negative outcomes. Viewing risk and resilience factors this way highlights the usefulness of considering the combination of factors (eg, if multiple risk factors are "piling up" for a given patient, in the absence of some resilience factors) rather than assessing each factor in isolation. Additionally, strengthening protective factors, even when risk factors are currently minimal, can serve as a valuable prevention tool against future risks.

Affective problems such as depression and anxiety may be more difficult to diagnose in older adults, owing to unclear differentiation between normative experiences (eg, bereavement and uncomplicated grief) and maladaptive syndromes (eg, complicated grief), differences in symptom presentation in this age group, and comorbid physical and cognitive conditions. It is critical for those working with older adults to use criteria and assessment instruments that are tailored to the unique needs and presentations of older adults, rather than depending on criteria and instruments that do not reflect this age group. The most important factor in determining diagnosis and the need for treatment is the impact on the individual's everyday functioning. If treatment is needed, implementation of or referral for appropriate treatments that are evidence based in older adults (eg, cognitive behavioral therapy,[59] problem solving therapy,[59,60] antidepressant treatment[61]) may significantly improve mood and quality of life.

CLINICS CARE POINTS

- Use of criteria and assessment instruments validated in older adults is necessary. The Geriatric Depression Scale (https://consultgeri.org/try-this/general-assessment/issue-4.pdf) and Geriatric Anxiety Inventory are examples of such instruments.
- The Patient Health Questionnaire-9 and P4 screener (https://gerocentral.org/wp-content/uploads/2013/04/P4-Suicide-Risk-Screener.pdf), in conjunction with a detailed clinical interview, may be used to assess risk for suicide.
- Safety planning (https://www.mirecc.va.gov/visn16/collaborative-safety-planning-manual.asp) is a brief, effective intervention that can help to manage suicide risk in a clinical setting.

DISCLOSURE

The authors have nothing to disclose. This work was supported by an NIMH National Research Service Award Postdoctoral Fellowship (T32MH20061; Conwell, PI).

REFERENCES

1. Charles ST, Carstensen LL. Social and emotional aging. Annu Rev Psychol 2010; 61:383–409.
2. Fiske A, Wetherell JL, Gatz M. Depression in older adults. Annu Rev Clin Psychol 2009;5:363–89.

3. Centers for Disease Control and Prevention NCfIPaC. Web-based Injury Statistics Query and Reporting System (WISQARS). 2019. Available at: https://www.cdc.gov/injury/wisqars/index.html. Accessed June 22, 2020.

4. World Health Organization. Preventing suicide: a global imperative. Geneva (Switzerland): World Health Organization; 2014.

5. Wuthrich VM, Johnco CJ, Wetherell JL. Differences in anxiety and depression symptoms: comparison between older and younger clinical samples. Int Psychogeriatr 2015;27(9):1523–32.

6. Haigh EAP, Bogucki OE, Sigmon ST, et al. Depression among older adults: a 20-year update on five common myths and misconceptions. Am J Geriatr Psychiatry 2018;26(1):107–22.

7. Uncapher H, Arean PA. Physicians are less willing to treat suicidal ideation in older patients. J Am Geriatr Soc 2000;48(2):188–92.

8. Nelson TD. Promoting healthy aging by confronting ageism. Am Psychol 2016; 71(4):276–82.

9. American Psychiatric Association. Diagnostic and statistical manual of mental disorders. 5th edition. Arlington (VA): American Psychiatric Association; 2013.

10. World Health Organization. The ICD-10 classification of mental and behavioural disorders: clinical descriptions and diagnostic guidelines. Geneva (Switzerland): World Health Organization; 1992.

11. Carstensen LL, Turan B, Scheibe S, et al. Emotional experience improves with age: evidence based on over 10 years of experience sampling. Psychol Aging 2011;26(1):21–33.

12. Carstensen LL, Isaacowitz DM, Charles ST. Taking time seriously. A theory of socioemotional selectivity. Am Psychol 1999;54(3):165–81.

13. Charles ST. Strength and vulnerability integration: a model of emotional well-being across adulthood. Psychol Bull 2010;136(6):1068–91.

14. Mather M. The emotion paradox in the aging brain. Ann N Y Acad Sci 2012; 1251(1):33–49.

15. Gonzalez HM, Tarraf W, Whitfield KE, et al. The epidemiology of major depression and ethnicity in the United States. J Psychiatr Res 2010;44(15):1043–51.

16. Mackenzie CS, El-Gabalawy R, Chou KL, et al. Prevalence and predictors of persistent versus remitting mood, anxiety, and substance disorders in a national sample of older adults. Am J Geriatr Psychiatry 2014;22(9):854–65.

17. Byers AL, Yaffe K, Covinsky KE, et al. High occurrence of mood and anxiety disorders among older adults: The National Comorbidity Survey Replication. Arch Gen Psychiatry 2010;67(5):489–96.

18. Bryant C. Anxiety and depression in old age: challenges in recognition and diagnosis. Int Psychogeriatr 2010;22(4):511–3.

19. Simons K, Van Orden K, Conner KR, et al. Age differences in suicide risk screening and management prior to suicide attempts. Am J Geriatr Psychiatry 2019;27(6):604–8.

20. Hegeman JM, Kok RM, van der Mast RC, et al. Phenomenology of depression in older compared with younger adults: meta-analysis. Br J Psychiatry 2012;200(4):275–81.

21. Laborde-Lahoz P, El-Gabalawy R, Kinley J, et al. Subsyndromal depression among older adults in the USA: prevalence, comorbidity, and risk for new-onset psychiatric disorders in late life. Int J Geriatr Psychiatry 2015;30(7):677–85.

22. Gould CE, Gerolimatos LA, Beaudreau SA, et al. Older adults report more sadness and less jealousy than young adults in response to worry induction. Aging Ment Health 2018;22(4):512–8.

23. Mohlman J, Bryant C, Lenze EJ, et al. Improving recognition of late life anxiety disorders in Diagnostic and Statistical Manual of Mental Disorders, Fifth Edition: observations and recommendations of the Advisory Committee to the Lifespan Disorders Work Group. Int J Geriatr Psychiatry 2012;27(6):549–56.
24. Yesavage JA, Brink TL, Rose TL, et al. Development and validation of a geriatric depression screening scale: a preliminary report. J Psychiatr Res 1983;17(1): 37–49.
25. Pachana NA, Byrne GJ, Siddle H, et al. Development and validation of the geriatric anxiety inventory. Int Psychogeriatr 2007;19(1):103–14.
26. Shear MK, Ghesquiere A, Glickman K. Bereavement and complicated grief. Curr Psychiatry Rep 2013;15(11):406.
27. Holland JM, Graves S, Klingspon KL, et al. Prolonged grief symptoms related to loss of physical functioning: examining unique associations with medical service utilization. Disabil Rehabil 2016;38(3):205–10.
28. Kersting A, Brahler E, Glaesmer H, et al. Prevalence of complicated grief in a representative population-based sample. J Affect Disord 2011;131(1–3):339–43.
29. Newson RS, Boelen PA, Hek K, et al. The prevalence and characteristics of complicated grief in older adults. J Affect Disord 2011;132(1–2):231–8.
30. Shah SN, Meeks S. Late-life bereavement and complicated grief: a proposed comprehensive framework. Aging Ment Health 2012;16(1):39–56.
31. Iglewicz A, Seay K, Zetumer SD, et al. The removal of the bereavement exclusion in the DSM-5: exploring the evidence. Curr Psychiatry Rep 2013;15(11):413.
32. Nielsen MK, Carlsen AH, Neergaard MA, et al. Looking beyond the mean in grief trajectories: a prospective, population-based cohort study. Soc Sci Med 2019; 232:460–9.
33. Dessonville C, Thompson LW, Gallagher D. The role of anticipatory bereavement in older women's adjustment to widowhood. Gerontologist 1988;28(6):792–6.
34. Thompson LW, Gallagher-Thompson D, Futterman A, et al. The effects of late-life spousal bereavement over a 30-month interval. Psychol Aging 1991;6(3):434–41.
35. Bruce LD, Wu JS, Lustig SL, et al. Loneliness in the United States: a 2018 national panel survey of demographic, structural, cognitive, and behavioral characteristics. Am J Health Promot 2019;33(8):1123–33.
36. Pikhartova J, Bowling A, Victor C. Is loneliness in later life a self-fulfilling prophecy? Aging Ment Health 2016;20(5):543–9.
37. Dickens AP, Richards SH, Greaves CJ, et al. Interventions targeting social isolation in older people: a systematic review. BMC Public Health 2011;11:647.
38. Qualter P, Vanhalst J, Harris R, et al. Loneliness across the life span. Perspect Psychol Sci 2015;10(2):250–64.
39. Cacioppo JT, Cacioppo S, Boomsma DI. Evolutionary mechanisms for loneliness. Cogn Emot 2014;28(1):3–21.
40. Baumeister RF, Leary MR. The need to belong: desire for interpersonal attachments as a fundamental human motivation. Psychol Bull 1995;117(3):497–529.
41. Han B, Compton WM, Gfroerer J, et al. Prevalence and correlates of past 12-month suicide attempt among adults with past-year suicidal ideation in the United States. J Clin Psychiatry 2015;76(3):295–302.
42. Drapeau CW, McIntosh JL. U.S.A. suicide 2017: official final data. Washington, DC: American Association of Suicidology; 2018.
43. Van Orden K, Conwell Y. Suicides in late life. Curr Psychiatry Rep 2011;13(3): 234–41.
44. Conwell Y. Suicide and suicide prevention in later life. Focus 2013;11(1):39–47.

45. Gesser G, Wong PTP, Reker GT. Death attitudes across the life-span: the development and validation of the death attitude profile (DAP). OMEGA - Journal of Death and Dying 1988;18(2):113–28.

46. De Raedt R, Koster EH, Ryckewaert R. Aging and attentional bias for death related and general threat-related information: less avoidance in older as compared with middle-aged adults. J Gerontol B Psychol Sci Soc Sci 2013; 68(1):41–8.

47. Maxfield M, Pyszczynski T, Kluck B, et al. Age-related differences in responses to thoughts of one's own death: mortality salience and judgments of moral transgressions. Psychol Aging 2007;22(2):341–53.

48. Bonnewyn A, Shah A, Bruffaerts R, et al. Are religiousness and death attitudes associated with the wish to die in older people? Int Psychogeriatr 2016;28(3): 397–404.

49. Dong L, Kalesnikava VA, Gonzalez R, et al. Beyond depression: estimating 12-months prevalence of passive suicidal ideation in mid- and late-life in the health and retirement study. Am J Geriatr Psychiatry 2019;27(12):1399–410.

50. Van Orden KA, O'Riley AA, Simning A, et al. Passive suicide ideation: an indicator of risk among older adults seeking aging services? Gerontologist 2015;55(6): 972–80.

51. Van Orden KA, Simning A, Conwell Y, et al. Characteristics and comorbid symptoms of older adults reporting death ideation. Am J Geriatr Psychiatry 2013;21(8): 803–10.

52. Szanto K, Reynolds CF 3rd, Frank E, et al. Suicide in elderly depressed patients: is active vs. passive suicidal ideation a clinically valid distinction? Am J Geriatr Psychiatry 1996;4:197–207.

53. Luoma JB, Martin CE, Pearson JL. Contact with mental health and primary care providers before suicide: a review of the evidence. Am J Psychiatry 2002;159: 909–16.

54. Stene-Larsen K, Reneflot A. Contact with primary and mental health care prior to suicide: a systematic review of the literature from 2000 to 2017. Scand J Public Health 2019;47(1):9–17.

55. Raue PJ, Ghesquiere AR, Bruce ML. Suicide risk in primary care: identification and management in older adults. Curr Psychiatry Rep 2014;16(9):466.

56. McDowell AK, Lineberry TW, Bostwick JM. Practical suicide-risk management for the busy primary care physician. Mayo Clin Proc 2011;86(8):792–800.

57. Dube P, Kurt K, Bair MJ, et al. The p4 screener: evaluation of a brief measure for assessing potential suicide risk in 2 randomized effectiveness trials of primary care and oncology patients. Prim Care Companion J Clin Psychiatry 2010; 12(6):PCC.

58. Conti EC, Jahn DR, Simons KV, et al. Safety planning to manage suicide risk with older adults: case examples and recommendations. Clin Gerontol 2020;43(1): 104–9.

59. Renn BN, Arean PA. Psychosocial treatment options for major depressive disorder in older adults. Curr Treat Options Psychiatry 2017;4(1):1–12.

60. Kirkham JG, Choi N, Seitz DP. Meta-analysis of problem solving therapy for the treatment of major depressive disorder in older adults. Int J Geriatr Psychiatry 2016;31(5):526–35.

61. Kok RM, Reynolds CF 3rd. Management of depression in older adults: a review. JAMA 2017;317(20):2114–22.

Mindfulness, Stress, and Aging

Katarina Friberg Felsted, PhD

KEYWORDS

- Mindfulness • MBSR • Older adults • Chronic conditions

KEY POINTS

- Mindfulness is an effective treatment for a variety of chronic conditions in older adults, because it is simple, inexpensive, and continues to show improvement over time.
- Mindfulness reduces stress and improves mental function in older adults, including cognitive function, anxiety, depression, sleep quality, loneliness, and posttraumatic stress disorder.
- Mindfulness reduces stress and improves physical function, including cardiovascular conditions, diabetes, rheumatoid arthritis, Parkinson disease, urge urinary incontinence, and chronic pain.

INTRODUCTION

As our population seeks to age optimally, the role of stress must be factored into the quest. Chronic stressors decrease the body's ability to recover from stress, creating mental and physical vulnerabilities. Mentally, stresses influence otherwise normative aging in the immune system, and its effects with age are interactive.[1] Physically, chronic stress suppresses both cellular (intracellular pathogens) and humoral (parasites and bacteria) immunity and affects functional measures; the older the age of participants studied, the more pronounced their decreases were.[2,3]

Although mindfulness meditation (MM) has its roots in Buddhism, traced back several thousand years, it has been introduced into scientific circles over the last several decades as a treatment for stress, particularly chronic stress. Modern mindfulness was pioneered in the late 1970s by Dr Jon Kabat-Zinn at the University of Massachusetts Medical School. Mindfulness is defined as paying attention to the present moment in a purposeful, nonjudgmental way. Dr Kabat-Zinn created the Mindfulness-Based Stress Reduction (MBSR) program, an 8-week program with a 2.5-hour session once a week for 8 weeks, with a daylong retreat between weeks 6 and 7.[4] Participants are encouraged to practice their mindfulness through audio recordings and specific

This article originally appeared in *Clinics in Geriatric Medicine*, Volume 36, Issue 4, November 2020.

University of Utah College of Nursing, 10 South Connor Road, #3655, Salt Lake City, UT 84112, USA

E-mail address: katarina.felsted@nurs.utah.edu

Twitter: @katarinafelsted (K.F.F.)

https://doi.org/10.1016/j.ccol.2020.12.047
2352-7986/21/© 2020 Elsevier Inc.

skills they learn in sessions. MBSR is applied to a variety of concerns and does not need to be modified to fit a specific condition.

This program has been modified in a myriad of ways in the last several decades. Another evidence-based MM program, which incorporates mindfulness training as well as cognitive therapy, is Mindfulness-Based Cognitive Therapy (MBCT).[5] MBCT was originally created to treat depression and has been used across other chronic conditions since its inception. Beyond MBSR and MBCT, other versions of MM programs are often referred to simply as mindfulness. Mindfulness programs may and do differ greatly from one another in the way that they are offered: variations in duration, frequency, practice options, location, and ways of transmission. In research it also is applied to a variety of populations: age, race and ethnicity, heterogeneity in physical and mental circumstances. The constant within each mindfulness program, regardless of its adaptations, is that it trains participants in a skill that allows the mind to be "calm, clear, open-hearted, and devoid of suffering."[6] Becoming aware and accepting of the present moment allows participants to respond authentically to their current experience, which is preferable to reflexively letting the mind be reactive and judgmental and which can potentially worsen the person's situation instead.

CONTENT
Why Older Adults Are Excellent Candidates for Mindfulness

Mindfulness and self-compassion have been shown to improve older adults' coping capabilities as well as their adaptation to stressful situations. Recent research has shown that mindfulness may improve resilience and positive reappraisal while reducing anxiety and stress as well as negative self-focus.[7] The research by Sorrell[8] on MM specifically in an older adult population found that mindfulness results in changed brain structure as it is related to stress and memory. As such, she suggests that health care professionals should consider mindfulness as "a helpful intervention for older adults with problems such as depression, anxiety, chronic pain, loneliness, and caregiver burden."

Mindfulness is particularly efficacious for older adults with chronic conditions. Self-management of chronic conditions has much to do with health-related behaviors, because compliance with recommendations has a large effect on how much of the chronic condition is controlled. These conditions include stress, anxiety, and depression as well as cardiovascular disease, diabetes, and more. Mindfulness has been shown to positively affect health-related behaviors in older adult participants and significantly reduce stress.[9,10] Older adults coping with various chronic mental and physical health conditions often present with anxiety. A recent review of 7 randomized controlled trials (RCTs) using mindfulness in a specifically geriatric population supported the use of MBSR and MBCT to reduce geriatric anxiety.[11]

Mindfulness as a buffer between stress and health-related quality of life was examined in a cross-sectional study of community-dwelling healthy older adults. Results identified an inverse relationship between stress and both mental and physical health. de Frias and Whyne[12] suggest that "mindfulness is a powerful, adaptive strategy that may protect older adults from the well-known harmful effects of stress on mental health."

Stress research also indicates that immune function decreases with stress and normal aging. Older adults are prone to late life stressors in the form of loss of spouse or close friends, relocation from independent living, and managing chronic conditions/comorbidities. Stress in older adults may speed the effects aging has on immune system function.[2] Given this link between stress, aging, and the immune system, mindfulness may prove particularly germane for older adults, because it helps reduce emotional reactivity, which occurs through "cognitive and affective mechanisms of action and neural activation of the cingulate cortex, amygdala, and hippocampus."[13]

Other reasons make mindfulness an encouraging course for older adult interventions. Older adults exhibit a higher than usual adherence rate to mindfulness programs. This impressive adherence rate is seen not only during the intervention but also at follow-up, with some follow-up points being at 6 and 12 months.[10,14–16] High adherence may be explained by the fact that older adults have rich life experience to bring to meditation, and being introduced to a "reflective, stationary intervention" could be an engaging modality.[17] As correlation, older adults may be more skilled at effective learning, the concept of how practice helps one respond better and better to a treatment.[18]

Older adults are also a population that may benefit more than younger adults by using an integrative, nonpharmacologic treatment. Age is significantly associated with negative pharmacologic side effects, and these can be more disconcerting in older adults. Furthermore, older adults may have fewer funds available for prescription and nonprescription drugs. Certain medications also show reduced efficacy with time. Given these reasons, using mindfulness to treat chronic conditions in older adults may be an important way to prepare for better health care in the growing older adult population.[19]

Mindfulness Application to Chronic Mental Health Conditions in Older Adults

Cognitive impairment

Several studies examine mindfulness' role in addressing issues related to cognitive impairment in older adults. For example, MBSR has been shown to increase executive function, with significance persistent at a 21-week follow-up.[20] Sustained findings regarding cognitive impairment in older adults are particularly noteworthy, because aging is generally associated with cognitive detriment and cannot be assumed to remain stable.[21,22]

MBSR has shown improved clinical outcomes on memory composite scores in older adults with neurocognitive difficulties in a multisite trial using a health education control condition. At a 3-month follow-up, improvement in worry, depression, and anxiety was evident.[23] As mentioned, MBSR tends to show sustained and even stronger outcomes at later follow-up.

In another study, participants showed improvements in memory, reduced worry severity, and increased mindfulness. The multisite trial offered an elongated 12-session MBSR group, containing the same components and using additional repetition. The extended version (12-week) provided no additional gains with regards to clinical or cognitive outcomes, satisfaction, or continued practice as compared with the 8-week version. These findings indicated that older adults are able to achieve significant improvement using the standardized, manualized 8-week session protocol, and most were continuing to practice at a 6-month follow-up.[24] Researchers noted that a mindfulness intervention may prove to hold a high value in public health, because anxiety and cognitive impairment are often found in the older adult population.

It has been assumed that older adults with more advanced stages of dementia are unable to benefit from mindfulness practices, because they require awareness of the present moment and a capacity to identify and accept one's feelings or reactions. However, a recent study was the first to include older adults in long-term care with dementia ranging from moderate to severe in a mindfulness versus cognitive activity to explore outcomes. Researchers used a crossover design, and "significant short-term changes in agitation, discomfort, anger, and anxiety" were found in the mindfulness group versus the cognitive activity group.[13] Residents in long-term care, as well those providing their care, may benefit from a reduced emotional reactivity in the resident.

Sleep quality
Cognitive daytime impairment has been linked to poor sleep quality. The population with the highest percentage of sleep problems is older adults: more than half of those 55 and older have some type of sleep disturbance, which holds true when assessed with biological measures as well as self-report measures.[25] A RCT with a mindfulness awareness practice and an active sleep hygiene education comparison group showed significantly superior improvements in the mindfulness group compared with the sleep hygiene education group in both biological and self-report measures.[26] Furthermore, improvements in the mindfulness group in sleep-related daytime impairment measures of anxiety, depression, fatigue, and stress were all statistically significant between groups.[26]

A qualitative study by Hubbling and colleagues[27] using MBSR as treatment for chronic insomnia uncovered the 4 following themes: the impact of mindfulness on sleep and motivation to adopt a healthy sleep lifestyle; benefits of mindfulness on aspects of life beyond sleep; challenges and successes in adopting mindfulness-based practices; and the importance of group sharing and support. MBSR proves as effective as prescription sedatives in treating chronic insomnia, but has few or no side effects.[28,29] The bypassing of pharmacologic negative side effects may be even more important in older adults.

A secondary analysis of an MBSR study and associated sleep changes in older adults (65 years and older) showed significant effect sizes in improved sleep.[30] It is notable that higher effect sizes correlated with poorer sleep quality scores at baseline, indicating that those with the worst sleep quality to begin with gained the most improvement. These significant findings remained at 6-month follow-up. A second sleep quality RCT, recruiting older adults (75 and older) with chronic insomnia to participate in an MBSR program, assessing its effectiveness on insomnia as well as combined anxiety or depressive symptoms also found significant effect on both insomnia and depression.[31] It is notable that MBSR was found to be a useful intervention for chronic insomnia, even when the insomnia is combined with anxious or depressive symptoms.

Older adults are more susceptible to depression as a result of stress, and the relationship between sleep quality and depression continues to be strong. A recent pilot study comparing MM with vacation time as a control examined variables related to depression. Participants were aged 55 to 90 years, and mindfulness showed improvements in sleep quality as well as other depression variables, including severity of pain.[32]

Loneliness
Along with sleep difficulties, older adults often experience loneliness in later life. Moving away from an independent living situation, loss of spouse or partner, and mortality affecting friendships and close ties are all potential causes. Researchers have found that loneliness is correlated with an increased proinflammatory gene expression,[33] which in turn may initiate the development and progression of acute and chronic conditions that contribute to comorbidities and mortality.[34] Given this potential cascade, addressing loneliness in older adults holds considerable value.

Prior studies of MBSR have shown its capacity to reduce inflammatory protein biomarkers.[35] A recent trial sought to examine MBSR's effectiveness in reducing loneliness and its concurrent biological threat to health in older adults. As predicted by researchers, a standardized 8-week MBSR program reduced loneliness, whereas it increased in the control group. It also evidenced a reduction of "downregulated NF-κB-associated gene expression profile" as well as C-reactive protein.[33] The downregulation of these 2 gene expressions in the mindfulness group evidenced a reduction in the inflammatory protein, indicating a protective effect on immunity as loneliness decreased. It is noteworthy that loneliness in the control group did not remain the same but worsened and may have been accompanied by exacerbated inflammation as a result.

Posttraumatic stress disorder

Posttraumatic stress disorder (PTSD) is an all too common concern in older adults, with one likely correlation being the veteran older population. According to the Pew Research Center, two-thirds of the veteran population are older adults. Unfortunately, the veteran population often does not receive sufficient PTSD treatment from their primary care provider and continue to suffer from functional impairment, poorer mental and physical health, and higher suicide rates.[36] Possemato and colleagues[37] conducted an RCT using primary care brief mindfulness training, an abbreviated 4-session mindfulness based on MBSR, compared with treatment as usual. Exploratory analyses revealed that "the describing, nonjudging, and acting with awareness facets of mindfulness may account for decreases in PTSD." This conclusion is often drawn from research results, describing why mindfulness is found efficacious and effective with such a variety of conditions.

Patients with subclinical levels of PTSD may still suffer PTSD-like symptoms. Cortisol levels tend to correlate with PTSD symptoms and are thus a useful indicator of PTSD. An RCT using semiweekly mindfulness-based stretching and deep breathing exercise (MBX) against a control group in an 8-week intervention sought to establish whether this type of mindfulness could normalize cortisol levels and thus reduce PTSD symptoms in older adult veterans.[38] Symptoms were measured at baseline, 4 weeks, 8-week completion, and 16-week follow-up. MBX outcomes were superior to the control group severity of symptoms and serum cortisol and were sustained at the 16-week follow-up mark.[38] Again, outcomes of mindfulness training continued to be significant at a follow-up point beyond intervention completion, indicating the persisting efficacy of mindfulness interventions.

A misconception exists that mindfulness may not be a feasible treatment option for a veteran PTSD population, because the focus on the present moment could be psychologically triggering in increased symptoms. However, an MM intervention in a veteran PTSD population found that veterans engaged at a higher level than called for and that no adverse reactions were reported. Furthermore, the MM was statistically significantly superior to the psychoeducational comparison arm in reducing PTSD symptoms in participants, in self-reported as well as clinician-administered measures.[39]

The effects of mindfulness have been studied in other related vulnerable older adult populations. A recent study examined older adult Nigerian Fulani herdsmen, who are often vulnerable to attacks from farmers as the herdsmen move their cattle from 1 spot to another. The role of positive reappraisal was examined within the relationship between mindfulness and well-being. According to researchers' findings, mindfulness interventions are valuable in promoting well-being in later life, because mindfulness was found to be independently associated with "better life satisfaction, lower perceived stress, and fewer depressive symptoms."[40]

Mindfulness Application to Chronic Physical Conditions in Older Adults

Cardiovascular disease

Two-thirds of older adults have hypertension, a risk factor for cardiovascular disease, which is the leading cause of death.[41] For this reason, hypertension is often referred to as the silent killer. Mindfulness interventions to reduce blood pressure have been shown effective in specific comorbid populations of patients with prostate cancer, patients with breast cancer, cancer survivors, and type II diabetics.[42–44] Palta and colleagues[17] examined diastolic and systolic blood pressure in a sample of older adult African Americans with high blood pressure at baseline. Although the social support control group showed increased diastolic blood pressure at intervention completion, statistically significant reductions in both systolic and diastolic blood pressure were shown in the MBSR group. Furthermore, attendance rates were 98%, indicating high acceptability. Because many older adults remain unaware and undiagnosed, mindfulness may be a particularly important treatment for other comorbidities, because it would potentially positively affect conditions the older adult is unaware they have.

Hypertension in a sample of older adult participants with chronic kidney disease (CKD) has also been explored. MM, a brief technique to reduce stress, was tested in CKD patients and compared with an education intervention. Study participants received 3 separate interventions: a 14-minute MM and a 14-minute education session in random order at 2 separate visits. MM resulted in statistically significant reduction in both systolic and diastolic blood pressure, reduced heart rate, and reduced arterial pressure, a striking finding because the entire intervention occurred in less than 15 minutes.[45] A small subset of the participants in the study was given a controlled breathing intervention to determine if the slowed breathing of MM was the mechanism for these significant improvements. No changes in hemodynamics were observed with sole controlled breathing, signifying that the breathing component alone will not alter cardiovascular measures.

Diabetes

Diabetes carries an emotional burden with its management, because the disease can be a harbinger of additional serious comorbidities, such as cardiovascular disease, neuropathy, and kidney disease.[46] Fisher and colleagues[47] estimate that up to 40% of diabetics are subject to emotional distress and impaired well-being. Using cross-sectional data, Son and colleagues[46] examined the relationship of mindfulness with anxious and depressive symptoms in 666 diabetic participants; analyses showed significant associations with mindfulness being inversely proportional with both anxiety and depressive symptoms in people with diabetes. Researchers concluded that mindfulness "shows promise as a potentially protective characteristic against the influence of stressful events on emotional well-being."[46]

A related study sought to explore whether an adapted MBSR training would prove effective in reducing distress and improving diabetes self-efficacy, self-management, and A1C scores. Training included a 90-minute session during an education class on diabetes. Study participants were instructed to perform 10-minute daily home practices over the 3-month study period. Statistically significant improvements were shown in A1C scores, self-management, and self-efficacy as related to diabetes from baseline to 3-month completion.[48] Retention and satisfaction measures also proved feasible and acceptable.

Rheumatoid arthritis

Mindfulness has also been shown to affect both distress and disease activity in rheumatoid arthritis (RA) populations. Two studies have recently demonstrated mindfulness' statistically significant role in reducing psychological distress, not only at study completion but also at 6- and 12-month follow-up.[49,50] Clinician-assessed RA disease activity also demonstrated reductions in stiffness, pain, tender joints, and patient global assessments.[50] No significant findings were found regarding swollen joints or C-reactive protein levels.

Parkinson's disease

Parkinson's disease is the most common movement disorder and the second most common neurodegenerative disease of aging.[51] Current treatment is pharmacologic, and the negative side effects can be severe. According to Advocat and colleagues,[52] this has created a trend to apply holistic approaches that includes mindfulness. As such, their RCT examined mindfulness with a wait-list control group and its effects on both function and well-being. Although changes at completion were not significant, by the 6-month follow-up, both function and well-being had reached statistical significance.[53] These findings underscore the long-term benefits of a mindfulness intervention on Parkinson disease function and well-being.

MBSR has also been examined for its benefits on nonmotor symptoms in Parkinson's patients. Participants received the standard 8-week MBSR course with a 16-week follow-up. Depression levels, anxiety, and stress were all statistically significantly decreased at intervention completion and at the 16-week follow-up.[54]

Urge urinary incontinence

Urge urinary incontinence (UUI) is a chronic condition that affects as many as half of older adult women. Few seek treatment; UUI is either seen as a stigma and too sensitive of a topic to raise with one's primary care provider, or it is assumed to be a normal part of aging. Studies have shown mindfulness may be effective in treating older adult women's UUI, with reduced bother and severity symptoms, as well as a reduction in perceived stress.[14–16] Results for various measures were statistically sustained at diverse intervals, including as long as 1 year.

Chronic pain

Chronic pain is another condition in which nonpharmacologic treatments are becoming more urgent. The original MBSR protocol was created to address chronic pain.[55] Mindfulness is being used to address nonspecific chronic pain, and results are staying significant through the 6-month follow-up, highlighting how mindfulness continues to effectively address conditions long after the participant's intervention.[56]

Low back pain (LBP) treatment in older adults is limited because of the negative side effects of analgesics in this population. Many older adults deal with chronic LBP, and several mindfulness studies have been administered to explore its efficacy. A mindfulness intervention for chronic LBP in older adults improved short-term function as well as long-term pain. The improved function did not remain at follow-up.[57] However, an RCT using MBSR to treat CLBP found reduced pain and improved function, which was sustained at 1-year follow-up and still noted at a 2-year follow-up.[58,59] A qualitative, grounded theory study of MM on older adults with CLBP found MM to result in "less pain, improved attention, better sleep, and enhanced well-being, and improved quality of life."[60]

SUMMARY
Wide Application

Substantial research has shown MM's strong significant results in the treatment of both mental and physical chronic conditions in older adults. It appears to be a simple, elegant tool for meeting complex conditions in the geriatric population and does not dilute when applied to more severe conditions. In fact, research has shown that the more stressed the participant at baseline, the greater the improvement at completion and follow-up.[23] Furthermore, it does not need to be tailored to a specific condition to be effective.

Improvement Across Several Areas

A common result that weaves through these studies on mental and physical conditions often found in older adults is that mindfulness improves many items at once. It is rare to effectively isolate 1 measure and see improvement in only that measure, making it even more valuable as a potential treatment, because multiple chronic conditions and comorbidities are likely to exist in older adulthood. Applications of mindfulness may address high blood pressure and depression at once or may address diabetic symptoms and improve sleep quality at the same time. Large RCTs find support for the uses of MBSR and MBCT specifically with older adults on a wide variety of conditions: chronic LBP, chronic insomnia, improved sleep quality, enhanced positive affect, reduced symptoms of anxiety and depression, and improved memory and executive functioning.[11]

Cost-Effective

Mindfulness is quite inexpensive, because it is learned within 1 course. No refresher classes or skill updates are needed. Medications and other treatments may bring decreased efficacy with time; mindfulness treatment does the exact opposite, with efficacy continuing to increase over time. Furthermore, this capability may allow for less prescription medication to be administered, an important development because medications tend to prove more dangerous in the older adult population, where polypharmacy and contraindications between medications are commonplace.

Future Research

For these reasons, it is crucial that further large-scale trials be conducted. Mindfulness research is a current funding priority of the National Center for Complementary and Integrative Health at the National Institutes of Health.[61] As health care providers work with an increasing aging population, additional mindfulness research is also recommended to study clusters of chronic conditions. Mindfulness may be uniquely suited to address several symptom clusters at once.

DISCLOSURE

The Hartford Center for Geriatric Nursing Excellence Jonas Center for Nursing and Veterans Healthcare Gamma Rho Chapter of Sigma Theta Tau International Office of the Associate Vice President for Health Equity and Inclusion, University of Utah College of Nursing Research Support Grant, University of Utah.

REFERENCES

1. Graham JE, Christian LM, Kiecolt-Glaser JK. Stress, age, and immune function: toward a lifespan approach. J Behav Med 2006;29(4):389–400.
2. Hawkley LC, Cacioppo JT. Stress and the aging immune system. Brain Behav Immun 2004;18(2):114–9.
3. Segerstrom SC, Miller GE. Psychological stress and the human immune system: a meta-analytic study of 30 years of inquiry. Psychol Bull 2004;130(4):601–30.
4. Kabat-Zinn J. Mindfulness-based stress reduction (MBSR). Constructivism in the Human Sciences 2003;8(2):73–107.
5. Segal ZV, Teasdale JD, Williams JMG. Mindfulness-based cognitive therapy: theoretical rationale and empirical status. In: Hayes SC, Follette VM, Linehan MM, editors. Mindfulness and acceptance: expanding the cognitive-behavioral tradition. New York: Guilford Press; 2004. p. 45–65.

6. Shastri PS. Mindfulness and older adults: reviewing the historical foundations of mindfulness in practice and the development of a mindful meditation program for older adults. Ann Arbor(MI): ProQuest Information & Learning; 2016.

7. Perez-Blasco J, Sales A, Meléndez JC, et al. The effects of mindfulness and self-compassion on improving the capacity to adapt to stress situations in elderly people living in the community. Clin Gerontol 2016;39(2):90–103.

8. Sorrell JM. Meditation for older adults: a new look at an ancient intervention for mental health. J Psychosoc Nurs Ment Health Serv 2015;53(5):15–9.

9. Salmoirago-Blotcher E, Hunsinger M, Morgan L, et al. Mindfulness-based stress reduction and change in health-related behaviors. J Evid Based Complement Altern Med 2013;18(4):243–7.

10. Ribeiro L, Atchley RM, Oken BS. Adherence to practice of mindfulness in novice meditators: practices chosen, amount of time practiced, and long-term effects following a mindfulness-based intervention. Mindfulness (N Y) 2018;9(2):401–11.

11. Greenawalt KE, Orsega-Smith E, Turner JL, et al. The impact of "The Art of Happiness" class on community dwelling older adults: a positive psychology intervention. Act Adapt Aging 2019;43(2):118–32.

12. de Frias CM, Whyne E. Stress on health-related quality of life in older adults: the protective nature of mindfulness. Aging Ment Health 2015;19(3):201–6.

13. Kovach CR, Evans C-R, Sattell L, et al. Feasibility and pilot testing of a mindfulness intervention for frail older adults and individuals with dementia. Res Gerontol Nurs 2018;11(3):137–50.

14. Felsted KF, Supiano KP. Mindfulness-based stress reduction versus a health enhancement program in the treatment of urge urinary incontinence in older adult women: a randomized controlled feasibility study. Res Gerontol Nurs 2019;12(6):285–97.

15. Baker J, Costa D, Guarino JM, et al. Comparison of mindfulness-based stress reduction versus yoga on urinary urge incontinence: a randomized pilot study. With 6-month and 1-year follow-up visits. Female Pelvic Med Reconstr Surg 2014;20(3):141–6.

16. Baker J, Costa D, Nygaard I. Mindfulness-based stress reduction for treatment of urinary urge incontinence: a pilot study. Female Pelvic Med Reconstr Surg 2012;18(1):46–9.

17. Palta P, Page G, Piferi RL, et al. Evaluation of a mindfulness-based intervention program to decrease blood pressure in low-income African-American older adults. J Urban Health 2012;89(2):308–16.

18. Gaylord SA, Palsson OS, Garland EL, et al. Mindfulness training reduces the severity of irritable bowel syndrome in women: results of a randomized controlled trial. Am J Gastroenterol 2011;106(9):1678–88.

19. Rowe JW, Fulmer T, Fried L. Preparing for better health and health care for an aging population. JAMA 2016;316(16):1643–4.

20. Moynihan JA, Chapman BP, Klorman R, et al. Mindfulness-based stress reduction for older adults: effects on executive function, frontal alpha asymmetry and immune function. Neuropsychobiology 2013;68(1):34–43.

21. Aine CJ, Sanfratello L, Adair JC, et al. Development and decline of memory functions in normal, pathological and healthy successful aging. Brain Topogr 2011;24(3–4):323–39.

22. Wang M, Gamo NJ, Yang Y, et al. Neuronal basis of age-related working memory decline. Nature 2011;476(7359):210–3.

23. Wetherell JL, Hershey T, Hickman S, et al. Mindfulness-based stress reduction for older adults with stress disorders and neurocognitive difficulties: a randomized controlled trial. J Clin Psychiatry 2017;78(7):e734–43.

24. Lenze EJ, Hickman S, Hershey T, et al. Mindfulness-based stress reduction for older adults with worry symptoms and co-occurring cognitive dysfunction. Int J Geriatr Psychiatry 2014;29(10):991–1000.

25. Ancoli-Israel S, Ayalon L. Diagnosis and treatment of sleep disorders in older adults. Am J Geriatr Psychiatry 2006;14(2):95–103.

26. Black DS, O'Reilly GA, Olmstead R, et al. Mindfulness meditation and improvement in sleep quality and daytime impairment among older adults with sleep disturbances: a randomized clinical trial. JAMA Intern Med 2015;175(4):494–501.

27. Hubbling A, Reilly-Spong M, Kreitzer MJ, et al. How mindfulness changed my sleep: focus groups with chronic insomnia patients. BMC Complement Altern Med 2014;14:50.

28. Winbush NY, Gross CR, Kreitzer MJ. The effects of mindfulness-based stress reduction on sleep disturbance: a systematic review. Explore (NY) 2007;3(6): 585–91.

29. Bootzin RR, Epstein DR. Understanding and treating insomnia. Annu Rev Clin Psychol 2011;7:435–58.

30. Gallegos AM, Moynihan J, Pigeon WR. A secondary analysis of sleep quality changes in older adults from a randomized trial of an MBSR Program. J Appl Gerontol 2018;37(11):1327–43.

31. Zhang J-X, Liu X-H, Xie X-H, et al. Mindfulness-based stress reduction for chronic insomnia in adults older than 75 years: a randomized, controlled, single-blind clinical trial. Explore (NY) 2015;11(3):180–5.

32. Wahbeh H, Nelson M. iRest meditation for older adults with depression symptoms: a pilot study. Int J Yoga Therap 2019;29(1):9–17.

33. Creswell JD, Irwin MR, Burklund LJ, et al. Mindfulness-Based Stress Reduction training reduces loneliness and pro-inflammatory gene expression in older adults: a small randomized controlled trial. Brain Behav Immun 2012;26(7): 1095–101.

34. Hackett RA, Hamer M, Endrighi R, et al. Loneliness and stress-related inflammatory and neuroendocrine responses in older men and women. Psychoneuroendocrinology 2012;37(11):1801–9.

35. Lengacher CA, Kip KE, Barta MK, et al. A pilot study evaluating the effect of mindfulness-based stress reduction on psychological status, physical status, salivary cortisol, and interleukin-6 among advanced-stage cancer patients and their caregivers. J Holist Nurs 2012;30(3):170–87.

36. Pew Research Center. The changing face of America's veteran population. FACTANK 2019. Available at: https://www.pewresearch.org/fact-tank/2017/11/10/the-changing-face-of-americas-veteran-population/. Accessed December 3, 2019.

37. Possemato K, Bergen-Cico D, Treatman S, et al. A randomized clinical trial of primary care brief mindfulness training for veterans with PTSD. J Clin Psychol 2016; 72(3):179–93.

38. Kim SH, Schneider SM, Bevans M, et al. PTSD symptom reduction with mindfulness-based stretching and deep breathing exercise: randomized controlled clinical trial of efficacy. J Clin Endocrinol Metab 2013;98(7):2984–92.

39. Niles BL, Klunk-Gillis J, Ryngala DJ, et al. Comparing mindfulness and psychoeducation treatments for combat-related PTSD using a telehealth approach. Psychol Trauma 2012;4(5):538–47.

40. Aliche JC, Onyishi IE. Mindfulness and wellbeing in older adults' survivors of herdsmen attack the mediating effect of positive reappraisal. Aging Ment Health 2020;24(7):1132–40.

41. Bragg SW. Hypertension in older adults. Ann Longterm Care: Clinical Care and Aging 2015;23(12):42–3.

42. Carlson LE, Speca M, Faris P, et al. One year pre-post intervention follow-up of psychological, immune, endocrine and blood pressure outcomes of mindfulness-based stress reduction (MBSR) in breast and prostate cancer outpatients. Brain Behav Immun 2007;21(8):1038–49.

43. Matchim Y, Armer JM, Stewart BR. Effects of mindfulness-based stress reduction (MBSR) on health among breast cancer survivors. West J Nurs Res 2011;33(8): 996–1016.

44. Rosenzweig S, Reibel DK, Greeson JM, et al. Mindfulness-based stress reduction is associated with improved glycemic control in type 2 diabetes mellitus: a pilot study. Altern Ther Health Med 2007;13(5):36–8.

45. Park J, Lyles RH, Bauer-Wu S. Mindfulness meditation lowers muscle sympathetic nerve activity and blood pressure in African-American males with chronic kidney disease. Am J Physiol Regul Integr Comp Physiol 2014;307(1):R93–101.

46. Son J, Nyklíček I, Nefs G, et al. The association between mindfulness and emotional distress in adults with diabetes: could mindfulness serve as a buffer? Results from Diabetes MILES: the Netherlands. J Behav Med 2015;38(2):251–60.

47. Fisher L, Skaff MM, Mullan JT, et al. A longitudinal study of affective and anxiety disorders, depressive affect and diabetes distress in adults with Type 2 diabetes. Diabet Med 2008;25(9):1096–101.

48. DiNardo M, Saba S, Greco CM, et al. A mindful approach to diabetes self-management education and support for veterans. Diabetes Educ 2017;43(6): 608–20.

49. Nyklíček I, Hoogwegt F, Westgeest T. Psychological distress across twelve months in patients with rheumatoid arthritis: the role of disease activity, disability, and mindfulness. J Psychosom Res 2015;78(2):162–7.

50. Fogarty FA, Booth RJ, Gamble GD, et al. The effect of mindfulness-based stress reduction on disease activity in people with rheumatoid arthritis: a randomised controlled trial. Ann Rheum Dis 2015;74(2):472–4.

51. Mhyre TR, Boyd JT, Hamill RW, et al. Parkinson's disease. Subcell Biochem 2012; 65:389–455.

52. Advocat J, Russell G, Enticott J, et al. The effects of a mindfulness-based lifestyle programme for adults with Parkinson's disease: protocol for a mixed methods, randomised two-group control study. BMJ Open 2013;3(10):e003326.

53. Advocat J, Enticott J, Vandenberg B, et al. The effects of a mindfulness-based lifestyle program for adults with Parkinson's disease: a mixed methods, wait list controlled randomised control study. BMC Neurol 2016;16(1):166.

54. Birtwell K, Dubrow-Marshall L, Dubrow-Marshall R, et al. A mixed methods evaluation of a mindfulness-based stress reduction course for people with Parkinson's disease. Complement Ther Clin Pract 2017;29:220–8.

55. Kabat-Zinn J. An outpatient program in behavioral medicine for chronic pain patients based on the practice of mindfulness meditation: theoretical considerations and preliminary results. Gen Hosp Psychiatry 1982;4(1):33–47.

56. la Cour P, Petersen M. Effects of mindfulness meditation on chronic pain: a randomized controlled trial. Pain Med 2015;16(4):641–52.

57. Morone NE, Greco CM, Moore CG, et al. A mind-body program for older adults with chronic low back pain: a randomized clinical trial. JAMA Intern Med 2016; 176(3):329–37.

58. Cherkin DC, Anderson ML, Sherman KJ, et al. Two-year follow-up of a randomized clinical trial of mindfulness-based stress reduction vs cognitive behavioral therapy or usual care for chronic low back pain. JAMA 2017;317(6):642–4.

59. Cherkin DC, Sherman KJ, Balderson BH, et al. Effect of mindfulness-based stress reduction vs cognitive behavioral therapy or usual care on back pain and functional limitations in adults with chronic low back pain: a randomized clinical trial. JAMA 2016;315(12):1240–9.

60. Morone NE, Lynch CS, Greco CM, et al. I felt like a new person." The effects of mindfulness meditation on older adults with chronic pain: qualitative narrative analysis of diary entries. J Pain 2008;9(9):841–8.

61. US Dept of Health and Human Services. NCCIH's funding priorities and research focus 2017. Modified 9/17/2019. Accessed September 26, 2019.